# Pharmaceutical Calculations

# Pharmaceutical Calculations

MITCHELL J. STOKLOSA, A.M., Sc.D.
*Professor of Pharmacy Emeritus,*
*Massachusetts College of Pharmacy*
*and Allied Health Sciences,*
*Boston, Massachusetts*

and

HOWARD C. ANSEL, Ph.D.
*Professor and Dean,*
*College of Pharmacy*
*University of Georgia,*
*Athens, Georgia*

*Eighth Edition*

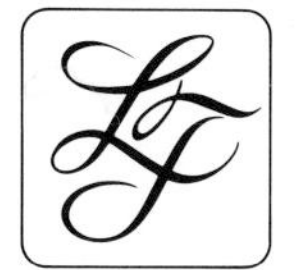

Lea & Febiger

Philadelphia 1986

Lea & Febiger
600 Washington Square
Philadelphia, PA 19106-4198
U.S.A.
(215) 922-1330



**Library of Congress Cataloging in Publication Data**

Stoklosa, Mitchell J.
Pharmaceutical calculations.

Includes index.
1. Pharmaceutical arithmetic. I. Ansel, Howard C., 1933– . II. Title. [DNLM: 1. Mathematics. 2. Pharmacy. QV 16 S874p]
RS57.S86 1986 615'.14'01513 85-15858
ISBN 0-8121-1007-2

**PHARMACEUTICAL CALCULATIONS**

Bradley and Gustafson 1st edition, 1945
Bradley, Gustafson and Stoklosa 2nd edition, 1952
3rd edition, 1957
4th edition, 1963
5th edition, 1968
Stoklosa 6th edition, 1974
Stoklosa and Ansel 7th edition, 1980
8th edition, 1986



Printed in the United States of America

Print number: 3 2 1

# *Preface*

In preparing the Eighth Edition of *Pharmaceutical Calculations* we have emphasized those calculations that serve the clinical needs of the student in preparation for professional practice. The successful format of previous editions and an appropriate balance between the applied and theoretical concepts have been maintained throughout this new edition. Theoretical discussion has been kept at a minimum and has been included only for the purposes of clarity and understanding of the problems and their solutions.

New practice problems have been added and older ones deleted, and new examples of medication orders from institutional practice sites have been introduced throughout the text. Problems at the end of the book that are available for review purposes have been revised to include new ones, and for the first time, the answers to half of the review problems have been included for purposes of checking.

The introductory material has been critically reviewed, and the section on number systems has been deleted; but the material dealing with certain fundamentals of measurement and calculation has been retained because it is thought to be desirable for the purpose of serving as a review of basic arithmetic principles. The main body of the text thereafter provides a logical development of topics which allows an arrangement of study that suits the requirements of separate or integrated courses dealing with pharmaceutical calculations in the professional curriculum.

Two new appendices have been added to render the text more reflective of today's professional requirements; they are: "Graphical Methods," and "Some Calculations Associated with Drug Availability and Pharmacokinetics." The first of these new appendices presents methods to plot experimental data, interpret graphic material and equations, and manipulate the relationships between curves and their equations. Linear relationships are defined and examples presented of experimental data utilizing regular and semilogarithmic graph paper. The second new appendix presents some elementary calculations associated with drug availability and pharmacokinetics. Included are examples to: plot and interpret drug dissolution data, calculate the amount of drug which is bioavailable from a dosage form, plot and interpret a blood drug concentration-time curve, calculate the plasma concentration of unbound versus bound drugs, calculate the apparent volume of distribution of a drug substance, determine the elimination half-life and elimination rate constant, and calculate dosage based on creatinine clearance.

In addition to the two new appendices, other expanded areas include:

simple conversion techniques of product concentration to "mg/mL"; calculations involving electrolyte solutions; and the use of nomograms in determining flow rate of infusion solutions.

We acknowledge with gratitude the helpful comments and suggestions of our colleagues in academic pharmacy, and express appreciation to the pharmacy practitioners who provided many examples of prescriptions and medication orders for use in the text as examples and practice problems.

*Boston, Massachusetts*
*Athens, Georgia*

Mitchell J. Stoklosa
Howard C. Ansel

# *Contents*

# 1

# Some Fundamentals of Measurement and Calculation

## NUMBERS AND NUMERALS

A *number* is a total quantity, or amount, of units. A *numeral* is a word or sign, or a group of words or signs, expressing a number.

For example, *3, 6,* and *48* are arabic numerals expressing numbers that are respectively *three times, six times,* and *forty-eight times* the unit *1.*

## KINDS OF NUMBERS

In *arithmetic,* which is the science of calculating with positive, real numbers, a number will usually be (a) a natural or *whole* number, or *integer,* such as *549;* (b) a *fraction,* or subdivision of a whole number, such as $\frac{4}{7}$; or (c) a *mixed* number, consisting of a whole number plus a fraction such as $3\frac{7}{8}$.

A number such as *4, 8,* or *12,* taken by itself, without application to anything concrete, is called an *abstract* or *pure* number. It merely designates how many times the unit *1* is contained in it, without implying that anything else is being counted or measured. An abstract number may be added to, subtracted from, multiplied by, or divided by any other abstract number. The result of any of these operations is always an abstract number designating a new total of units.

But a number that designates a quantity of objects or units of measure, such as *4 grams, 8 ounces, 12 grains,* is called a *concrete* or *denominate* number. It designates the total quantity of whatever has been measured. A denominate number may be added to or subtracted from any other number of the same denomination; but a denominate number may be multiplied or divided only by a pure number. The result of any of these operations is always a number *of the same denomination.*

*Examples:*

*10 grams + 5 grams = 15 grams*
*10 grams − 5 grams = 5 grams*
*300 grains × 2 = 600 grains*
*12 ounces ÷ 3 = 4 ounces*

If any one rule of arithmetic may take first place in importance, this is it: *Numbers of different denominations have no direct numerical connection with each other and cannot be used together in any arithmetical operation.* We shall see again and again that if quantities are to be added, or if one quantity is to be subtracted from another, they must be expressed in the same denomination. And when we apparently multiply or divide a denominate number by a number of different denomination, we are in fact using the multiplier or divisor as an abstract number. If, for example, *1 ounce* costs *5 cents* and we want to find the cost of *12 ounces,* we do not multiply *5 cents* by 12 *ounces,* but by the abstract number *12.*

## ARABIC NUMERALS

The so-called "arabic" system of notation is properly called a *decimal system.* With only *ten figures*—a *zero* and *nine digits* (1, 2, 3, 4, 5, 6, 7, 8, 9)—any number can be expressed by an ingenious system in which different values are assigned to the digits according to the *place* they occupy in a row. The central place in the row is usually identified by a sign placed to its right called the *decimal point.* Any digit occupying this place expresses its own value—in other words, a certain number of *ones;* but the former value of a digit is increased tenfold each time it moves one place to the left; and, conversely, its value is one-tenth of its preceding value each time it moves one place to the right. *Zero* serves to mark a place not occupied by one of the digits.

The simplicity of the system is further evidenced by the fact that these *ten figures* serve all our needs in dealing with positive integers, and with the aid of a few signs, are adequate for expressing fractions, negative numbers, and irrational and imaginary numbers.

The practical range of the system is represented by the following scheme (which can be extended, of course, to the left or right into even higher or lower reaches):

*Scheme of the decimal system:*

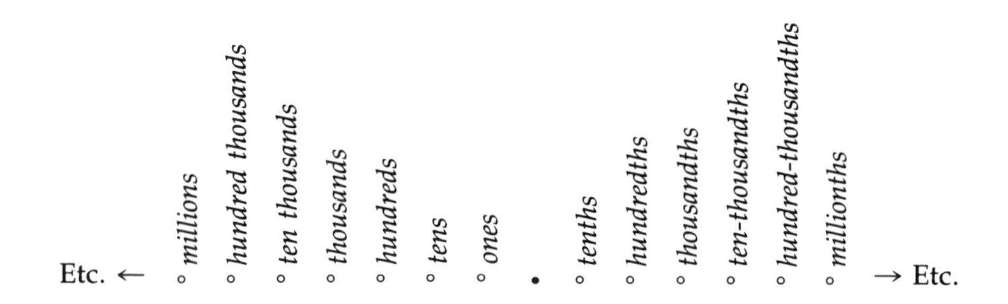

The total value of any number expressed in the arabic (decimal) system, then, is the sum of the values of its digits as determined by their position.

*Example:*

*5,083.623 means:*

| | |
|---|---|
| 5,000.000 or | 5 thousands |
| + 000.000 | plus 0 hundreds |
| + 080.000 | plus 8 tens |
| + 003.000 | plus 3 ones |
| + 000.600 | plus 6 tenths |
| + 000.020 | plus 2 hundredths |
| + 000.003 | plus 3 thousandths |

The universal use of this system has resulted from the ease with which it can be adapted to the various purposes of arithmetical calculations.

## ROMAN NUMERALS

The roman system of notation expresses a fairly large range of numbers by the use of a few letters of the alphabet in a simple "positional" notation indicating adding to or subtracting from a succession of bases extending from *one* through *five, ten, fifty, one hundred, and five hundred* to *one thousand.*

Roman numerals can merely record quantities: they are of no use in computation. They customarily designate quantities on prescriptions when ingredients are measured by the common or apothecaries' systems.

To express quantities in the roman system, these eight letters of fixed values are used:[1]

| | | | |
|---|---|---|---|
| ss = ½ | V or v = 5 | L or l = 50 | D or d = 500 |
| I or i = 1 | X or x = 10 | C or c = 100 | M or m = 1000 |

Other quantities are expressed by combining these letters by the general rule that when the second of two letters has a value equal to or smaller than that of the first, their values are to be added; but when the second has a value greater than that of the first, the smaller is to be subtracted from the larger. This rule may be illustrated as follows:

[1] On prescriptions physicians tend to use capitals except for the letter *i*, which they dot for the sake of clarity; and may use *j* for a final *i*. Following the Latin custom, they put the symbol for the denomination first and the roman numeral second (e.g., gr $\overline{\dot{\text{i}}\text{v}}$). Dates are customarily expressed in capitals.

(1) Two or more letters express a quantity that is the *sum* of their values *if they are successively equal or smaller in value:*

| | | | |
|---|---|---|---|
| ii = 2 | xx = 20 | ci = 101 | dc = 600 |
| iii = 3 | xxii = 22 | cv = 105 | mi = 1001 |
| vi = 6 | xxxiii = 33 | cx = 110 | mv = 1005 |
| vii = 7 | li = 51 | cl = 150 | mx = 1010 |
| viii = 8 | lv = 55 | cc = 200 | ml = 1050 |
| xi = 11 | lx = 60 | di = 501 | mc = 1100 |
| xii = 12 | lxvi = 66 | dv = 505 | md = 1500 |
| xiii = 13 | lxxvii = 77 | dx = 510 | mdclxvi = 1666 |
| xv = 15 | lxxxviii = 88 | dl = 550 | mm = 2000 |

(2) Two or more letters express a quantity that is the *sum* of the values remaining *after the value of each smaller letter has been substracted from that of a following greater:*

| | | | |
|---|---|---|---|
| iv = 4 | xxxix = 39 | xcix = 99 | cdxc = 490 |
| ix = 9 | xl = 40 | cd = 400 | cm = 900 |
| xiv = 14 | xli = 41 | cdi = 401 | cmxcix = 999 |
| xix = 19 | xliv = 44 | cdxl = 440 | MCDXCII = 1492 |
| xxiv = 24 | xc = 90 | cdxliv = 444 | MCMLXXXV = 1985 |

**Practice Problems**

1. Write the following in roman numerals:

(*a*) 18. (*d*) 126. (*g*) 84.
(*b*) 64. (*e*) 99. (*h*) 48.
(*c*) 72. (*f*) 37. (*i*) 1984.

2. Write the following in arabic numerals:

(*a*) Part IV. (*c*) MCMLIX.
(*b*) Chapter XIX. (*d*) MDCCCXIV.

3. Interpret the *quantity* in each of these phrases taken from prescriptions:

(*a*) Caps. no. xlv.
(*b*) Gtts. M.
(*c*) Tabs no. xlviii.
(*d*) Pil. no. lxiv.
(*e*) Pulv. no. xvi.
(*f*) Caps. no. lxxxiv.

4. Interpret the *quantities* in each of these prescriptions:

(*a*) ℞ Zinc Oxide part. v
Wool Fat part. xv
Petrolatum part. lxxx
Disp. ℥iv
Sig. Apply.

| | | | |
|---|---|---|---|
| *(b)* | ℞ | Dilaudid | gr iss |
| | | Ammonium Chloride | gr xl |
| | | Syrup ad | ℥vi |
| | | Sig. ʒss pro tuss. | |

## COMMON AND DECIMAL FRACTIONS

Much of the arithmetic of pharmacy requires facility in the handling of common fractions and decimal fractions. Even if the student already has a good working knowledge of their use, the following brief review of certain principles and rules governing them should be helpful, and the practice problems should provide a means of gaining accuracy and speed in their manipulation.

### Common Fractions

A number in the form $\frac{1}{8}$, $\frac{3}{16}$, and so on, is called a *common fraction,* or very often simply a *fraction.* Its *denominator,* or second or lower figure, always indicates the number of aliquot parts into which *1* is divided; and its *numerator,* or first or upper figure, specifies the number of those parts with which we are concerned.

The *value* of a fraction is the quotient when its numerator is divided by its denominator. If the numerator is smaller than the denominator, the fraction is called *proper,* and its value is less than *1.* If the numerator and denominator are alike, its value is *1.* If the numerator is larger than the denominator, the fraction is called *improper,* and its value is greater than *1.*

Now, two principles must be understood by anyone attempting to calculate with common fractions.

*First Principle.* Multiplying the numerator increases the value of a fraction, and multiplying the denominator decreases the value; but *when both numerator and denominator are multiplied by the same number, the value does not change.*

$$\frac{2}{7} = \frac{3 \times 2}{3 \times 7} = \frac{6}{21}$$

This principle allows us to reduce two or more fractions to a common denomination when necessary. We usually want the *lowest common denominator,* which is the smallest number divisible by all the given denominators. It is most easily found by testing successive multiples of the largest given denominator until we reach a number divisible by all the other given denominators. Then we multiply both numerator and denominator of each fraction by the number of times its denominator is contained in the common denominator.

*Example:*

*Reduce the fractions $\frac{3}{4}$, $\frac{4}{5}$, and $\frac{1}{3}$ to a common denomination.*

By testing successive multiples of 5, we discover that 60 is the smallest number divisible by 4, 5, and 3.
4 is contained 15 times in 60; 5, 12 times; and 3, 20 times.

$$\left.\begin{aligned}\frac{3}{4} &= \frac{15 \times 3}{15 \times 4} = \frac{45}{60},\\ \frac{4}{5} &= \frac{12 \times 4}{12 \times 5} = \frac{48}{60},\\ \frac{1}{3} &= \frac{20 \times 1}{20 \times 3} = \frac{20}{60},\end{aligned}\right\} \text{answers.}$$

*Second Principle.* Dividing the numerator decreases the value of a fraction, and dividing the denominator increases the value; but *when both numerator and denominator are divided by the same number, the value does not change.*

$$\frac{6}{21} = \frac{6 \div 3}{21 \div 3} = \frac{2}{7}$$

This principle allows us to reduce an unwieldy fraction to more convenient lower terms, either at any time during a series of calculations or when recording a final result. To reduce a fraction to its *lowest terms,* divide both the numerator and the denominator by the largest common divisor.

*Example:*

*Reduce $\frac{36}{2880}$ to its lowest terms.*

The largest common divisor is 36.

$$\frac{36}{2880} = \frac{36 \div 36}{2880 \div 36} = \frac{1}{80}, \text{ answer.}$$

These principles often suggest direct solutions to practical problems.

*Examples:*

*A prescription calls for $\frac{3}{50}$ grain of atropine sulfate. How many $\frac{1}{200}$-grain tablets will supply the required amount?*

50 is contained 4 times in 200.

$$\frac{3}{50} \text{ gr} = \frac{4 \times 3}{4 \times 50} \text{ gr} = \frac{12}{200} \text{ gr}$$

Twelve $\frac{1}{200}$-grain tablets would supply $\frac{12}{200}$ gr which equals the $\frac{3}{50}$ gr required, *answer.*

*Justify the assertion that nine $\frac{1}{150}$-grain tablets would supply the $\frac{3}{50}$ grain of atropine sulfate called for.*

Nine $\frac{1}{150}$-grain tablets would supply $\frac{9}{150}$ gr

50 is contained 3 times in 150.

$$\frac{9}{150}\text{ gr} = \frac{9 \div 3}{150 \div 3}\text{ gr} = \frac{3}{50}\text{ gr required, } \textit{answer.}$$

Besides developing a firm grasp of these two principles, the student should follow two rules before indulging in any short cuts.

*Rule 1.* Before performing any arithmetical operation involving fractions, *reduce every mixed number to an improper fraction.* To do so, multiply the integer, or whole number, by the denominator of the fractional remainder, add the numerator, and write the result over the denominator.

For example, before attempting to multiply $\frac{3}{4}$ by $1\frac{1}{5}$, first reduce the $1\frac{1}{5}$ to an improper fraction:

$$1\frac{1}{5} = \frac{(1 \times 5) + 1}{5} = \frac{6}{5}$$

If the final result of a calculation is an improper fraction, you may, if you like, reduce it to a mixed number. To do so, simply divide the numerator by the denominator and express the remainder as a common, not a decimal fraction:

$$\frac{6}{5} = 6 \div 5 = 1\frac{1}{5}$$

*Rule 2.* When performing an operation involving a fraction and a whole number, *express (or at least visualize) the whole number as a fraction having 1 for its denominator.*

Think of 3, as $\frac{3}{1}$, 42 as $\frac{42}{1}$, and so on.

As will be seen, this visualization is desirable when a fraction is subtracted from a whole number, and it is necessary when a fraction is divided by a whole number.

**To add fractions:**

To add common fractions, reduce them to a common denomination, add the numerators, and write the sum over the common denominator. If whole and mixed numbers are involved, the safest (though not the quickest) procedure is first to apply *Rules 1* and *2*. If the sum is an improper fraction, you may want to reduce it to a mixed number.

*Examples:*

*A prescription for a capsule contains* $\frac{3}{80}$ *grain of ingredient A,* $\frac{1}{200}$ *grain of ingredient B,* $\frac{1}{50}$ *grain of ingredient C, and* $\frac{3}{16}$ *grain of ingredient D. What is the total weight of these four ingredients?*

The lowest common denominator of the four fractions is 400.

Reducing to a common denomination:

$\frac{3}{80} = \frac{15}{400}$, $\frac{1}{200} = \frac{2}{400}$, $\frac{1}{50} = \frac{8}{400}$, and $\frac{3}{16} = \frac{75}{400}$

Adding the numerators:

$$\frac{15 + 2 + 8 + 75}{400} \text{ gr} = \frac{100}{400} \text{ gr}$$

Reducing the sum to its simplest terms:

$\frac{100}{400}$ gr $= \frac{1}{4}$ gr, *answer.*

*A patient receives the following doses of a certain drug:* $\frac{1}{4}$ *grain,* $\frac{1}{12}$ *grain,* $\frac{1}{8}$ *grain, and* $\frac{1}{6}$ *grain. Calculate the total amount of the drug received by the patient.*

The lowest common denominator of the fractions is 24.

$\frac{1}{4} = \frac{6}{24}$, $\frac{1}{12} = \frac{2}{24}$, $\frac{1}{8} = \frac{3}{24}$, and $\frac{1}{6} = \frac{4}{24}$

$$\frac{6 + 2 + 3 + 4}{24} \text{ gr} = \frac{15}{24} \text{ gr}$$

$\frac{15}{24}$ gr $= \frac{5}{8}$ gr, *answer.*

**To subtract fractions:**

To subtract one fraction from another, reduce them to a common denomination, subtract, and write the difference over the common denominator. If a whole or mixed number is involved, first apply *Rule 1* or 2. If the difference is an improper fraction, you may want to reduce it to a mixed number.

*Examples:*

*A patient's medication chart shows that he has received a total of* $\frac{7}{12}$ *grain of morphine sulfate. If he had not been given the last dose of* $\frac{1}{8}$ *grain, what quantity would he have received?*

The lowest common denominator is 24.

$\frac{7}{12} = \frac{14}{24}$ and $\frac{1}{8} = \frac{3}{24}$

$$\frac{14 - 3}{24} \text{ gr} = \frac{11}{24} \text{ gr, } \textit{answer.}$$

*A capsule is to weigh 3 grains. If it contains $\frac{1}{24}$ grain of ingredient A, $\frac{1}{4}$ grain of ingredient B, and $\frac{1}{3}$ grain of ingredient C, how much diluent should be added?*

The lowest common denominator of the fractions is 24.

$\frac{1}{24} = \frac{1}{24}$, $\frac{1}{4} = \frac{6}{24}$, and $\frac{1}{3} = \frac{8}{24}$

$$\frac{1 + 6 + 8}{24} \text{ gr} = \frac{15}{24} \text{ gr} = \frac{5}{8} \text{ gr}$$

Interpreting the given 3 grains as $\frac{3}{1}$ grains, and reducing it to a fraction with 8 for a denominator:

$\frac{3}{1}$ gr $= \frac{24}{8}$ gr

Subtracting:

$$\frac{24 - 5}{8} \text{ gr} = \frac{19}{8} \text{ gr}$$

Changing the difference to a mixed number:

$\frac{19}{8}$ gr $= (19 \div 8)$ gr $= 2\frac{3}{8}$ gr, *answer.*

**To multiply fractions:**

To multiply fractions, multiply the numerators and write the product over the product of the denominators. If either is a mixed number, first apply *Rule 1.* If the multiplier is a whole number, simply multiply the numerator of the fraction and write the product over the denominator.

*Examples:*

*How much active ingredient is represented in 24 tablets each containing $\frac{1}{320}$ grain of the ingredient?*

$$24 \times \frac{1}{320} \text{ gr} = \frac{24 \times 1}{320} \text{ gr} = \frac{24}{320} \text{ gr} = \frac{3}{40} \text{ gr, } \textit{answer.}$$

*The adult dose of a drug is $\frac{3}{20}$ grain. Calculate the dose for a child if it is $\frac{1}{12}$ of the adult dose.*

$$\frac{1}{12} \times \frac{3}{20} \text{ gr} = \frac{1 \times 3}{12 \times 20} \text{ gr} = \frac{3}{240} \text{ gr} = \frac{1}{80} \text{ gr, } \textit{answer.}$$

**To divide fractions:**

In the division of fractions, it is important for the student to grasp the meaning of *reciprocal*. By definition, the *reciprocal* of a number is *1* divided by the number. For example, the reciprocal of 3 is $\frac{1}{3}$. If you apply *Rule 2* above and regard 3 as the same as the fraction $\frac{3}{1}$, then its reciprocal equals the inversion of this fraction. In general, therefore, when *a* is a fraction, its reciprocal is $1/a$ and proves to have the same value as the fraction inverted. So, the reciprocal of $1/4$ is $4/1$ or 4, and the reciprocal of $2\frac{1}{2}$ or $5/2$ is $2/5$.

Now, if the fraction $3/4$ is interpreted as meaning 3 divided by 4, then it should be emphasized that dividing by 4 is exactly the same as multiplying by the reciprocal of 4, or $1/4$. This method of handling division when fractions are involved is called the *reciprocal method,* and it points out the reciprocal relation, or inverse relation, between multiplication and division.

To divide by a fraction, then, simply invert its terms and multiply. And when a fraction is to be divided by a whole number, first interpret the whole number as a fraction having 1 for its denominator, invert to gets its reciprocal, and multiply.

*Examples:*

*If $1/2$ ounce is divided into 4 equal parts, how much will each part contain?*

Interpreting 4 as $4/1$:

$$\frac{1}{2}\text{ oz} \div \frac{4}{1} = \frac{1}{2}\text{ oz} \times \frac{1}{4} = \frac{1 \times 1}{2 \times 4}\text{ oz} = \frac{1}{8}\text{ oz, } \textit{answer.}$$

*The dose of a drug is $1/60$ grain. How many doses can be made from $1/5$ grain?*

$$\frac{1}{5} \div \frac{1}{60} = \frac{1}{5} \times \frac{60}{1} = \frac{1 \times 60}{5 \times 1} = 12 \text{ doses, } \textit{answer.}$$

*A child is given $5/8$ grain of a drug. If this represents $1/16$ of the adult dose, what is the adult dose?*

If $1/16$ of (that is, *times*) the adult dose is $5/8$ grain, then $5/8$ grain divided by $1/16$ must equal the adult dose.

$$\frac{5}{8}\text{ gr} \div \frac{1}{16} = \frac{5}{8}\text{ gr} \times \frac{16}{1} = \frac{5 \times 16}{8 \times 1}\text{ gr} = 10 \text{ gr, } \textit{answer.}$$

## Decimal Fractions

A fraction whose denominator is 10 or any power of ten is called a *decimal fraction,* or simply a *decimal.* The denominator of a decimal fraction is never written, since the decimal point serves to indicate the place value of the numerals. The numerator and the decimal point are sufficient to express the fraction. So, $1/10$ is written 0.1, $45/100$ is written 0.45, and $65/1000$ is written 0.065.

All operations with decimal fractions are carried out in the same manner as with whole numbers, but care must be exercised in putting the decimal point in its proper place in the results.

Three familiar operations are worth recalling.

(1) As a direct consequence of the place value in the decimal notation, moving the decimal point one place to the right multiplies a number by 10, two places to the right multiplies it by 100, and so on. Likewise, moving the point one place to the left divides a number by 10, two places to the left divides it by 100, and so on.

(2) A decimal fraction may be changed to a common fraction by writing the numerator over the denominator and (if desired) reducing to lowest terms:

$$0.125 = {}^{125}/_{1000} = {}^{1}/_{8}$$

(3) A common fraction may be changed to a decimal by dividing the numerator by the denominator (note that the result may be a repeating or endless decimal fraction):

$$^{3}/_{8} = 3 \div 8 = 0.375$$

$$^{1}/_{3} = 1 \div 3 = 0.3333 \ldots.$$

### Practice Problems

1. Add each of the following:
   (*a*) $^{5}/_{8}$ gr + $^{9}/_{32}$ gr + $^{1}/_{4}$ gr
   (*b*) $^{1}/_{150}$ gr + $^{1}/_{200}$ gr + $^{1}/_{100}$ gr
   (*c*) $^{1}/_{60}$ gr + $^{1}/_{20}$ gr + $^{1}/_{16}$ gr + $^{1}/_{32}$ gr

2. Find the difference:

   (*a*) $3^{1}/_{2}$ grain − $^{15}/_{64}$ grain.
   (*b*) $^{1}/_{30}$ grain − $^{1}/_{40}$ grain.
   (*c*) $2^{1}/_{3}$ grain − $1^{1}/_{2}$ grain.

3. Find the product:

   (*a*) $^{30}/_{75} \times {}^{15}/_{32} \times 25$.
   (*b*) $2^{1}/_{2} \times 12 \times {}^{7}/_{8}$.
   (*c*) $^{1}/_{125} \times {}^{9}/_{20}$.

4. What is the reciprocal of each of the following?
   (*a*) $^{1}/_{10}$.
   (*b*) $3^{1}/_{3}$.
   (*c*) $^{12}/_{1}$.
   (*d*) $^{3}/_{2}$.
   (*e*) $1^{7}/_{8}$.
   (*f*) $^{1}/_{64}$.

5. Find the quotient:
   (*a*) $^{2}/_{3} \div {}^{1}/_{24}$.
   (*b*) $^{1}/_{5000} \div 12$.
   (*c*) $6^{1}/_{4} \div {}^{1}/_{2}$.

6. Solve each of the following:
   (*a*) $(\frac{1}{120} \div \frac{1}{150}) \times 50 = ?$
   (*b*) $\frac{1\frac{1}{2}}{100} \times 1000 = ?$
   (*c*) $\frac{3}{4} \times ? = 48.$
   (*d*) $\frac{\frac{1}{500}}{5} \times ? = 5.$

7. What fractional part:
   (*a*) of 64 is 2?
   (*b*) of $\frac{1}{16}$ is $\frac{1}{20}$?
   (*c*) of $\frac{1}{32}$ is 2?

8. A prescription contains $\frac{5}{8}$ grain of ingredient A, $\frac{1}{4}$ grain of ingredient B, $\frac{1}{100}$ grain of ingredient C, and $\frac{3}{50}$ grain of ingredient D. Calculate the weight of the four ingredients in the prescription.

9. How many $\frac{1}{2000}$-grain doses can be obtained from $\frac{3}{80}$ grain of a certain drug?

10. A patient received the following doses of a drug:
    3 doses each containing $\frac{1}{20}$ grain
    3 doses each containing $\frac{1}{24}$ grain
    2 doses each containing $\frac{1}{32}$ grain
    2 doses each containing $\frac{1}{64}$ grain

Calculate the total amount of the drug received by the patient.

11. A capsule contains $\frac{1}{40}$ grain of ingredient A, $\frac{1}{4}$ grain of ingredient B, $\frac{1}{120}$ grain of ingredient C, and enough of ingredient D to make 4 grains. How many grains of ingredient D are in the capsule?

12. The adult dose of a certain drug is $\frac{1}{120}$ grain. If the child dose is $\frac{1}{6}$ of the adult dose, what fraction of a grain will be given if 8 doses are administered to a child?

13. Calculate the fractional difference between a $\frac{1}{100}$-grain tablet and a $\frac{1}{150}$-grain tablet of atropine sulfate.

14. The dose of a drug is $\frac{1}{120}$ grain. How many doses can be made from $\frac{2}{3}$ grain?

15. What decimal fraction:

    (*a*) of 18 is $2\frac{1}{4}$?
    (*b*) of 25 is 0.005?
    (*c*) of 7000 is 437.5?

16. Write the following as decimals and add:

    $\frac{3}{1000}$, $\frac{75}{100}$, $\frac{3}{20}$, $\frac{5}{8}$, $\frac{13}{25}$

17. Write the following as decimals and add:

$\frac{3}{5}$, $\frac{1}{20}$, $\frac{65}{1000}$, $\frac{19}{40}$, $\frac{3}{8}$

18. How many 0.000065-gram doses can be made from 0.130 gram of a drug?

19. Calculate the fractional difference between a $\frac{1}{400}$-grain and a $\frac{1}{150}$-grain tablet of nitroglycerin.

20. Calculate the fractional difference between $\frac{1}{400}$-grain and $\frac{1}{600}$-grain tablets of digitoxin.

21. A patient received the following doses of a drug:

4 doses each containing $\frac{1}{120}$ grain
4 doses each containing $\frac{1}{100}$ grain
2 doses each containing $\frac{1}{150}$ grain
4 doses each containing $\frac{1}{200}$ grain

Calculate the total amount of the drug received by the patient.

22. A pharmacist had three grains of hydromorphone hydrochloride. He used it in preparing the following:

8 capsules each containing $\frac{1}{32}$ grain
8 capsules each containing $\frac{1}{24}$ grain
20 capsules each containing $\frac{1}{48}$ grain

How many grains of hydromorphone hydrochloride were left after he prepared the capsules?

23. A patient received the following doses of a drug:

6 doses each containing 0.0065 gram
6 doses each containing 0.00325 gram
4 doses each containing 0.005 gram

Calculate the total amount of the drug received by the patient.

24. A pharmacist had 5 grams of codeine phosphate. He used it in preparing the following:

8 capsules each containing 0.0325 gram
12 capsules each containing 0.015 gram
18 capsules each containing 0.008 gram

How many grams of codeine phosphate were left after he had prepared the capsules?

25. Norlestrin tablets are available as a combination containing $\frac{1}{60}$ grain of norethindrone acetate and $\frac{1}{1200}$ grain of ethinyl estradiol per tablet.

(*a*) Calculate the total amount, as a fraction of a grain, of drugs in each tablet.
(*b*) Calculate the number of tablets which may be prepared from 7000 grains (1 pound) of ethinyl estradiol, assuming an adequate supply of norethindrone acetate.

## RATIO, PROPORTION, VARIATION

### Ratio

The relative magnitude of two like quantities is called their *ratio*. Ratio is sometimes defined as *the quotient of two like numbers*. But in order not to lose sight of the fact that *two* quantities are being *compared*, this quotient is always expressed as an *operation*, not as a *result:* in other words, it is expressed as a *fraction*, and the fraction is interpreted as indicating the operation of dividing the numerator by the denominator. Thus, a ratio presents us with the concept of a common fraction as expressing the relation of its two numbers.

The ratio of *20* and *10*, for example, is not expressed as *2* (that is, the quotient of *20* divided by *10*), but as the fraction $^{20}/_{10}$. And when this fraction is to be interpreted as a ratio, it is traditionally written *20:10* and always read *twenty to ten*. Similarly, when the fraction ½ is to be interpreted as a ratio, it is traditionally written *1:2*, and it is read not as *one-half* but as *one to two*.

All the rules governing common fractions equally apply to a ratio. Of particular importance is the principle that *if the two terms of a ratio are multiplied or are divided by the same number, the value is unchanged*—the *value*, of course, being the quotient of the first term divided by the second.

For example, the ratio *20:4* or $^{20}/_{4}$ has a value of *5*. Now, if both terms are multiplied by *2*, the ratio becomes *40:8* or $^{40}/_{8}$, still with a value of *5;* and if both terms are divided by *2*, the ratio becomes *10:2* or $^{10}/_{2}$, again with a value of *5*.

The terms of a ratio must be of the same kind, for the *value* of a ratio is an abstract number expressing how many *times* greater or smaller the first term (or numerator) is than the second term (or denominator).[1] The terms may themselves be abstract numbers, or else they may be concrete numbers of the same denomination. Thus, we can have a ratio of *20* to *4* ($^{20}/_{4}$) or *20 grains* to *4 grains* ($\frac{20 \text{ grains}}{4 \text{ grains}}$). To recognize this relationship clearly, it is useful to interpret a ratio as expressing in its *denominator* a number of parts that a certain quantity (used for comparison) is conveniently

[1]The ratio of *1* gallon to *3* pints is surely not *1:3*, for the gallon contains *8* pints, and the ratio therefore is *8:3*. To ignore this principle is to invite disaster in our calculations.

taken to contain, and in its *numerator* the number of *those parts* that the quantity we are measuring is found to contain.[1]

When two ratios have the same value they are *equivalent*. An interesting fact about equivalent ratios is this: *the product of the numerator of the one and the denominator of the other always equals the product of the denominator of the one and the numerator of the other.* That is to say, *the cross products are equal:*

$$\text{Since } 2/4 = 4/8,$$

$$2 \times 8 \text{ (or 16)} = 4 \times 4 \text{ (or 16)}.$$

It is also true that *if two ratios are equal, their* reciprocals are equal:

$$\text{Since } 2/4 = 4/8, \text{ then } 4/2 = 8/4.$$

We discover further that the *numerator of the one fraction equals the product of its denominator and the other fraction:*

$$\text{If } 6/15 = 2/5,$$

$$\text{then } 6 = 15 \times 2/5 \text{ (or } \tfrac{15 \times 2}{5}) = 6,$$

$$\text{and } 2 = 5 \times 6/15 \text{ (or } \tfrac{5 \times 6}{15}) = 2.$$

*And the denominator of the one equals the quotient of its numerator divided by the other fraction:*

$$15 = 6 \div 2/5 \text{ (or } 6 \times 5/2) = 15,$$

$$\text{and } 5 = 2 \div 6/15 \text{ (or } 2 \times 15/6) = 5.$$

An extremely useful practical application of these facts is found in *proportion.*

## Proportion

A *proportion* is the expression of the equality of two ratios. It may be written in any one of three standard forms:

(1) $a:b = c:d$
(2) $a:b :: c:d$
(3) $\frac{a}{b} = \frac{c}{d}$

---

[1]Ratios are expressed or implied everywhere in mathematics, "the science of measure." A common fraction may always be understood to designate in its denominator the number of equal parts into which *1* is divided, and in its numerator the number of those parts we are concerned with. Decimal fractions are ratios with a fixed series of denominators: *10, 100, 1000,* and so on. We have observed that every whole number implies a ratio with *1*, our unit of counting. Percentage is a convenient ratio that expresses a number of parts in every hundred of the same kind.

Each of these expressions is read: *a is to b as c is to d,* and $a$ and $d$ are called the *extremes* (meaning "outer members") and $b$ and $c$ the *means* ("middle members").

In any proportion *the product of the extremes is equal to the product of the means.* This principle allows us to find the missing term of any proportion when the other three terms are known. If the missing term is a *mean,* it will be *the product of the extremes divided by the given mean:* and if it is an *extreme,* it will be *the product of the means divided by the given extreme.* And from this we may derive the following fractional equations:

If $\frac{a}{b} = \frac{c}{d}$, then

$$a = \frac{bc}{d},\ b = \frac{ad}{c},\ c = \frac{ad}{b},\ \text{and } d = \frac{bc}{a}.$$

Most experienced calculators are indifferent to the order of terms in the proportions they devise. For the sake of the greater mechanical accuracy gained by routine discipline, some teachers still prefer the old pattern of putting the unknown term in the fourth place— that is, in the denominator of the second fraction.

There are few arithmetic problems, save for the simplest, that cannot most directly be solved by proportion. Provided that we correctly interpret the relationships implied by the data, *given any three terms of a proportion, by appeal to the facts set forth above we may easily calculate the value of the fourth.* Since the missing fourth is usually the desired answer, proportion takes us to it without any intermediate steps.

*Examples:*

*If 3 tablets contain 15 grains of aspirin, how many grains should be contained in 12 tablets?*

$$\frac{3\ \text{(tablets)}}{12\ \text{(tablets)}} = \frac{15\ \text{(grains)}}{\text{x (grains)}}$$

$$\text{x} = \frac{12 \times 15}{3}\ \text{grains} = 60\ \text{grains, } \textit{answer.}$$

*If 3 tablets contain 15 grains of aspirin, how many tablets should contain 60 grains?*

$$\frac{3\ \text{(tablets)}}{\text{x (tablets)}} = \frac{15\ \text{(grains)}}{60\ \text{(grains)}}$$

$$\text{x} = \frac{3 \times 60}{15}\ \text{tablets} = 12\ \text{tablets, } \textit{answer.}$$

*If 12 tablets contain 60 grains of aspirin, how many grains should 3 tablets contain?*

$$\frac{12 \text{ (tablets)}}{3 \text{ (tablets)}} = \frac{60 \text{ (grains)}}{x \text{ (grains)}}$$

$$x = \frac{3 \times 60}{12} \text{ grains} = 15 \text{ grains, } \textit{answer.}$$

*If 12 tablets contain 60 grains of aspirin, how many tablets should contain 15 grains?*

$$\frac{12 \text{ (tablets)}}{x \text{ (tablets)}} = \frac{60 \text{ (grains)}}{15 \text{ (grains)}}$$

$$x = \frac{12 \times 15}{60} \text{ tablets} = 3 \text{ tablets, } \textit{answer.}$$

Some calculators will set up "mixed" ratios in their proportions, invoking the principle that if the ratios are regarded as abstract numbers *the means or the extremes may be interchanged without destroying the validity of the equation.*[1] However true this principle may be of abstract numbers, it is nevertheless illogical (and never necessary) to make a ratio between, say, a number of tablets and a number of grains. It is very risky to ignore the rule that *ratios should express the relationship of denominate numbers of the same kind.* In many problems we find that the quantities given must be reduced or converted to a common denomination before we can proceed with the solution.

Proportions need not contain whole numbers. If common or decimal fractions are supplied in the data, they may be included in the proportion without changing the method.

---

[1] So that if:

$$\frac{3 \text{ (tablets)}}{12 \text{ (tablets)}} = \frac{15 \text{ (grains)}}{60 \text{ (grains)}}$$

then:

$$\frac{3 \text{ (tablets)}}{15 \text{ (grains)}} = \frac{12 \text{ (tablets)}}{60 \text{ (grains)}}$$

and:

$$\frac{60 \text{ (grains)}}{12 \text{ (tablets)}} = \frac{15 \text{ (grains)}}{3 \text{ (tablets)}}$$

and:

$$\frac{60 \text{ (grains)}}{15 \text{ (grains)}} = \frac{12 \text{ (tablets)}}{3 \text{ (tablets)}}$$

But, since calculating with common fractions is more complicated than with whole numbers or decimal fractions, it is useful to know—and wherever possible to apply—these two facts:

(1) *Two fractions having a common denominator are directly proportional to their numerators.*

$$\frac{60/100}{50/100} = \frac{60}{50}$$

$$\text{Proof: } \frac{60}{100} \div \frac{50}{100} = \frac{60}{100} \times \frac{100}{50} = \frac{60}{50}$$

(2) *Two fractions having a common numerator are inversely proportional to their denominators.*

$$\frac{2/3}{2/7} = \frac{7}{3}$$

$$\text{Proof: } 2/3 \div 2/7 = 2/3 \times 7/2 = 7/3$$

*Examples:*

*If $1\frac{1}{2}$ grains of a drug represent 18 doses, how many doses are represented in $\frac{1}{4}$ grain?*

$$1\tfrac{1}{2} \text{ grains} = 3/2 \text{ grains} = 6/4 \text{ grains}$$

$$\frac{6/4 \text{ (grains)}}{1/4 \text{ (grain)}} = \frac{18 \text{ (doses)}}{x \text{ (doses)}}$$

$$\text{Or: } \frac{6}{1} = \frac{18}{x} \text{ (doses)}$$

$$x = \frac{1 \times 18}{6} \text{ doses} = 3 \text{ doses, } \textit{answer.}$$

*If 30 milliliters represent $\frac{1}{6}$ of the volume of a prescription, how many milliliters will represent $\frac{1}{4}$ of the volume?*

$$\frac{1/6 \text{ (volume)}}{1/4 \text{ (volume)}} = \frac{30 \text{ (mL)}}{x \text{ (mL)}}$$

$$\text{Or: } \frac{4}{6} = \frac{30}{x} \text{ (mL)}$$

$$x = \frac{6 \times 30}{4} \text{ mL} = 45 \text{ mL, } \textit{answer.}$$

## Variation

In the examples above involving tablets and grains, the relationship was clearly *proportional*—that is, the variation between number of tablets and number of grains was known to be consistent and regular. In every proportion the "cause" must have a *constant rate* of "effect" if the equation is to be valid.

Most pharmaceutical calculations deal with simple, *direct* relationships: twice the cause, double the effect, and so on. Occasionally they deal with *inverse* relationships: twice the cause, half the effect, and so on—as when you *decrease* the strength of a solution by *increasing* the amount of diluent.[1]

Here is a typical problem involving inverse proportion:

*If 10 pints of a 5% solution are diluted to 40 pints, what is the percentage strength of the dilution?*

$$\frac{10 \text{ (pints)}}{40 \text{ (pints)}} = \frac{x\ (\%)}{5\ (\%)}$$

$$x = \frac{10 \times 5}{40}\% = 1.25\%, \textit{ answer.}$$

The use of proportion in pharmaceutical problems is abundantly illustrated in the text. The following miscellany reveals a variety of applications of the method.

### Practice Problems

1. *Make valid ratios between these familiar quantities:*

   (*a*) 3 gallons and 2 quarts.
   (*b*) 1 yard and 2 feet.
   (*c*) ½ mile and 1760 feet.
   (*d*) 4 hours and 120 minutes.
   (*e*) 2 feet and 6 inches.

[1]In expressing an inverse proportion we must not forget that *every* proportion asserts the equivalence of two fractions, and therefore the numerators must both be smaller or both larger than their respective denominators.

*Solve by proportion:*

2. If 250 pounds of a chemical cost $480, what will be the cost of 135 pounds?

3. If 75 pounds of a chemical cost $250, what will be the cost of 95 pounds?

4. A formula for 1250 tablets contains 3.25 grams of diazepam. How much diazepam should be used in preparing 350 tablets?

5. If 100 capsules contain $\frac{3}{8}$ grain of an active ingredient, how much of the ingredient will 48 capsules contain?

6. If 450 pounds of Green Soap costs $310.50, what will be the cost of 33 pounds?

7. If 50 tablets contain 0.625 gram of an active ingredient, how many tablets can be prepared from 31.25 grams of the ingredient?

8. If 24 pounds of a chemical cost $46.80, how many pounds can be bought for $78.00?

9. If 15 gallons of a certain liquid cost $36.25, how much will 4 gallons cost?

10. If 125 gallons of a mouth rinse contain 20 grams of a coloring agent, how many grams will 160 gallons contain?

11. If 50 tablets contain 1.5 grams of active ingredient, how much of the ingredient will 1,375 tablets contain?

12. If a diarrhea mixture contains 3.7 mL of paregoric in each 30 mL of mixture, how many milliliters of paregoric would be contained in a teaspoonful (5 mL) dose of the mixture?

13. If 1.625 grams of a coloring agent are used to color 250 liters of a certain solution, how many liters could be colored by using 0.750 gram?

14. How many grains of a substance are needed for 350 tablets if 75 tablets contain 3 grains of the substance?

15. Ipecac Syrup contains the equivalent of 32 grains of ipecac in each fluidounce (480 minims) of the syrup. How many minims would provide the equivalent of 20 grains of ipecac?

16. A pediatric vitamin drug product contains the equivalent of 0.5 milligram of fluoride ion in each milliliter. How many milligrams of fluoride ion would be provided by a dropper which delivers 0.6 milliliter?

17. If 1000 grams of an ointment contain 0.875 gram of a certain ingredient, how much of the ingredient will 625 grams contain?

18. An elixir of aprobarbital contains 40 milligrams of aprobarbital in each 5 milliliters. How many milligrams would be used in preparing 4,000 milliliters of the elixir?

19. An elixir of ferrous sulfate contains 220 milligrams of ferrous sulfate in each 5 milliliters. If each milligram of ferrous sulfate contains the equivalent of 0.2 milligram of elemental iron, how many milligrams of elemental iron would be represented in each 5 milliliters of the elixir?

20. At a constant temperature, the volume of a gas varies inversely

with the pressure. If a gas occupies a volume of 1000 milliliters at a pressure of 760 millimeters, what is its volume at a pressure of 570 millimeters?

21. If 150 milliliters of a $\frac{1}{10}$% solution are diluted to 750 milliliters, what is the percentage strength of the resulting product?

22. How many $\frac{1}{120}$-grain tablets will yield the same amount of atropine sulfate as 50 tablets each containing $\frac{1}{150}$ grain?

23. A solution contains $\frac{1}{4}$ grain of morphine sulfate per 15 minims. How many minims will contain $\frac{1}{6}$ grain of morphine sulfate?

24. A penicillin V potassium preparation provides 400,000 units of activity in each 250-milligram tablet. How many total units of activity would a patient receive from taking four tablets a day for 10 days?

25. A solution of digitoxin contains 0.2 milligram per milliliter. How many milliliters will contain 0.03 milligram of digitoxin?

26. A pharmacist prepared a solution containing 5 million units of penicillin per 10 milliliters. How many units of penicillin will 0.25 milliliter contain?

27. If a 5.0-gram packet of a potassium supplement provides 20 milliequivalents of potassium ion and 3.34 milliequivalents of chloride ion, *(a)* how many grams of the powder would provide 6 milliequivalents of potassium ion, and *(b)* how many milliequivalents of chloride ion would be provided by this amount of powder?

28. If an intravenous fluid is adjusted to deliver 15 milligrams of medication to a patient per hour, how many milligrams are delivered per minute?

29. If a potassium chloride elixir contains 20 milliequivalents of potassium ion in each 15 milliliters of elixir, how many milliliters will provide 25 milliequivalents of potassium ion to the patient?

30. If an insulin injection contains 100 U.S.P. Units of insulin per milliliter, how many milliliters would be required to administer 40 U.S.P. Units of insulin?

31. If a syringe contains 5 milligrams of medication in each 10 milliliters of solution, how many milligrams would be administered when 4 milliliters of solution are injected?

## SIGNIFICANT FIGURES

When we *count* objects accurately, *every* figure in the numeral expressing the total number of objects must be taken at its face value. Such figures may be said to be *absolute.*

But when we record a *measurement,* the last figure to the right must be taken to be an *approximation,* an admission that the limit of possible precision or of necessary accuracy has been reached, and that any further figures to the right would be non-significant—that is, either meaningless or, for a given purpose, needless.

We should learn to interpret a denominate number like *325 grams* as follows: The *3* means *300 grams,* neither more nor less, and the *2* means *exactly 20 grams more;* but the final *5* means *approximately 5 grams more*—that is, *5 grams plus or minus some fraction of a gram.* Whether this fraction is, for a given purpose, negligible depends upon how precisely the quantity was (or is to be) weighed.

*Significant figures,* then, are consecutive figures that express the value of a denominate number accurately enough for a given purpose. The accuracy varies with the number of significant figures, which are all absolute in value except the last—and this is properly called *uncertain.*

Two-figure accuracy is liable to a deviation as high as 5% from the theoretic absolute measurement. For example, if a substance is reported to weigh *10 grams* to the nearest *gram,* its actual weight may be anything between *9.5 grams* and *10.5 grams.*

Three-figure accuracy is liable to a deviation as high as 0.5%; four-figure accuracy may deviate 0.05%; and five-figure accuracy, 0.005%.

Any of the digits in a valid denominate number must be regarded as significant. Whether *zero* is significant, however, depends upon its position or upon known facts about a given number. The interpretation of *zero* may be summed up as follows:

1. *Any zero between digits is significant.*
2. *Initial zeros to the left of the first digit are never significant: they are included merely to show the location of the decimal point and thus give place value to the digits that follow.*
3. *One or more final zeros to the right of the decimal point may be taken to be significant.*
4. *One or more final zeros in a whole number—that is, immediately to the left of the decimal point—sometimes merely serve to give place value to digits to the left, but the data may show them to be significant.*

*Examples:*

*Assuming that the following numbers are all denominate—*

(1) In *12.5* there are *three* significant figures; in *1.256, four* significant figures; and in *102.56, five* significant figures.

(2) In *0.5* there is *one* significant figure. The digit *5* tells us how many *tenths* we have. The non-significant *0* simply calls attention to the decimal point.

(3) In *0.05* there is still only *one* significant figure, and again in *0.005.*

(4) In *0.65* there are *two* significant figures, and likewise *two* in *0.065* and *0.0065.*

(5) In *0.0605* there are *three* significant figures. The first *0* calls

attention to the decimal point; the second *0* shows the number of places to the right of the decimal point occupied by the remaining figures; and the third *0* significantly contributes to the value of the number. In *0.06050* there are *four* significant figures, since the final *0* also contributes to the value of the number.

(6) In *20000* there are *five* significant figures; but *20000* $\pm$*50* (or, to express the same quantity another way, *20000 to the nearest 100)* contains only *three* significant figures.

As already pointed out, one of the factors determining the degree of approximation to perfect measurement is the precision of the instrument used. It would be absurd to claim that *7.76 milliliters* had been measured in a graduate calibrated in units of *1 milliliter;* or that *25.562 grains* had been weighed on a balance sensitive to *1/10 grain.*

*Other Examples:*

(1) If a substance weighs *0.06 gram* according to a balance sensitive to *0.001 gram,* we may record the weight as *0.060 gram.* But if the balance is sensitive only to *0.01 gram,* the value should be recorded as *0.06 gram,* and a record of *0.060 gram* would be invalid.

(2) Again, when recording a length of *10 millimeters* found by use of an instrument accurate to *0.1 millimeter,* the value may be recorded as *10.0 millimeters.*

(3) And again, if a volume of *5 milliliters* is measured with an instrument calibrated in *10ths of a milliliter,* the volume may be recorded as *5.0 milliliters.*

We must clearly distinguish *significant figures* from *decimal places.* When recording a measurement, the number of decimal places we include indicates *the degree of precision with which the measurement has been made,* whereas the number of significant figures retained indicates *the degree of accuracy* that is sufficient for a given purpose.

Sometimes we are asked to record a value "correct to (so-many) decimal places"; and we should never confuse this familiar expression with the expression "correct to (so-many) significant figures."

*Examples:*

(1) If the value of *27.625918* is rounded off to *five decimal places,* it is written *27.62592;* but when rounded off to *five significant figures* it is written *27.626.*

(2) The value *54.3265,* when rounded off to *54.3,* is precise to *one decimal place* but accurate to *three significant figures.*

The *principle* that *the result of any calculation involving an approximate number should be rounded off so as to contain only one uncertain figure* holds for quotients and products as well for sums anddifferences.

With this principle in mind, we can get valid results, and save a good deal of time, by obeying the following rules for (a) recording measurements, (b) calculating with approximate numbers, and (c) recording the results of such calculations.

> 1. *When recording a measurement, retain as many figures as will give only one uncertain figure.*

The uncertain figure will sometimes represent an estimate between graduations on a scale. Thus, if you use a ruler calibrated in centimeters, you might record a measurement as approximately 11.3 *centimeters*, but not as approximately 11.32 *centimeters*. Since the 3 is uncertain, no other figure should follow it.

> 2. *When rejecting superfluous figures in the result of a calculation, add 1 to the last figure retained if the following figure is 5 or more.*

Thus, 2.43 may be rounded off to 2.4, but 2.46 should be rounded off to 2.5. Note that if a number like 2.597 is rounded off to three significant figures, the 1 added to the 9 makes 10, and 0 should be recorded, for it is significant: 2.60.

> 3. *When adding or subtracting approximate numbers, include only as many decimal places as there are in the number with the least decimal places.*

*Example:*

*Add these approximate weights: 162.4 grams, 0.489 gram, 0.1875 gram, and 120.78 grams.*

| *Incorrect* | *Correct* |
|---|---|
| 162.4 | 162.4 |
| 0.489 | 0.5 |
| 0.1875 | 0.2 |
| 120.78 | 120.8 |
| 283.8565, *answer.* | 283.9, *answer.* |

It is important to note that in filling a prescription, the pharmacist *must* assume that the physician means each quantity to be measured with *the same degree of precision*. Hence, if we add these quantities taken from a prescription:

*5.5 grams*
*0.01 gram*
*0.005 gram*

we must *not* round off the total to one decimal place. Rather we must retain at least *three* decimal places in the total by interpreting the given quantities to mean 5.500 *grams,* 0.010 *gram,* and 0.005 *gram.* Where greater precision is required, we may interpret the given quantities to mean 5.5000, 0.0100, and 0.0050, etc.

4. *When multiplying or dividing one approximate number by another approximate number, round off the component with the greater number of significant figures to the number contained in the component having fewer significant figures. Retain no more significant figures in the product or quotient than in the number with the least significant figures.*

*Example:*

*Multiply* 1.65370 *grams by* 0.26.

1.65370 grams is rounded off to 1.65 grams

1.65 grams × 0.26 = 0.4290 or
0.43 gram, *answer.*

When multiplying or dividing with denominate numbers taken from a prescription or official formula, since we must assume that each quantity is meant to be measured with the same degree of accuracy, we must interpret each quantity as having at least as many significant figures as appear in the quantity containing the greatest number of significant figures. So, if the quantities 0.25 *gram,* 0.5 *gram,* and 5 *grams* are included in a prescription, they should be interpreted as 0.25 *gram,* 0.50 *gram,* and 5.0 *grams* for purposes of multiplication or division (as when we enlarge or reduce a formula); and results should be rounded off to contain two significant figures. Where greater accuracy is required, we may interpret the given quantities to mean 0.2500, 0.5000, and 5.000, etc.[1]

It should be noted that in multiplication and division we are concerned with the number of significant figures, whereas in addition and subtraction it is the number of decimal places that is important.

5. *After multiplying or dividing an approximate number by an absolute number, round off the result to the same number of significant figures as are contained in the approximate number.*

This is consistent with #4, for the denominate number contains fewer significant figures if the absolute number is interpreted as being followed by significant zeros to an infinite number of decimal places.

---

[1]When converting from one system of measurement to another, we are expressly ordered by the *United States Pharmacopeia* as follows: ". . . to calculate quantities required in pharmaceutical formulas, use the exact equivalents. For prescription compounding, use the exact equivalents rounded to three significant figures."

*Example:*

*If a patient has taken 96 doses, each containing 2.54 milligrams of active ingredient, how much of the active ingredient has he taken in all?*

$$\begin{array}{r} 2.54 \text{ milligrams} \\ \times\ 96 \\ \hline 1524 \\ 2286\phantom{0} \\ \hline 24384 \text{ or} \end{array}$$

244 milligrams, *answer.*

**Practice Problems**

1. State the number of significant figures in each of the *italicized* quantities:

(*a*) One gram equals *15.4324* grains.
(*b*) One liter equals *1000* milliliters.
(*c*) One inch equals *2.54* centimeters.
(*d*) The chemical costs *$1.05* a pound.
(*e*) One gram equals *1,000,000* micrograms.
(*f*) One microgram equals *0.001* milligram.

2. Assuming these numbers to be denominate, how many significant figures has each?

(*a*) 35
(*b*) 609
(*c*) 2.7
(*d*) 9004
(*e*) 506.03
(*f*) 0.0047
(*g*) 40.07
(*h*) 350 (to nearest 1).
(*i*) 350 (to nearest 10).
(*j*) 5000 (to the nearest 100).

3. Round off each of the following to three significant figures:

(*a*) 32.75
(*b*) 200.39
(*c*) 0.03629
(*d*) 21.635
(*e*) 0.00944
(*f*) 1.0751
(*g*) 27.052
(*h*) 0.86249
(*i*) 3.14159
(*j*) 1.00595632

4. Round off each of the following to three decimal places:

(*a*) 0.00083
(*b*) 34.79502
(*c*) 0.00494
(*d*) 6.12963
(*e*) 14.8997
(*f*) 1.00595632

5. If a mixture of seven ingredients contains the following approximate weights, what can you validly record as the approximate total combined weight of the ingredients?

26.83 grains, 275.3 grains, 2.752 grains, 4.04 grains, 5.197 grains, 16.64 grains, and 0.085 grain.

6. If each of a batch of tablets contains 0.050 grain of active ingredient, what approximate weight of active ingredient will be contained in 750 tablets?

7. If each tablet contains 0.05 grain of active ingredient, what will be the approximate weight of active ingredient in 750 tablets?

8. Perform the following computations and retain only significant figures in the results:

*(a)* 6.39 − 0.008
*(b)* 7.01 − 6.0
*(c)* 97.1 − 6.9368
*(d)* 5.0 × 48.3 grains
*(e)* 24 × 0.25 gram
*(f)* 350 × 0.60156 gram
*(g)* 0.720 × 0.095 grain
*(h)* 0.056 × 0.9626 gram
*(i)* 56.824 ÷ 0.0905
*(j)* 250 ÷ 1.109
*(k)* 5.0001 ÷ 1.9
*(l)* 0.00729 ÷ 0.2735
*(m)* 71.455 ÷ 0.512
*(n)* 71.955 ÷ 3.0

9. What is the difference in meaning between a volume recorded as 473 milliliters and one that is recorded as 473.0 milliliters?

10. What is the difference in meaning between a weight recorded as 0.65 gram and one that is recorded as 0.6500 gram?

11. The answers in the following computations are arithmetically correct. In each case, if the answer does not contain the proper number of significant figures, rewrite it so that all the figures retained are significant.

*(a)* 15.432 grains × 0.26 = 4.01232 grains
*(b)* 0.2350 grain ÷ 0.55 = 0.42727 grain
*(c)* 1.25500 grams + 0.650 gram + 0.125 gram + 12.78900 grams = 14.81900 grams
*(d)* 16.23 minims × 0.75 = 12.1725 minims
*(e)* 437.5 grains ÷ 1.25 = 350.000 grains

## ESTIMATION

One of the best checks of the reasonableness of a numerical computation is an estimation of the answer. If we have arrived at a wrong answer by use of a wrong method, a thoughtless, mechanical final verification of our figuring may not show up the error. But an absurd result, such as occurs when the decimal point is put in the wrong place, will not likely slip past if we check it against a preliminary estimation of what the result should be.

Since it is imperative that pharmacists insure the accuracy of their calculations by every possible means, pharmacy students are urged to adopt *estimation* as one of those means. Since proficiency in estimating comes only from constant practice, pharmacy students are urged to acquire the habit of estimating the answer to every problem encountered before attempting to solve it. Estimation not only will serve as a means for judging the reasonableness of the final result but also will very often serve as a guide in the solution of the problem.

*Checking* the accuracy of every calculation, of course, such as by adding a column first upwards and then downwards, is very important. Hence the student should follow this invariable procedure: (1) *estimate,* (2) *compute,* (3) *check.*

The estimating process is basically very simple. First the numbers given in a problem are mentally rounded off to slightly larger or smaller numbers containing fewer significant figures. So, the number *59* would be rounded off to *60,* and the number *732* to *700.* Then the required computations are performed, as far as possible mentally, and the result, although known to be somewhat greater or smaller than the exact answer, is close enough to serve as an estimate.

No set rules for estimating can be given to cover all the computations in arithmetic. But examples can illustrate some of the methods that can be used.

In *addition,* one way to obtain a reasonable estimate of the total is first to add the figures in the leftmost column. But the neglected remaining figures of each number are equally likely to express more or less than one-half the value of a unit of the order we have just added, and hence to the sum of the leftmost column should be added ½ for every number—or *1* for every two numbers—in the column.

*Examples:*

*Add the following numbers: 7428, 3652, 1327, 4605, 2791, and 4490.*

| *Estimation:* | *Calculation:* |
|---|---|
| The figures in the thou- | 7428 |
| sands column add up to | 3652 |
| 21000, and with each | 1327 |
| number on the average | 4605 |
| contributing 500 more, | 2791 |
| or every pair 1000 more, | 4490 |
| we get 21000 + 3000 = | —— |
| 24000, *estimated answer.* | 24293, *answer.* |

*Add the following numbers: 2556, 449, 337, 1572.*

| *Estimation:* | *Calculation:* |
|---|---|
| The figures of the thousands | 2556 |
| column add up to 3000, and | 449 |
| with each pair of numbers | 337 |
| contributing approximately | 1572 |
| another 1000, we get 3000 + | —— |
| 2000 = 5000, *estimated answer.* | 4914, *answer.* |

In *multiplication,* the product of the two leftmost digits plus a sufficient number of *zeros* to give the right place value will serve as a fair estimate. The number of *zeros* supplied must equal the total number of all discarded figures to the left of the decimal point. A closer approximation to the correct answer will result if the discarded figures are used to round off the value of those retained.

*Examples:*

*Multiply 612 by 413.*

| *Estimation:* | *Calculation:* |
|---|---|
| | 612 |
| 4 × 6 = 24, and | × 413 |
| since we have dis- | ——— |
| carded four fig- | 1836 |
| ures, four zeros | 612 |
| must be supplied, | 2448 |
| giving 240,000, | ——— |
| *estimated answer.* | 252756, *answer.* |

*Multiply 2889 by 209.*

| *Estimation:* | *Calculation:* |
|---|---|
| | 2889 |
| The given numbers | × 209 |
| round off to 3000 | ——— |
| and 200. 3 × 2 = 6, | 26001 |
| and supplying five | 5778 |
| zeros we get 600,000, | ——— |
| *estimated answer.* | 603801, *answer.* |

The correct place value is easier to keep track of if relatively insignificant decimal fractions are ignored. When the multiplier is a decimal fraction, the possibility of error is reduced if we first convert it to a common fraction of approximately the same value.

*Examples:*

*Multiply 41.76 by 20.3.*
Estimate: $42 \times 20 = 840$.

*Multiply 730.5 by 321.*
Estimate: $700 \times 300 = 210{,}000$.

*Multiply 314.2 by 0.18*
Estimate: Since 0.18 or $^{18}/_{100}$ lies between $^1/_6$ and $^1/_5$, the answer will lie between 50 and 60.

*Multiply 48.16 by 0.072.*
Estimate: $^7/_{100}$ equals about $^1/_{15}$, and $^1/_{15}$ of 48 is about 3.

In *division,* the given numbers may be rounded off to convenient approximations, but here again care must be exercised to preserve correct place values.

*Example:*

*Divide 2456 by 5.91.*
Estimate: The numbers may be rounded off to 2400 and 6. We may divide 24 by 6 mentally; but we must not forget the two zeros substituted for the given 56 in 2456, and our estimated answer will be 400.

The use of short cuts and variations in arithmetical computations contributes to both speed and accuracy in mental calculation. Facility in the use of short cuts can be developed only if we select or devise variations that appeal to us and practice them constantly. Here are some short cuts that may suggest other possibilities:

(1) To multiply by 10, 100, 1000, etc., move the decimal place one, two, three places to the right, etc. To divide by 10, 100, 1000, etc., move the decimal place one, two, three places to the left, etc.

(2) To multiply by 200, 300, 500, etc., multiply by 2, 3, 5, etc., and then multiply by 100. To divide by the same numbers, divide by 2, 3, 5, etc., and divide by 100.

(3) To multiply by 2000, 4000, 6000, etc., multiply by 2, 4, 6, etc., and then multiply by 1000. To divide by these numbers, divide by 2, 4, 6, etc., and divide by 1000.

(4) To multiply by 75, which is $^3/_4$ of a hundred, multiply by 300 and divide by 4. To divide by 75, multiply by 4 and divide by 300.

(5) To multiply by $66^2/_3$, which is $^2/_3$ of a hundred, multiply by 200 and divide by 3. To divide by $66^2/_3$, multiply by 3 and divide by 200.

(6) To multiply by 50, which is $\frac{1}{2}$ of a hundred, multiply by 100 and divide by 2. To divide by 50, multiply by 2 and divide by 100.

(7) To multiply by $33\frac{1}{3}$, which is $\frac{1}{3}$ of a hundred, multiply by 100 and divide by 3. To divide by $33\frac{1}{3}$, multiply by 3 and divide by 100.

(8) To multiply by 25, which is $\frac{1}{4}$ of a hundred, multiply by 100 and divide by 4. To divide by 25, multiply by 4 and divide by 100.

(9) To multiply by $12\frac{1}{2}$, which is $\frac{1}{8}$ of a hundred, multiply by 100 and divide by 8. To divide by $12\frac{1}{2}$, multiply by 8 and divide by 100.

(10) To multiply any *two-digit* number by 11, first add the two digits. If the sum is less than ten, place it between the digits; if the sum is ten or more, place the unit figure between the digits and add 1 to the left digit.

$11 \times 43$: $4 + 3 = 7$, hence 473
$11 \times 83$: $8 + 3 = 11$, hence 913

To multiply *any* number by eleven, multiply by 10 and add the multiplicand.

### Practice Problems

1. In estimating the result of multiplying 8,329 by 7,242 how many zeros will follow 56?
2. In estimating the result of dividing 811,500 by 16.23, how many zeros will follow 5?
3. How many terminal zeros are there in the product obtained by multiplying 5.100 by 90,000?
4. How many terminal zeros are there in the quotient obtained by dividing 8.100 by 0.009?

*Estimate the sums:*

| 5. | 7. | 9. |
|---|---|---|
| 5641 | 3298 | $ 75.82 |
| 2177 | 368 | 37.92 |
| 294 | 5192 | 14.69 |
| 8266 | 627 | 45.98 |
| 3503 | 4835 | 28.91 |
| | | 49.87 |

| 6. | 8. | 10. |
|---|---|---|
| 9874 | 7466 | $ 49.55 |
| 6018 | 5288 | 9.75 |
| 459 | 9013 | 12.98 |
| 1297 | 8462 | 53.36 |
| 3361 | 716 | 29.79 |
| 396 | 4369 | 14.56 |

*Estimate the products:*

11. $17 \times 22 =$
12. $28 \times 31 =$
13. $8 \times 48 =$
14. $19 \times 38 =$
15. $28 \times 62 =$
16. $39 \times 77 =$
17. $42 \times 39 =$
18. $125 \times 92 =$
19. $365 \times 98 =$
20. $473 \times 102 =$
21. $596 \times 204 =$
22. $604 \times 122 =$
23. $675 \times 19 =$
24. $998 \times 13 =$
25. $6549 \times 830 =$
26. $1073 \times 972 =$
27. $8431 \times 9760 =$
28. $7183 \times 19 =$
29. $5106 \times 963 =$
30. $2349 \times 5907 =$
31. $2\tfrac{1}{2} \times 14\tfrac{1}{2} =$
32. $\tfrac{2}{3} \times 400 =$
33. $21\tfrac{1}{3} \times 6\tfrac{2}{3} =$
34. $\tfrac{3}{4} \times 816 =$
35. $\tfrac{2}{3} \times 425.65 =$
36. $5.8 \times 7165 =$
37. $2.04 \times 705.3 =$
38. $0.016 \times 589.4 =$
39. $0.0726 \times 6951 =$
40. $98 \times 0.0031 =$
41. $6.1 \times 67.39 =$
42. $7569 \times 0.0963 =$

*Estimate the quotients:*

43. $171 \div 19 =$
44. $165 \div 15 =$
45. $184 \div 2300 =$
46. $3080 \div 144 =$
47. $160 \div 3200 =$
48. $36900 \div 41 =$
49. $86450 \div 72 =$
50. $1078 \div 98 =$
51. $98000 \div 49 =$
52. $17015 \div 57 =$
53. $1.0745 \div 500 =$
54. $18.954 \div 0.39 =$
55. $1.9214 \div 0.026 =$
56. $19.223 \div 47 =$
57. $458.4 \div 8 =$
58. $448.32 \div 0.048 =$

*Estimate the final results:*

59. $\dfrac{272103 \times 300}{901} =$

60. $\dfrac{750 \times 300 \times 380.5}{760 \times 375} =$

61. $\dfrac{270\ (15 - 10)}{91 \times 5} =$

62. $\tfrac{1}{120} \times \tfrac{1}{10} \times 11.95 =$

63. $\dfrac{437.5}{8.05} \times \tfrac{1}{16} =$

64. $\dfrac{809 \times (35 - 25)}{4.01 \times 20} =$

65. $\dfrac{\tfrac{1}{100}}{\tfrac{1}{2}} \times 5123 =$

66. $\dfrac{627 \times (25 - 10)}{30 \times 15} =$

67. $\dfrac{750 \times 380 \times 319.53}{760 \times 750} =$

68. What should be the approximate total cost of 625,250 tablets at $\frac{3}{5}$ cent each?

69. Estimate the approximate cost of 32,560 capsules at $12.50 per M.

70. Estimate the approximate cost of 30,125 capsules at $1.50 per hundred.

71. What should be the approximate cost of 120,050 tablets at 66$\frac{2}{3}$ cents per C?

72. A formula for 1,250 capsules contains 3.635 grams of a medicament. Estimate the amount of medicament that should be used in preparing 325 capsules.

73. Approximately how many teaspoonful- (5 milliliter-) doses can be obtained from 1 gallon (3,784 milliliters) of a liquid?

74. The cost of 1000 capsules is $15.00. If they are sold at the rate of $1.50 for 48 capsules, estimate the profit that can be realized from the sale of 1000 capsules.

75. The cost of 5000 capsules is $56.00. If they are sold at the rate of 75 cents for 24 capsules, estimate the profit that can be realized from the sale of 500 capsules.

## PERCENTAGE OF ERROR

Since measurements are never absolutely accurate, it is important for the pharmacist to recognize the limitations of his measuring instruments and to know the magnitude of the errors that may be incurred when he uses them.

When he weighs a substance on a torsion prescription balance, for instance, he may record the weight as a single quantity, such as *80 milligrams;* but he should be aware that a truer record of the weight should include two quantities, expressing (1) the apparent weight and (2) the possible excess or deficiency calculated from the known *sensitivity* or from the *sensitivity requirement* of the balance.[1] The second quantity is called the *maximum potential error.* So, if the pharmacist weighs *"80 milligrams"* on a torsion prescription balance having a *sensitivity requirement* of *4 milligrams,* he has actually weighed something between *76* and *84 milligrams,* for the maximum potential error is ± *4 milligrams.* This potential error may be used to calculate the percentage of possible error in order to determine whether an error of this magnitude may be allowed.

*Percentage of error* may be defined as *the maximum potential error multiplied by 100 and divided by the quantity desired.* The calculation may be formulated as follows:

$$\frac{\text{Error} \times 100\%}{\text{Quantity desired}} = \text{Percentage of error}$$

This formula is valid only if the error and the quantity desired are expressed in the same denomination.

---

[1]The *sensitivity* of a balance may be defined in several ways. Balance manufacturers use the term to designate the smallest weight that will just cause a perceptible movement of the balance indicator. Chemists define the *sensitivity* of an analytical balance as (1) the number of indicator scale divisions by which the zero point is displaced by a weight of 1 milligram or (2) the fraction of a milligram (expressed in tenths) necessary to produce a deflection of one scale division.

The term *sensitivity* as it applies to a prescription balance may be defined as the smallest weight that will disturb its equilibrium. This designation of the *sensitivity* of a prescription balance is not to be confused with the term *sensitivity requirement (SR)* which is defined in the United States Pharmacopeia as "the maximum change in load that will cause a specified change, one subdivision on the index plate, in the position of rest of the indicating element or elements of the balance."

In view of the fact that the term *sensitivity* has been variously interpreted, the United States Pharmacopeia has adopted the term *sensitivity requirement* to designate the sensitiveness of a balance. In accordance with this adoption the designation *sensitivity requirement* will be used herein when reference is made to the sensitiveness of a prescription balance.

The *sensitivity requirement* may be determined by the following procedure:

1. Level the balance.
2. Determine the rest point of the balance.
3. Determine the smallest weight which causes the rest point to shift one division on the index plate.

NOTE: The smaller the weight which is required to move the indicating element one division, the more sensitive is the balance.

In pharmacy practice, the pharmacist utilizes a "Class A" prescription balance which has a *sensitivity requirement (SR)* of 6 mg with no load and with a load of 10 g in the center of each pan. The United States Pharmacopeia states that "In order to avoid errors of 5 percent or more that might be due to the limit of sensitivity of the Class A prescription balance, do not weigh less than 120 mg (2 grains) of any material. If a smaller weight of dry material is required, mix a larger known weight of the ingredient with a known weight of dry diluent, and weigh an aliquot portion of the mixture for use."

*Example:*

*When the maximum potential error is ± 4 milligrams in a total of 100 milligrams, what is the percentage of error?*

$$\frac{4 \times 100\%}{100} = 4\%, \textit{ answer.}$$

Now, if the sensitivity of an instrument of dubious accuracy is not known, its performance may be checked with that of an instrument of known high accuracy. If the two instruments are used to measure the same thing, the difference between the two results will not be a potential error but a close approximation of an actual error; and given this, we may calculate the percentage of error actually committed by the less accurate instrument.

*Example:*

*A prescription calls for 800 milligrams of a substance. After weighing this amount on a balance, the pharmacist decides to check by weighing it again on a much more sensitive balance. Now he finds that he has only 750 milligrams. Since the first weighing was 50 milligrams short of the desired amount, what was the percentage of error?*

$$\frac{50 \times 100\%}{800} = 6.25\%, \textit{ answer.}$$

Finally, if a certain percentage of error is not to be exceeded, and the maximum potential error of an instrument is known, it is possible to calculate the smallest quantity that can be measured within the desired accuracy. Here is a convenient formula:

$$\frac{100 \times \text{maximum potential error}}{\text{Permissible percentage of error}} = \text{Smallest quantity}$$

*Example:*

*What is the smallest quantity that can be weighed with a potential error of not more than 5% on a balance sensitive to 6 milligrams?*

$$\frac{100 \times 6 \text{ milligrams}}{5} = 120 \text{ milligrams, } \textit{answer.}$$

**Practice Problems**

1. A pharmacist attempts to weigh 120 milligrams of atropine sulfate on a balance having a sensitivity requirement of 6 milligrams. Calculate the maximum potential error in terms of percentage.

2. In compounding a prescription, a pharmacist weighed 0.050 gram

of a substance on a balance insensitive to quantities smaller than 0.004 gram. What was the maximum potential error in terms of percentage?

3. A pharmacist wants to weigh 5 grains of a substance on a balance having a sensitivity requirement of ¼ grain. Calculate the maximum potential error in terms of percentage.

4. A pharmacist weighed 825 milligrams of a substance. When checked on another balance, the weight was found to be 805 milligrams. Calculate the deviation from the original weighing in terms of percentage.

5. A pharmacist weighed 475 milligrams of a substance on a balance of dubious accuracy. When checked on a balance of high accuracy, the weight was found to be 445 milligrams. Calculate the percentage of error in the first weighing.

6. A 10-milliliter graduate weighs 42.745 grams. When 5 milliliters of distilled water are measured in it, the combined weight of graduate and water is 47.675 grams. By definition, 5 milliliters of water should weigh 5 grams. Calculate the weight of the measured water and express any deviation from 5 grams as percentage of error.

7. A graduate weighs 35.825 grams. When 10 milliliters of water are measured in it, the weight of the graduate and water is 45.835 grams. Calculate the weight of the water and express any deviation from 10 grams as percentage of error.

8. In preparing a certain ointment, a pharmacist used 45.5 grains of zinc oxide instead of the 48 grains called for. Calculate the percentage of error on the basis of the desired quantity.

9. A pharmacist attempts to weigh 0.375 gram of morphine on a balance of dubious accuracy. When checked on a highly accurate balance, the weight is found to be 0.400 gram. Calculate the percentage of error in the first weighing.

10. On a prescription balance having a sensitivity requirement of 0.012 gram, what is the smallest amount that can be weighed with a maximum potential error of not more than 5%?

11. On a torsion prescription balance having a sensitivity requirement of $\frac{1}{16}$ grain, what is the smallest amount that can be weighed with a potential error of not more than 2%?

12. If an accuracy of 2% is desired, what is the minimum amount that should be weighed on a torsion prescription balance having a sensitivity requirement of 0.004 gram?

13. A pharmacist measured 60 milliliters of glycerin by difference,

starting with 100 milliliters. After completing the measurement, he noted that the graduate which he used contained 45 milliliters of glycerin. Calculate the percentage of error that was incurred in the measurement.

14. A pharmacist failed to place the balance in equilibrium before weighing three grains of codeine. Later, he discovered that the balance was out of equilibrium and that a 20% error was incurred. If the balance pan on which he placed the codeine was heavy, how many grains of codeine did he actually weigh?

15. In compounding a prescription for a nasal spray, a pharmacist weighed $\frac{1}{2}$ grain of menthol on a balance having a sensitivity requirement of $\frac{1}{20}$ grain. Calculate the percentage of error that may have been incurred.

16. Assuming a torsion balance having a sensitivity requirement of 4 milligrams (or $\frac{1}{16}$ grain), state which of the following weights could be made on it with a dispensing error not greater than plus or minus 5 percent:

(*a*) $\frac{5}{8}$ grain
(*b*) 0.085 gram
(*c*) $1\frac{1}{2}$ grains
(*d*) 50,000 micrograms
(1 microgram = 0.001 milligram)
(*e*) 65 milligrams
(*f*) $1\frac{1}{4}$ grains

17. A certain prescription balance is not to be used in weighing loads of less than 648 milligrams. Assuming that its sensitivity requirement is 30 milligrams, calculate the percentage of error that might be incurred in weighing the minimum specified load.

18. The sensitivity requirement of a Class A prescription balance is 0.006 gram. Calculate the percentage of error that might be incurred in weighing 0.1 gram on this balance.

19. A pharmacist measures 900 milliliters in a 1000-milliliter cylindrical graduate calibrated in units of 10 milliliters. Calculate the percentage of error that might be incurred in the measurement.

20. When substances are to be "accurately weighed" in an assay or a test, the *United States Pharmacopeia* directs that a quantity of 50 milligrams is to be weighed to the nearest 0.05 milligram. Calculate the percentage of error in the weighing.

21. You are directed to weigh 10 grams of a substance so as to limit the error to 0.2%. Calculate the maximum potential error, in terms of grams, that you would not be permitted to exceed.

22. In a certain assay, 100 milligrams of a substance are to be weighed so as to limit the error to 0.1%. Calculate the maximum potential error, in terms of milligrams, which the analyst must not exceed.

## ALIQUOT METHOD OF MEASURING

When a degree of precision in measurement is required that is beyond the capacity of the instrument at hand, the pharmacist may achieve the desired precision by measuring and calculating in terms of aliquot parts.

An *aliquot part* may be defined as any part that is contained a whole number of times in a quantity. Thus, *2* is an aliquot part of *10;* and since *10 ÷ 2 = 5, 2* is called the *fifth aliquot* of *10.* Again, *4* is an aliquot part of *16;* and since *16 ÷ 4 = 4, 4* is the *fourth aliquot* of *16.*

**To weigh by the aliquot method:**

*The aliquot method of weighing* is a method by which small quantities of a substance may be obtained within the degree of accuracy desired. The procedure may be summed up as follows:

*Step 1.* Select some multiple of the desired quantity that can be weighed with the required precision. Weigh this multiple.

*Step 2.* Using an inert substance that is compatible with the given preparation, dilute the multiple quantity.

*Step 3.* Weigh the aliquot part of the dilution that contains the desired quantity.

*To select the multiple quantity in Step 1,* first calculate the smallest quantity of the substance that can be weighed with the required precision (see Percentage of Error, pp. 33). To insure an error no greater than 5%, for instance, a quantity at least twenty times the sensitivity requirement of the balance must be weighed; and hence, if the sensitivity requirement of a balance is *4 milligrams, 20 × 4 milligrams,* or *80 milligrams,* is the smallest amount that can be weighed. If *50 milligrams* were weighed on such a balance, the maximum potential error would be 8% (see pp. 34). Convenience in multiplying, availability of weights, and the cost of the substance are other factors that help determine the choice of the multiple quantity.

*The amount of inert diluent used in Step 2* is determined by the fact that the aliquot part of the dilution to be weighed in *Step 3* must be a quantity large enough to be weighed within the desired degree of accuracy. In *Step 1* we have already calculated the minimum quantity that satisfies this condition. The aliquot must weigh as least as much as the multiple quantity weighed in *Step 1;* and to reduce the potential error its weight should usually be somewhat greater. So, if the multiple quantity weighs *80 milligrams,* the aliquot must weigh at least *80 milligrams,* but preferably

*100 milligrams* or more. When we multiply the chosen aliquot by the multiple selected in *Step 1*, we get the quantity of the dilution, and have only to add sufficient diluent to the multiple quantity to equal this weight of dilution.

*The aliquot weighed in Step 3* will contain the quantity originally desired, for if, say, *20* times the original quantity is diluted, $\frac{1}{20}$ of the dilution will contain the original quantity. And by arbitrarily selecting a sufficiently large multiple quantity and a sufficiently large dilution, we can be sure that we have measured within the required degree of precision.

*Example:*

*A torsion prescription balance has a sensitivity requirement of 4 milligrams. Explain how you would weigh 5 milligrams of atropine sulfate with an accuracy of ± 5%, using lactose as the diluent.*

Since 4 milligrams (mg) is the potential balance error, 80 milligrams is the smallest amount that should be weighed to achieve the required precision.

If 100 milligrams, or 20 times the desired amount of atropine sulfate, is chosen as the multiple quantity to be weighed in Step 1, and if 150 milligrams is set as the aliquot to be weighed in Step 3, then—

(1) Weigh 20 × 5 mg, or 100 mg of atropine sulfate
(2) Dilute with 2900 mg of lactose
  to make 3000 mg of dilution
(3) Weigh $\frac{1}{20}$ of dilution, or 150 mg of dilution, which will contain 5 milligrams of atropine sulfate, *answer.*

In this example the weight of the aliquot was arbitrarily set as *150 milligrams* which exceeds the weight of the multiple quantity, as it preferably should. If *100 milligrams* had been set as the aliquot, the multiple quantity should have been diluted with *1900 milligrams* of lactose to get *2000 milligrams* of dilution, and its twentieth aliquot, or *100 milligrams,* would have contained *5 milligrams* of atropine sulfate. On the other hand, if *200 milligrams* had been set as the aliquot, the multiple quantity of atropine sulfate should have been diluted with *3900 milligrams* of lactose to get *4000 milligrams* of dilution.

*Another example:*

*A torsion prescription balance has a sensitivity requirement of $\frac{1}{10}$ grain. Explain how you would weigh $\frac{1}{4}$ grain of atropine sulfate with an accuracy of ± 5%, using lactose as the diluent.*

Since $\frac{1}{10}$ grain (gr) is the potential balance error, 2 grains is the smallest amount that should be weighed to achieve the required precision.

If 12 is chosen as the multiple, and if 3 grains is set as the weight of the aliquot, then—

(1) Weigh 12 × ¼ gr, or 3 gr of atropine sulfate
(2) Dilute with 33 gr of lactose
to make 36 gr of dilution
(3) Weigh $\frac{1}{12}$ of dilution, or 3 gr of dilution, which will contain ¼ grain of atropine sulfate, *answer.*

**To measure volume by the aliquot method:**

*The aliquot method of measuring volume,* which is identical in principle to the aliquot method of weighing, may be used when relatively small volumes must be measured with great precision:

*Step 1.* Select a multiple of the desired quantity that can be measured with the required precision.

*Step 2.* Dilute the multiple quantity with a compatible diluent (usually a solvent for the liquid to be measured) to an amount evenly divisible by the multiple selected.

*Step 3.* Measure the aliquot of the dilution that contains the quantity originally desired.

In conformity with the legal requirements for pharmaceutical graduates as stated in the National Bureau of Standards Handbook 44—Fourth Edition, it should be kept in mind that a graduate shall have an initial interval that is not subdivided, equal to not less than one-fifth and not more than one-fourth of the capacity of the graduate.

*Examples:*

*A prescription calls for 0.5 milliliter of hydrochloric acid. Using a 10-milliliter graduate calibrated from 2 to 10 milliliters in 1-milliliter divisions, explain how you would obtain the desired quantity of hydrochloric acid by the aliquot method.*

If 4 is chosen as the multiple, and if 2 milliliters (mL) is set as the volume of the aliquot, then—

(1) Measure 4 × 0.5 mL, or 2 mL of the acid
(2) Dilute with 6 mL of water
to make 8 mL of dilution
(3) Measure ¼ of dilution, or 2 mL of dilution, which will contain 0.5 milliliter of hydrochloric acid, *answer.*

*A prescription calls for 5 minims of clove oil. Using a 60-minim graduate calibrated from 15 to 60 minims in units of 5 minims, explain how you would obtain the clove oil by the aliquot method. Use alcohol as the diluent.*

If 3 is chosen as the multiple, and if 20 minims is set as the volume of the aliquot, then—

(1) Measure 3 × 5 minims, or 15 minims of clove oil
(2) Dilute with 45 minims of alcohol
 to make 60 minims of dilution
(3) Measure ⅓ of dilution, or 20 minims of dilution, which will contain 5 minims of clove oil, *answer.*

## LEAST WEIGHABLE QUANTITY METHOD OF WEIGHING

This method may be used as an alternative to the aliquot method of weighing to obtain small quantities of a drug substance.

**To weigh by the least weighable quantity method:**

After determining the quantity of drug substance desired and the smallest quantity that can be weighed on the balance with the desired degree of accuracy, the procedure is as follows:

*Step 1.* Weigh an amount of the drug substance that is *equal to or greater than* the least weighable quantity.

*Step 2.* Dilute the drug substance with a calculated quantity of inert diluent such that a predetermined quantity of the drug-diluent mixture will contain the desired quantity of drug.

*Example:*

*If 20 mg of a drug substance are needed to fill a prescription, explain how you would obtain this amount of drug with an accuracy of ± 5% using a balance having a sensitivity requirement of 6 mg. Use lactose as the diluent.*

In the example, 20 mg is the amount of drug substance needed. The least weighable quantity would be 120 mg. The amount of drug substance to be weighed, therefore, must be equal to or greater than 120 mg. In solving the problem, 120 mg of drug substance is weighed. In calculating the amount of diluent to use, a predetermined quantity of drug-diluent mixture must be selected to contain the desired 20 mg of drug substance. The quantity selected must be greater than 120 mg since the drug-diluent mixture will need to be obtained accurately through weighing on the balance. An amount of 150 mg may be arbitrarily selected. The total amount of diluent to use may then be determined through the calculation of the following proportion:

$$\frac{\text{20 mg (drug needed for ℞)}}{\text{150 mg (drug-diluent mixture to use in ℞)}} = \frac{\text{120 mg (total drug substance weighed)}}{\text{x mg (total amount of drug-diluent mixture prepared)}}$$

x = 900 mg of the drug-diluent mixture to prepare

Hence, 900 mg − 120 mg = 780 mg of diluent (lactose) to use, *answer*.

It should be noted that in this procedure, each weighing, including that of the drug substance, the diluent, and the drug-diluent mixture, must be determined to be equal to or greater than the least weighable quantity as determined for the balance used and accuracy desired.

### Practice Problems

1. If 1000 milliliters of a certain solution contain 30 milligrams of a dye, (a) what is the volume of the tenth aliquot and (b) how many milligrams of the dye will the tenth aliquot contain?

2. A prescription balance has a sensitivity requirement of 0.006 gram. Explain how you would weigh 0.012 gram of atropine sulfate with an error not greater than 5%, using lactose as the diluent.

3. A torsion prescription balance has a sensitivity requirement of 4 milligrams. Explain how you would weigh 5 milligrams of hydromorphone hydrochloride with an error not greater than 5%. Use lactose as the diluent.

4. The sensitivity requirement of a prescription balance is $\frac{1}{16}$ grain. Explain how you would weigh $\frac{1}{10}$ grain of atropine sulfate with an error not greater than 5%. Use milk sugar as the diluent.

5. A prescription balance has a sensitivity requirement of 6.5 milligrams. Explain how you would weigh 20 milligrams of a substance with an error not greater than 2%.

6. A prescription balance has a sensitivity requirement of $\frac{1}{6}$ grain. Explain how you would weigh 1 grain of a substance with an error not greater than 5%.

7. A torsion prescription balance has a sensitivity requirement of 0.004 gram. Explain how you would weigh 0.008 gram of a substance with an error not greater than 5%.

8. A prescription balance has a sensitivity requirement of $\frac{1}{8}$ grain. Explain how you would weigh $\frac{3}{4}$ grain of a substance with an error not greater than 5%.

9. A formula calls for 0.6 milliliter of a coloring solution. Using a 10-milliliter graduate calibrated from 2 to 10 milliliters in units of 1 milliliter, how could you obtain the desired quantity of the coloring solution by the aliquot method? Use water as the diluent.

10. A pharmaceutical formula calls for 0.4 mL of the surfactant polysorbate 80. Using water as the diluent and a 10-milliliter graduate calibrated in units of 1 milliliter, how could you obtain the desired quantity of polysorbate 80?

11. Using a 10-milliliter graduate calibrated in units of 1 milliliter, explain how you would measure 1.25 milliliters of a dye solution by the aliquot method. Use water as the diluent.

12. The formula for 100 mL of Pentobarbital Sodium Elixir calls for 0.75 mL of orange oil. Using alcohol as a diluent and a 10-milliliter graduate calibrated in units of 1 milliliter, how could you obtain the desired quantity of orange oil?

13. A prescription calls for 50 mg of chlorpheniramine maleate. Using a prescription balance having a sensitivity requirement of 6 mg, explain how you would obtain the required amount of chlorpheniramine maleate with an error not greater than 5%.

# 2

# Interpretation of the Prescription or Medication Order

By definition, a *prescription* is an order for medication issued by a physician, dentist, or other properly licensed medical practitioner. Prescriptions designate a specific medication and dosage to be prepared by a pharmacist and administered to a particular patient.

Prescriptions are usually written on preprinted forms containing the name, address, telephone number, and other pertinent information regarding the physician or other prescriber. In addition, there are blank spaces utilized by the prescriber in providing information about the patient, the medication desired, and the directions for use. The information generally found on a completed prescription is listed and shown in the figure below:

(1) JOHN M. BROWN, M.D.
100 Main Street
Libertyville, Maryland
Phone 333-5555

(2) NAME Mary L. Smith DATE July 1, 1980 (3)

ADDRESS 123 Broad Street

(4) ℞

(5) Codeine Phosphate Tablets, 30 mg.

(6) Dispense 12 tablets

(7) Sig. Take one (1) tablet every 6 hours as needed for pain.

(8) Do not refill

Label: Codeine Phosphate Tablets, 30 mg.

John M. Brown M.D. (1)

DEA No. AS22244455

Typical prescription.

(1) Prescriber Information and Signature
(2) Patient Information
(3) Date Prescription was written
(4) ℞ Symbol (the Superscription) meaning "take thou," "you take," or "recipe"
(5) Medication Prescribed (the Inscription)
(6) Dispensing Instructions to the Pharmacist (the Subscription)
(7) Direction to the Patient (the Signa)
(8) Special Instructions

In hospitals and other institutions, the forms are somewhat different and are referred to as *medication orders.* A typical medication order sheet is shown below:

John Doe
Hosp. #12-34-56

PHYSICIAN'S ORDERS

Location B25
Dr. Smith

| Date Ordered | Date Discontinued | ORDERS |
|---|---|---|
| 1/1/86 | | Digitoxin 0.1 mg. one at 7:00 a.m. |
| | | Hexavitamin Capsule one daily |
| 1/2/86 | | Secobarbital 100 mg. one h.s. prn |
| 1/3/86 | 1/5/86 | Potassium Chloride 1 g. one daily in a.m. |
| | | |
| | | |
| | | |

Typical Medication Order Sheet found in the patient's medical record. The orders shown here are typed. Under normal circumstances, these are written by the physician in ink. Adapted from *Hospital Pharmacy* by William E. Hassan, Jr., Lea & Febiger, 1981, 4th ed., p. 223.

Prescriptions and medication orders written for infants, children, and sometimes the elderly, may also include the age and/or weight of the patient. This information is frequently necessary in calculating the appropriate medication dosage.

In addition to the written form, prescription orders are frequently received by the pharmacist by telephone or by direct communication. In these instances, the pharmacist immediately reduces the order to properly written form.

It is not the purpose of this text to discuss all aspects of the prescription, but only those that are relevant to pharmaceutical calculations. It is important to recognize the following types of prescriptions: (1) those written for a single component or prefabricated product and *not requiring compounding* or admixture by the pharmacist, and (2) those written for more than a single component and *requiring compounding*. Prescriptions may utilize the chemical or non-proprietary name of the substance or the manufacturer's brand or trademark name. Prescriptions requiring compounding contain the quantities of each ingredient required.

*Examples:*

1. *Prescriptions not requiring compounding:*

℞ Phenobarbital Tablets, ½ gr
Dispense 24 tablets.

℞ Feosol Elixir
Dispense 12 fluidounces.

2. *Prescriptions requiring compounding:*

| ℞ | | |
|---|---|---|
| ℞ | Aspirin | 3.6 g |
| | Codeine | 0.4 g |
| | Mix and make 12 capsules | |

| ℞ | | |
|---|---|---|
| ℞ | Paregoric | 30 mL |
| | Kaopectate q.s. ad | 120 mL |
| | Mix well. | |

The quantities of ingredients to be used may be expressed on the prescription in the metric or apothecaries' systems of weights and measures. These systems are covered in detail in Chapters 3 and 4. In the use of the metric system the decimal is often replaced by a vertical line that may be imprinted on the prescription blank or drawn by the prescriber. In these instances whole or subunits of grams of weight and milliliters of volume are separated by the vertical line. Sometimes the abbreviations g (for gram) and mL (for milliliter) are absent and must be presumed. Examples of prescriptions written in the apothecaries' and metric systems are:

*Apothecaries'*

| ℞ | | |
|---|---|---|
| ℞ | Codeine Phosphate | gr iv |
| | Ammonium Chloride | ʒi |
| | Ephedrine Sulfate Syrup ad | f℥iii |
| | Sig. ʒi t.i.d. for cough. | |

| | | |
|---|---|---|
| ℞ | Aminophylline | ℈i |
| | Ephedrine Hydrochloride | gr iv |
| | Amobarbital | gr iv |
| | Lactose as needed | |
| | Mix and make capsules no. xii | |
| | Sig. One capsule every 3 hours. | |

*Metric*

| | | |
|---|---|---|
| ℞ | Acetylsalicylic Acid | 4.0 g |
| | Phenacetin | 0.8 g |
| | Codeine Phosphate | 0.5 g |
| | Mix and make capsules no. 20 | |
| | Sig. One capsule every 4 hours. | |

| | | | |
|---|---|---|---|
| ℞ | Phenobarbital | 0 | 6 |
| | Belladonna Tincture | 12 | 0 |
| | Aromatic Elixir ad | 120 | 0 |
| | Sig. 5 mL in water a.c. | | |

The portions of the prescription presenting directions to the pharmacist (the Subscription) and the directions to the patient (the Signa) commonly contain abbreviated forms of English or Latin terms as well as Roman numerals. The correct interpretation of these abbreviations and prescription notations plays an important part in pharmaceutical calculations and thus in the accurate filling and dispensing of medication.

*Examples of Prescription Directions to the Pharmacist:*

(a) *M. ft. ung.*
Mix and make an ointment.

(b) *Ft. sup. no xii*
Make 12 suppositories.

(c) *M. ft. cap. d.t.d. no. xxiv*
Mix and make capsules. Give 24 such doses.

*Examples of Prescription Directions to the Patient:*

(a) *Caps. i q.i.d. p.c. et h.s.*
Take one (1) capsule four (4) times a day after each meal and at bedtime.

(b) *gtt. ii o.d. q.d. a.m.*
Instill two (2) drops in the right eye every day in the morning.

(c) *tab. ii stat; tab. 1 q. 6 h. × 7 d.*
Take two (2) tablets immediately, then take one (1) tablet every 6 hours for 7 days.

A list of abbreviations commonly used in prescriptions and medication orders is presented in the following table.

## ABBREVIATIONS COMMONLY USED IN PRESCRIPTIONS AND MEDICATION ORDERS

| *Abbreviation* | *Meaning* |
|---|---|
| aa. or $\overline{aa}$ | of each |
| a.c. | before meals |
| ad | up to |
| a.d. | right ear |
| ad lib. | at pleasure, freely |
| a.m. | morning |
| amp. | ampul |
| aq. | water |
| a.s. | left ear |
| a.u. | each ear |
| b.i.d. | twice a day |
| BSA | body surface area |
| c. or $\bar{c}$ | with |
| cap. | capsule |
| cc. or cc | cubic centimeter |
| comp. | compound |
| dil. | dilute |
| disc or D.C. | discontinue |
| disp. | dispense |
| div. | divide |
| d.t.d. | give of such doses |
| DW | distilled water |
| $D_5W$ | dextrose 5% in water |
| elix. | elixir |
| e.m.p. | as directed |
| et | and |
| ex aq. | in water |
| fl or fld | fluid |
| ft. | make |
| g. or Gm. or g | gram |
| gr. or gr | grain |
| gtt. | drop |
| H | hypodermic |
| h. or hr. | hour |
| h.s. | at bedtime |
| IM | intramuscular |
| inj. | injection |
| IV | intravenous |
| IVP | intravenous push |
| IVPB | intravenous piggy back |
| M. | mix |
| $m^2$ or $M^2$ | square meter |
| mcg. or mcg | microgram |
| mEq | milliequivalent |
| mg. or mg | milligram |
| ml. | milliliter |
| N&V | nausea and vomiting |
| N.F. | National Formulary |
| noct. | night |
| non rep. | do not repeat |
| NPO | nothing by mouth |
| N.S. or NS or N/S | normal saline |
| ½NS | half-strength normal saline |
| O. | pint |
| o.d. | right eye |
| o.l. | left eye |
| o.s. | left eye |
| o.u. | each eye |
| $o_2$ | both eyes |
| p.c. | after meals |
| p.m. | afternoon; evening |
| p.o. | by mouth |
| p.r.n. | when required |
| pulv. | powder |
| q.d. | every day |
| q.h. | every hour |
| q.i.d. | four times a day |
| q.o.d. | every other day |
| q.s. | a sufficient quantity |
| q.s. ad | a sufficient quantity to make |
| R | rectal |
| R.L. or R/L | Ringer's Lactate |
| s. or $\bar{s}$ | without |
| Sig. | write on label |
| sol. | solution |
| s.o.s. | if there is need |
| ss. or $\overline{ss}$ | one-half |
| stat. | immediately |
| subc or subq or s.c. | subcutaneously |
| sup. | suppository |
| susp. | suspension |
| syr. | syrup |
| tab. | tablet |
| tal. | such |
| tal. dos. | such doses |
| tbsp. | tablespoonful |
| t.i.d. | three times a day |
| tr. | tincture |
| tsp. | teaspoonful |
| U or u | unit |
| u.d. | as directed |
| ung. | ointment |
| U.S.P. | United States Pharmacopeia |

## Practice Exercises

1. Interpret each of the following *Subscriptions* (directions to the pharmacist) taken from prescriptions:

(*a*) Disp. sup. rect. no. xii
(*b*) M. ft. isoton. sol. Disp. ℥i
(*c*) M. et div. in pulv. no. xl
(*d*) Disp. tal. dos. vi. Non rep.
(*e*) M. et ft. ung. Disp. 10 g
(*f*) M. et ft. sol. DTD xlviii
(*g*) M. et ft. sol. 1 g/tbsp.
(*h*) Ft. cap. #1. Disp. tal. no. xxxvi N.R.
(*i*) M. et ft. pulv. Div. in dos. #C
(*j*) M. et ft. inj. for I.V. use.

2. Interpret each of the following *Signas* (directions to the patient) taken from prescriptions:

(*a*) Gtt. ii o.u. q. 4 h. p.r.n. pain.
(*b*) Tbsp. i in ⅓ gl. aq. q. 6 h.
(*c*) Appl. am & pm for pain e.m.p.
(*d*) Gtt. iv a.d. m. & n.
(*e*) Tsp. i ex aq. q. 4 or 5 h. p.r.n. pain.
(*f*) Appl. ung. o.s. ad lib.
(*g*) Caps i c̄ aq. h.s. N.R.
(*h*) Gtt v a.u. 3x d. s.o.s.
(*i*) Tab. i sublingually, rep. p.r.n.
(*j*) Instill gtt. ii o.u. of neonate.
(*k*) Dil. c̄ = vol. aq. and use as gargle q. 5 h.
(*l*) Cap. ii 1 h. prior to departure, then cap. i after 12 h.

3. Interpret each of the following taken from medication orders.

(*a*) Secobarbital sodium gr iss p.o. q.d. h.s. repeat s.o.s.
(*b*) 1000 mL $D_5W$ q. 8 h. IV c 20 mEq KCl to every third bottle.
(*c*) Prochlorperazine 10 mg IM q. 3h. prn N&V
(*d*) Minocycline HCl susp. 1 tsp p.o. q.i.d. disc after 5 d.
(*e*) Propranolol HCl 10 mg p.o. t.i.d. a.c. & h.s.
(*f*) NPH U-100 insulin 40 U subc q.d. A.M.
(*g*) Cefamandole nafate 250 mg IM q. 12 h.
(*h*) Potassium chloride 15 mEq p.o. b.i.d. p.c.
(*i*) Vincristine sulfate 2 mg/m$^2$ BSA

# 3

# The Metric System

The *measure* of a quantity is the number of times that it contains a standard quantity taken as a *unit*. A 5-pound weight, for instance, contains five times the weight of a standard 1-pound unit. Some kinds of quantities measured are temperature, length, area, volume, and time—respectively measured in such familiar units as degrees, feet, square miles, gallons, and hours.

The standard subdivisions and multiples of the unit in any system of measurement are called *denominations,* as we have seen that figures specifying their number are called *denominate numbers.* So, in the expression "ten cents" the term "cents" designates a denomination in our monetary system, and "ten" is a denominate number. We find it convenient, as a rule, to express large quantities in terms of large denominations, and small quantities in small—as great distances are measured by the common system in miles, short intervals in inches. Denominations are understood to stand in a fixed ratio with the unit upon which the system is based—as a cent has a fixed value of $\frac{1}{100}$ of a dollar—and therefore they have a fixed ratio with each other. A statement of the mutual relationships of denominations of the same kind is called a *table of measure.*

The *metric system* of measure was formulated in France in the late 18th century. Its *use* in the United States was legalized in 1866. By act of Congress in 1893 it became our legal *standard* of measure, and all other systems are referred to it for official comparison.

Its acceptance by scientists the world over has resulted from these two merits: (1) its tables are simple, for they are based upon the decimal system of notation, and the greater of two consecutive denominations of the same kind is always ten times the less; (2) its tables of length, volume, and weight are conveniently correlated, for the meter is the fundamental unit of the system.

Each table of the metric system contains a definitive unit. The *meter* is the unit of length, the *liter* of volume, and the *gram* of weight.

Subdivisions and multiples of these principal units are indicated respectively by the following prefixes:

*pico-* to denote one trillionth ($10^{-12}$) of the basic unit,
*nano-* to denote one billionth ($10^{-9}$) of the basic unit,
*micro-* to denote one millionth of the basic unit,

| | |
|---|---|
| *milli-* | to denote one-thousandth of the basic unit, |
| *centi-* | to denote one-hundredth of the basic unit, |
| *deci-* | to denote one-tenth of the basic unit, |
| | |
| *deka-* | to denote ten times the basic unit, |
| *hekto-* | to denote one hundred times the basic unit, |
| *kilo-* | to denote one thousand times the basic unit, |
| *myria-* | to denote ten thousand times the basic unit. |

Anyone who wishes to become quickly used to the system should note that our money is "metrically" or decimally computed. The names of the chief fractions of the dollar unit are a clue to their value: a *mill* (for which we have no coin) is one-thousandth, a *cent* one-hundredth, and a *dime* one-tenth of the unit.

The abbreviations in the tables of metric length, volume, and weight are those commonly employed and include those adopted by the *United States Pharmacopeia.*

## MEASURE OF LENGTH

The meter is the fundamental unit of this system. It has been determined as approximately one ten-millionth part of the distance from the earth's equator to the North Pole, and is, in fact, a little over a yard long.

**Table of metric length:**

| | | |
|---|---|---|
| 1 kilometer (km) | = | 1000.000 meters |
| 1 hektometer (hm) | = | 100.000 meters |
| 1 dekameter (dam) | = | 10.000 meters |
| 1 meter (m) | = | 1.000 meter |
| 1 decimeter (dm) | = | 0.100 meter |
| 1 centimeter (cm) | = | 0.010 meter |
| 1 millimeter (mm) | = | 0.001 meter |
| 1 micrometer (μm) | = | 0.000,001 meter |
| 1 nanometer (nm) | = | 0.000,000,001 meter |

Formerly the abbreviation μ (for *micron*) was used in expressing a millionth of a meter (micrometer); and the abbreviation mμ (for *millimicron*) was used in designating a thousandth of a micron (nanometer).

A very small unit equal to one ten-thousandth of a micron is the *angstrom* (Å) which is used in expressing the length of light waves.

The table may also be written:

1 meter = 0.001 kilometer
= 0.01 hektometer
= 0.1 dekameter
= 10 decimeters
= 100 centimeters
= 1000 millimeters
= 1,000,000 micrometers
= 1,000,000,000 nanometers

The most commonly used denominations are the millimeter, centimeter, and meter, as if the table were:

1000 millimeters (mm) = 100 centimeters (cm)
100 centimeters (cm) = 1 meter (m)

## MEASURE OF VOLUME

The *liter* is the metric unit of volume. It represents the volume of the cube of one-tenth of a meter—that is, of one cubic decimeter.

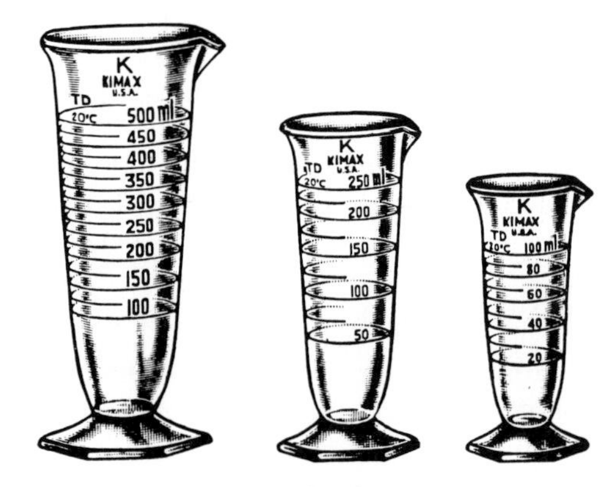


Metric Graduates.
(Courtesy of Kimble Glassware Co.)

**Table of metric volume:**

| | | |
|---|---|---|
| 1 kiloliter (kL) | = | 1000.000 liters |
| 1 hektoliter (hL) | = | 100.000 liters |
| 1 dekaliter (daL) | = | 10.000 liters |
| 1 liter (L) | = | 1.000 liter |
| 1 deciliter (dL) | = | 0.100 liter |
| 1 centiliter (cL) | = | 0.010 liter |
| 1 milliliter (mL) | = | 0.001 liter |
| 1 microliter (µL) | = | 0.000.001 liter |

This table may also be written:

| | | |
|---|---|---|
| 1 liter | = | 0.001 kiloliter |
| | = | 0.010 hektoliter |
| | = | 0.100 dekaliter |
| | = | 10 deciliters |
| | = | 100 centiliters |
| | = | 1000 milliliters |
| | = | 1,000,000 microliters |

Although in theory the liter was meant to have the volume of one cubic decimeter, or a thousand cubic centimeters, precise modern measurement has discovered that the standard liter contains slightly less than this volume. But the discrepancy is insignificant for most practical purposes; and since the milliliter has so very nearly the volume of a cubic centimeter, the *United States Pharmacopeia* states: "One milliliter (mL) is used herein as the equivalent of 1 cubic centimeter (cc)."

The most commonly used denominations are the milliliter and liter, as if the table were simply:

1000 milliliters (mL) = 1 liter (L)

## MEASURE OF WEIGHT

The unit of weight in the metric system is the *gram,* which is the weight of 1 cubic centimeter of water at 4° centigrade, its temperature of greatest density.

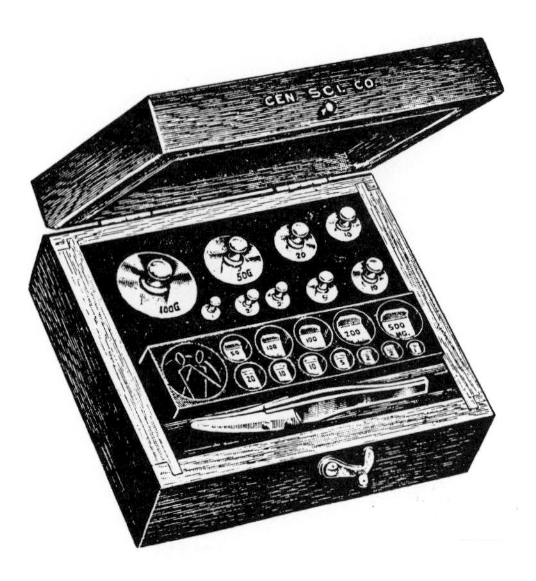


A set of Metric Weights.

**Table of metric weight:**

| | | |
|---|---|---|
| 1 kilogram (kg) | = | 1000.000 grams |
| 1 hektogram (hg) | = | 100.000 grams |
| 1 dekagram (dag) | = | 10.000 grams |
| 1 gram (g) | = | 1.000 gram |
| 1 decigram (dg) | = | 0.100 gram |
| 1 centigram (cg) | = | 0.010 gram |
| 1 milligram (mg) | = | 0.001 gram |
| 1 microgram (μg or mcg) | = | 0.000,001 gram |
| 1 nanogram (ng) | = | 0.000,000,001 gram |
| 1 picogram (pg) | = | 0.000,000,000,001 gram |

This table may also be written:

| | | |
|---|---|---|
| 1 gram | = | 0.001 kilogram |
| | = | 0.010 hektogram |
| | = | 0.100 dekagram |
| | = | 10 decigrams |
| | = | 100 centigrams |
| | = | 1000 milligrams |
| | = | 1,000,000 micrograms |
| | = | 1,000,000,000 nanograms |
| | = | 1,000,000,000,000 picograms |

The denominations most commonly used are the microgram, milligram, gram, and kilogram, as if the table were:

1000 micrograms (μg or mcg) = 1 milligram (mg)
1000 milligrams (mg) = 1 gram (g)
1000 grams (g) = 1 kilogram (kg)

The abbreviation *mcg* came into general use in pharmaceutical literature and labeling some years ago and was formerly used in Pharmacopeial monographs; however, the symbol μg now is more widely accepted and is presently used in the Pharmacopeia. The abbreviation *mcg* is still commonly employed to denote microgram(s) in labeling and prescription writing. The term *gamma,* symbolized by γ, is customarily used for microgram in biochemical literature.

When prescriptions are written in the metric system, arabic numerals are always used and are written *before* the abbreviations for the denominations, if such abbreviations are used. Quantities of weight are usually written as grams and *decimals* of a gram, and volumes as milliliters and *decimals* of a milliliter.

*Example:*

| | | |
|---|---|---|
| ℞ | Codeine Phosphate | 0.26 g |
| | Ammonium Chloride | 6.0 g |
| | Cherry Syrup ad | 120.0 mL |
| | Sig. 5 mL as directed. | |

## FUNDAMENTAL COMPUTATIONS

**To reduce to lower or higher denominations:**

The restatement of a given quantity in terms of a higher or lower denomination is called *reduction.* "Thirty minutes" may equally be expressed as a "half hour" or, if occasion requires, as "1800 seconds." The process of changing from higher to lower denominations is known as *reduction descending;* from lower to higher, *reduction ascending.*

A length, a volume, or a weight expressed in one denomination of the metric system may be expressed in another denomination by simply moving the decimal point. In doing this, it is often best to reduce the given quantity first to the *unit* and then to the required denomination.

To change a metric denomination to the next smaller denomination, move the decimal point one place to the right. To change to the next larger denomination, move the decimal point one place to the left as shown in the following figure.

METRIC WEIGHT SCALE

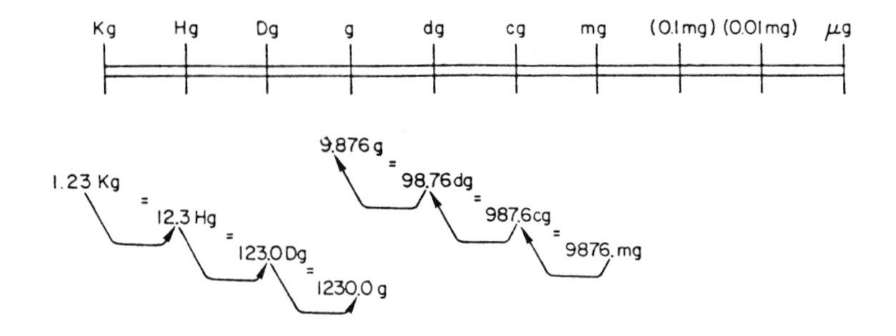


DECIMAL MOVEMENT

⊙→ TO CONVERT FROM LARGER TO SMALLER UNITS

←⊙ TO CONVERT FROM SMALLER TO LARGER UNITS

Adapted from *Introduction to Pharmaceutical Dosage Forms* by Howard C. Ansel, Lea & Febiger, 1985, 4th ed., p. 384.

*Examples:*

*Reduce 1.23 kilograms to grams.*
1.23 kg = 1230 g, *answer.*

*Reduce 9876 milligrams to grams.*
9876 mg = 9.876 g, *answer.*

In the first example, 1.23 kilograms (kg) are to be converted to grams (g). On the scale, the gram position is three decimal positions from the kilogram position. Thus, the decimal point is moved three places toward the right. In the second example, the conversion from milligrams (mg) also requires the movement of the decimal point three places, but this time to the left.

*Examples:*

*Reduce 85 micrometers to centimeters.*
85 μm = 0.085 mm = 0.0085 cm, *answer.*

*Reduce 2.525 liters to microliters.*
2.525 L = 2525 mL = 2,525,000 μL, *answer.*

**To add or subtract:**

To add or subtract quantities in the metric system, we must reduce them to a *common denomination*—preferably the unit of the table—and arrange their denominate numbers for addition or subtraction as ordinary decimals.

*Examples:*

*Add 1 kg, 250 mg, and 7.5 g. Express the total in grams.*

$$\begin{aligned} 1\text{ kg} &= 1000.\ \text{g} \\ 250\text{ mg} &= 0.250\text{ g} \\ 7.5\text{ g} &= \underline{7.5\ \ \text{g}} \\ & \quad 1007.750\text{ g or } 1008\text{ g, } \textit{answer.} \end{aligned}$$

*Add 4 L, 375 mL, and 0.75 L. Express the total in milliliters.*

$$\begin{aligned} 4\text{ L} &= 4000\text{ mL} \\ 375\text{ mL} &= 375\text{ mL} \\ 0.75\text{ L} &= \underline{750\text{ mL}} \\ & \quad 5125\text{ mL, } \textit{answer.} \end{aligned}$$

*A capsule contains the following amounts of medicinal substances: 0.075 g, 20 mg, 0.0005 g, 4 mg, and 500 μg. What is the total weight of the substances in the capsule?*

$$\begin{aligned} 0.075\text{ g} &= 0.075\ \text{g} \\ 20\text{ mg} &= 0.020\ \text{g} \\ 0.0005\text{ g} &= 0.0005\text{ g} \\ 4\text{ mg} &= 0.004\ \text{g} \\ 500\ \mu\text{g} &= \underline{0.0005\text{ g}} \\ & \quad 0.1000\text{ g or } 100\text{ mg, } \textit{answer.} \end{aligned}$$

*Subtract 2.5 mg from 4.850 g.*

$$\begin{aligned} 4.850\text{ g} &= 4.850\ \text{g} \\ 2.5\text{ mg} &= \underline{0.0025\text{ g}} \\ & \quad 4.8475\text{ g or } 4.848\text{ g, } \textit{answer.} \end{aligned}$$

*A prescription calls for 0.060 g of one ingredient, 2.5 mg of another, and enough of a third to make 0.5 g. How many milligrams of the third ingredient should be used?*

Interpreting all quantities as accurate to the nearest tenth of a milligram—

$$\begin{aligned} \text{1st ingredient: } 0.0600\text{ g} &= 0.0600\text{ g} \\ \text{2nd ingredient: } 2.5\text{ mg} &= \underline{0.0025\text{ g}} \\ & \quad 0.0625\text{ g} \end{aligned}$$

$$\begin{aligned} &\text{Total weight:} && 0.5000\text{ g} \\ &\text{Weight of 1st and 2nd:} && \underline{0.0625\text{ g}} \\ &\text{Weight of 3rd:} && 0.4375\text{ g or } 437.5\text{ mg, } \textit{answer.} \end{aligned}$$

**To multiply or divide:**

Since every measurement in the metric system is expressed in a single given denomination, problems involving multiplication and division are solved by the methods used for any decimal numbers.

*Examples:*

*Multiply 820 mL by 12.5 and express the result in liters.*

820 mL × 12.5 = 10250 mL = 10.25 L, *answer.*

*Divide 0.465 g by 15 and express the result in milligrams.*

0.465 g ÷ 15 = 0.031 g = 31 mg, *answer.*

### Practice Problems

1. Add 0.5 kg, 50 mg, and 2.5 g. Reduce the result to grams.

2. Add 7.25 L and 875 mL. Reduce the result to milliliters.

3. Reduce 25 μg to grams.

4. Reduce 1.256 g to micrograms, to milligrams, and to kilograms.

5. Multiply 255 mg by 380, divide the result by 0.85, and reduce the result to grams.

6. Divide 0.03 g by 8000 and reduce the result to milligrams.

7. Adhesive tape made from fabric has a tensile strength of not less than 20.41 kg per 2.54 cm of width. Reduce these quantities to grams and millimeters.

8. A liquid contains 0.25 mg of a substance per milliliter. How many milligrams of the substance will 3.5 L contain?

9. A vitamin capsule contains 6.25 μg of vitamin $B_{12}$. How many capsules can be prepared from 1 g of vitamin $B_{12}$?

10. A certain suppository contains the following:

| | |
|---|---|
| Ergotamine Tartrate | 2.0 mg |
| Caffeine | 100.0 mg |
| Cocoa Butter q.s. ad | 2.0 g |

(a) How many milligrams of cocoa butter are required in the formula?

(b) How many grams of caffeine would be required to make 24 such suppositories?

11. How many colchicine tablets, each containing 600 μg, may be prepared from 30 g of colchicine?

12. ℞ Codeine Sulfate

| | | | |
|---|---|---|---|
| Papaverine Hydrochloride | aa | 0 | 015 |
| Calcium Carbonate | ad | 0 | 3 |

M. ft. cap. no. i D.T.D. no. xv
Sig. Cap. i q.i.d. p.c. and h.s.

(a) How many milligrams of codeine sulfate would be contained in each capsule?

(b) How many grams of calcium carbonate should be used in filling the prescription?

(c) How many milligrams of papaverine hydrochloride would be taken daily?

13. Aspirin tablets generally contain 325 mg of aspirin. How many such tablets may be prepared from 5 kg of aspirin?

14. ℞

| | | |
|---|---|---|
| Codeine Phosphate | | 8.4 mg |
| Ephedrine Hydrochloride | | 4.2 mg |
| Calcium Iodide | | 152 mg |
| Aromatic Syrup | ad | 5 mL |

Disp. 60 mL
Sig. 5 mL t.i.d.

How many grams of calcium iodide should be used in filling the prescription?

15. Norgestrel and Ethinyl Estradiol Tablets usually available contain 0.5 mg of norgestrel and 50 μg of ethinyl estradiol. How many grams of each ingredient would be used in making 10,000 tablets?

16. ℞

| | | |
|---|---|---|
| Phenobarbital | | 0.540 g |
| Hyoscine Hydrobromide | | 0.34 mg |
| Atropine Sulfate | | 0.84 mg |
| Lactose | ad | 10.0 g |

M. Div. in caps. no. 36
Sig. One capsule q.i.d.

How many micrograms of hyoscine hydrobromide, milligrams of atropine sulfate and grams of phenobarbital would be contained in each capsule of the prescription?

17. How many grams of reserpine would be required to make 25,000 tablets each containing 250 μg of reserpine?

18. ℞ Paregoric 15.0 mL
Pectin 0.6 g
Kaolin 22.0 g
Alcohol 0.8 mL
Purified Water ad 120.0 mL
Mix and make a suspension.
Sig. 15 mL p.r.n. for diarrhea.

(a) How many milliliters of paregoric would be contained in each 15-mL dose?
(b) How many milligrams of pectin would be contained in each prescribed dose?
(c) How many microliters of alcohol would be contained in each dose?

19. If an injectable solution contains 25 μg of a drug substance in each 0.5 mL, how many milliliters will be required to provide a patient with 0.25 mg of the drug substance?

20. ℞ Ergonovine Maleate
200 μg Tablets
Disp. tabs. no. 16
Sig. One tab. 4 times daily.

How many milligrams of ergonovine maleate would the patient taking the prescription receive daily?

21. ℞ Hydrocodone Bitartrate 0.2 g
Phenacetin 3.6 g
Aspirin 6.0 g
Caffeine 0.6 g
M. ft. caps. no. 24
Sig. One capsule t.i.d. p.r.n. for pain.

(a) How many milligrams of hydrocodone bitartrate would be contained in each capsule?
(b) What is the total weight, in milligrams, of the ingredients in each capsule?
(c) How many milligrams of caffeine would be taken daily?

22. Digitoxin is available for parenteral pediatric use in a concentration of 0.1 mg per mL. How many milliliters would provide a dose of 40 micrograms?

23. ℞ Actifed Syrup 60 mL
Robitussin Syrup ad 120 mL
Sig. 5 mL p.r.n. for cough.

If a pharmacist had four 1-liter stock bottles of each of the ingredients, how many times could this prescription be filled?

24. If a 20-mL ampul contains 0.5 g of aminophylline, how many milliliters should be administered to provide a 25-mg dose of aminophylline?

25. ℞ Belladonna Tincture 10 mL
Alurate Elixir 60 mL
Maalox Suspension ad 120 mL
Sig. 5 mL t.i.d.

How many milliliters of Maalox Suspension would be contained in each dose?

26. An intravenous solution contains 500 μg of a drug substance in each milliliter. How many milligrams of the drug would a patient receive from the intravenous infusion of a liter of the solution?

27. If an intravenous solution containing 125 mg of a drug substance in each 250-mL bottle is to be administered at the rate of 200 μg of drug per minute, how many milliliters of the solution would be given per hour?

28. ℞ Decadron Elixir
Benadryl Elixir aa 20 mL
Triple Sulfas Suspension 80 mL
Sig. 10 mL stat., then 5 mL t.i.d.

How many milliliters of Decadron Elixir would be taken in the initial dose of the prescription?

29. The prophylactic dose of riboflavin is 2 mg. How many micrograms of riboflavin are in a multiple vitamin capsule containing ⅕ the prophylactic dose?

30. If 0.065 g of thyroid extract represents 170 μg of thyroxin, how many micrograms of thyroxin are represented in 5 mg of thyroid extract?

31. One mg of streptomycin sulfate contains the antibiotic activity of 650 μg of streptomycin base. How many grams of streptomycin sulfate would be the equivalent of 1 g of streptomycin base?

32. If 480 mL of a certain solution contain 0.24 g of a chemical, (a) what is the volume of the thirtieth aliquot? (b) how many milligrams of the chemical will the thirtieth aliquot contain? (c) how many micrograms of the chemical are in this aliquot?

33. A prefilled syringe of furosemide contains 20 mg of drug in 2 mL of solution. How many micrograms of drug would be administered by an injection of 0.5 mL of the solution?

34. A vial of tobramycin sulfate contains 80 mg of drug in 2 mL of injection. How many milliliters of the injection should be administered to obtain 0.02 g of tobramycin sulfate?

35. A half-liter of $D_5W$ contains 2000 μg of added drug. How many milliliters of the fluid would contain 0.5 mg of the drug?

36. A multidose vial of sulfisoxazole diolamine contains 2 g of drug per 5 mL. How many milliliters would be used to administer 400 mg of the drug to a patient?

# 4

# The Common Systems

In addition to the metric system, the avoirdupois and apothecaries' systems of measurement are used in the United States; and, in spite of the increasing use of the official metric system in pharmacy, some physicians continue to use the apothecaries' systems of measuring volume and weight in their prescriptions. The pharmacist, therefore, must have a practical knowledge of the so-called *common systems of measure.*

### APOTHECARIES' FLUID MEASURE

60 minims (♏) = 1 fluidrachm or fluidram (fʒ or ʒ)[1]
8 fluidrachms (480 minims) = 1 fluidounce (f℥ or ℥)[1]
16 fluidounces = 1 pint (pt or 0)
2 pints (32 fluidounces) = 1 quart (qt)
4 quarts (8 pints) = 1 gallon (gal or C)

This table may also be written:

| *gal* | *qt* | *pt* | f℥ | fʒ | ♏ |
|---|---|---|---|---|---|
| 1 | 4 | 8 | 128 | 1024 | 61440 |
| | 1 | 2 | 32 | 256 | 15360 |
| | | 1 | 16 | 128 | 7680 |
| | | | 1 | 8 | 480 |
| | | | | 1 | 60 |

### APOTHECARIES' MEASURE OF WEIGHT

20 grains (gr) = 1 scruple (℈)
3 scruples (60 grains) = 1 drachm or dram (ʒ)
8 drachms (480 grains) = 1 ounce (℥)
12 ounces (5760 grains) = 1 pound (℔)

[1]When there is no doubt that a liquid is to be measured, physicians commonly omit the *f* in this symbol.

This table may also be written:

| ℔ | ℥ | ʒ | ℈ | *gr* |
|---|---|---|---|---|
| 1 | 12 | 96 | 288 | 5760 |
| | 1 | 8 | 24 | 480 |
| | | 1 | 3 | 60 |
| | | | 1 | 20 |

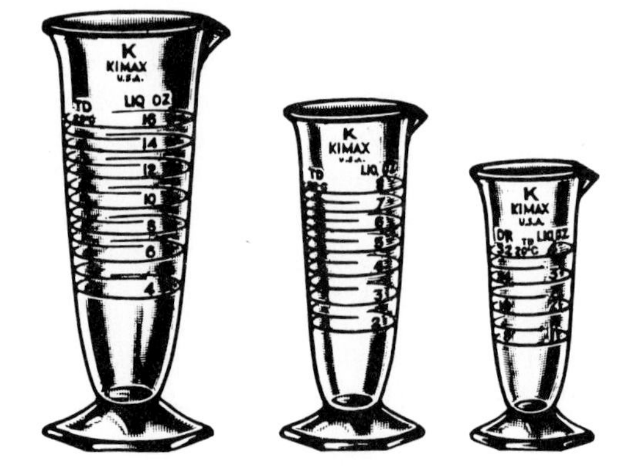


Apothecaries' Graduates.
(Courtesy of Kimble Glassware Co.)

A typical set of Apothecaries' Weights consists of the following units:

℥ii ℥i ℥ss ʒii ʒi ʒss ℈ii ℈i ℈ss
5-grain, 4-grain, 3-grain, 2-grain, 1-grain, ½-grain

## AVOIRDUPOIS MEASURE OF WEIGHT

437½ or 437.5 grain (gr) = 1 ounce (oz)
16 ounces (7000 grains) = 1 pound (lb)

This table may also be written:

| *lb* | *oz* | *gr* |
|---|---|---|
| 1 | 16 | 7000 |
| | 1 | 437.5 |

Only one denomination has a value common to the apothecaries' and avoirdupois systems of measuring weight, namely, the *grain*. The other denominations bearing the same name have quite different values.

The pharmacist buys by the avoirdupois system, for manufacturers and wholesalers customarily supply drugs and chemicals, when they are sold by weight, in avoirdupois units only. The pharmacist likewise sells in bulk "over the counter" by the avoirdupois system. However, when compounding prescriptions the pharmacist employs the apothecaries' and metric systems to weigh and measure ingredients.

In contrast with the invariable use of *simple* quantities in the metric system, in the common systems measurements are recorded whenever possible in *compound quantities*—that is, quantities expressed in two or more denominations. So, 20 f℥ may be used during the process of calculating, but as a final result it should be recorded as 1 pt 4 f℥. The process of reducing a quantity to a compound quantity beginning with the highest possible denomination is called *simplification.* Decimal fractions may be used in calculation, but the subdivision of a minim or a grain in a final result is recorded as a *common fraction.*

When prescriptions are written in the common system, the numbers are written in roman numerals and *follow* the abbreviations or symbols for the denominations.

*Examples:*

| ℞ | Codeine Phosphate | gr iv |
|---|---|---|
| | Ammonium Chloride | ʒ iss |
| | Cherry Syrup ad | f℥ iv |
| | Sig. ʒi as directed. | |

## FUNDAMENTAL COMPUTATIONS

**To reduce a compound quantity to a simple quantity:**

Before a compound quantity can be used in a calculation it must usually be expressed in terms of a single denomination. To do so, reduce each of the denominations in the compound quantity to the required denomination and add the results.

*Examples:*

*Reduce ℥ss ʒii ℈i to grains.*

℥ss = ½ × 480 gr = 240 gr
ʒii = 2 × 60 gr = 120 gr
℈i = 1 × 20 gr = 20 gr

380 gr, *answer.*

*Reduce f℥iv fʒiiss to fluidrachms.*

f℥iv = 4 × 8 fʒ = 32 fʒ
fʒiiss = 2½ fʒ

34½ fʒ, *answer.*

**To reduce simple quantities to weighable or measurable denominations:**

Before being weighed, a given quantity should be expressed in denominations equal to the actual weights on hand; and before a volume is measured, a given quantity should be expressed in denominations represented by the calibrations on the graduate.

*Examples:*

*Change 165 grains to weighable apothecaries' units.*

By selecting larger weight units to account for as many of the required grains as possible, beginning with the largest, we find that we may use the following weights:

ʒii, ʒss, ℈ss, 5 gr, *answer.*

*Check:* ʒii = 120 gr<br>
ʒss = 30 gr<br>
℈ss = 10 gr<br>
5 gr = 5 gr<br>
165 gr, *total.*

*In enlarging a formula, we find that we are to measure 90 fʒ of a liquid. Using two graduates, if necessary, in what denominations may we measure this quantity?*

11 f℥ and 2 fʒ, *answer.*

*Check:* 11 f℥ = 88 fʒ<br>
2 fʒ = 2 fʒ<br>
90 fʒ, *total.*

**To add or subtract:**

To add or subtract quantities in the common systems, reduce to a common denomination, add or subtract, and reduce the result (unless it is to be used in further calculations) to a compound quantity.

*Examples:*

*A formula contains ℈ii of Ingredient A, ʒi of Ingredient B, ʒiv of Ingredient C, and gr viiss of Ingredient D. Calculate the total weight of the ingredients.*

℈ii = 2 × 20 gr = 40 gr<br>
ʒi = 1 × 60 gr = 60 gr<br>
ʒiv = 4 × 60 gr = 240 gr<br>
gr viiss = 7½ gr<br>
347½ gr = 5 ʒ 2 ℈ 7½ gr, *answer.*

*A pharmacist had 1 gallon of alcohol. At different times he dispensed f℥iv, Oii, f℥viii, and fʒiv. What volume of alcohol was left?*

f℥iv = 4 f℥
Oii = 2 × 16 f℥ = 32 f℥
f℥viii = 8 f℥
fʒiv = ½ f℥
44½ f℥, *total dispensed.*

1 gal = 128 f℥
− 44½ f℥
83½ f℥ = 5 pt 3 f℥ 4 fʒ, *answer.*

**To multiply or divide:**

A *simple* quantity may be multiplied or divided by any *pure* number—as *12 × 10 oz = 120 oz* or *7 lb 8 oz.*

But if *both* terms in division are derived from denominate numbers (as when we express one quantity as a fraction of another) they must be reduced to a *common* denomination before division can be performed.

A *compound* quantity is most easily multiplied or divided, and with least chance of careless error, if it is first reduced to a *simple* quantity: *2 × 8 f℥ 6 fʒ = 2 × 70 fʒ = 140 fʒ or 17 f℥ 4 fʒ.*

The *result* of multiplication should be (1) left as it is, if it is to be used in further calculations, (2) simplified, or (3) reduced to weighable or measurable denominations.

*Examples:*

*A prescription for 24 powders calls for gr ¼ of Ingredient A, ℈ss of Ingredient B, and gr v of Ingredient C in each powder. How much of each ingredient should be used in compounding the prescription?*

24 × gr ¼ = 6 gr of Ingredient A,
24 × ½ ℈ = 12 ℈, or 4 ʒ of Ingredient B,
24 × gr v = 120 gr, or 2 ʒ of Ingredient C, *answers.*

*A formula for 24 capsules contains ℈ss of one ingredient, ʒi of another, and ʒiiss of a third. How many grains of each ingredient will be contained in each capsule?*

℈ss = 10 gr, and $\frac{10}{24}$ gr = $\frac{5}{12}$ gr,
ʒi = 60 gr, and $\frac{60}{24}$ gr = 2½ gr,
ʒiiss = 150 gr, and $\frac{150}{24}$ gr = 6¼ gr, *answers.*

*How many 15-minim doses can be obtained from a mixture containing f℥iii of one ingredient and fʒii of another?*

f℥iii = 3 × 480 ♏ = 1440 ♏
fʒii = 2 × 60 ♏ = 120 ♏

1560 ♏, *total.*

$^{1560}/_{15}$ doses = 104 doses, *answer.*

## RELATIONSHIP OF AVOIRDUPOIS AND APOTHECARIES' WEIGHTS

As noted above, the *grain* is the same in both the avoirdupois and apothecaries' systems of weight, but other denominations with the same names are not equal.

To convert from either system to the other, first reduce the given quantity to grains in the one system, and then reduce the result to any desired denomination in the other system.

The custom of buying drugs by avoirdupois weight and dispensing them by apothecaries' weight leads to problems many of which can be most conveniently solved by proportion.

*Examples:*

*Convert ℥ii ʒii to avoirdupois weight.*

℥ii = 2 × 480 gr = 960 gr
ʒii = 2 × 60 gr = 120 gr
Total: 1080 gr

1 oz = 437.5 gr

$\frac{1080}{437.5}$ oz = 2 oz, 205 gr, *answer.*

*How many grains of a chemical are left in a 1-oz bottle after ʒvii are dispensed from it?*

1 oz = 1 × 437.5 gr = 437.5 gr
ʒvii = 7 × 60 gr = 420.0 gr
Difference: 17.5 gr, *answer.*

*If a drug costs $1.75 per oz, what is the cost of 2 ʒ?*

1 oz = 437.5 gr, and 2 ʒ = 120 gr

$$\frac{437.5\ (\text{gr})}{120\ (\text{gr})} = \frac{1.75\ (\$)}{x\ (\$)}$$

x = $0.48, *answer.*

## Practice Problems

1. Reduce each of the following quantities to grains:

   (a) ʒii ℈iss.
   (b) ℥ii ʒiss.
   (c) ℥i ℥ss ℈i.
   (d) ʒi ℈i gr x.

2. Reduce 0i ℥ii to fluidrachms.

3. Reduce each of the following quantities to weighable apothecaries' denominations:

   (a) 158 gr
   (b) 175 gr
   (c) 210 gr
   (d) 75 gr
   (e) 96 gr

4. ℞ Phenobarbital gr ¼
   Aspirin gr iv
   Lactose ad gr vi
   D.T.D. cap. #48
   Sig. cap. i t.i.d.

What combination of individual apothecaries' weights from a standard set could a pharmacist use to weigh the amount of lactose required to fill the prescription?

5. A pharmacist had 1 gallon of phenobarbital elixir; at different times he dispensed 0i, f℥vi, fʒiv, 0ss, f℥iss, and f℥xii. What volume, in fluidounces, of the elixir was left?

6. How many f℥ii-bottles of cough syrup can be obtained from 5 gal of the cough syrup?

7. How many ¼-gr tablets of morphine sulfate can be made from ⅛-oz (avoir.) bottle of morphine sulfate?

8. How many grains of a chemical are left in a 1-oz (avoir.) bottle after enough of it has been used to make 2000 tablets each containing 1/200 gr of the chemical?

9. If a chemical costs $1.75 per oz (avoir.), what is the cost of ʒiii?

10. How many 1/120-gr doses of atropine sulfate can be obtained from a manufacturer's ⅛-oz bottle of atropine sulfate?

11. A cough syrup contains ℈ss of ammonium chloride in fʒiv. How many grains should be used in preparing 1 gallon of the syrup?

12. In checking a narcotic file, a pharmacist found that the following quantities of codeine phosphate had been used from a bottle originally containing 1 oz:

℞1—gr v
℞2—℈i
℞3—ʒss
℞4—℈ss
℞5—gr iiss

How many grains of codeine phosphate were left in the bottle?

13. ℞ Salicylamide gr viiss
Aspirin gr iiss
M. ft. caps. no. i d.t.d. no. xl
Sig. One capsule q. 4 h. for arthritis pain.

*(a)* What compound quantity of salicylamide and aspirin should be used in filling the prescription?
*(b)* How many grains of aspirin would be taken daily?

14. ℞ Codeine Phosphate gr iii
Aspirin ʒiss
Phenacetin ʒi
Caffeine ℈i
M. ft. caps. no. xxiv
Sig. One capsule p.r.n. pain.

How many grains of each ingredient would be contained in each capsule?

15. ℞ Colchicine Tablets gr $\frac{1}{100}$
Disp. no. xii
Sig. Two tablets q. 2 h. as directed.

How many such tablets can be made from a 1-oz (avoir.) package of colchicine?

16. ℞ Aminophylline ʒss
Ephedrine Hydrochloride gr vi
Amobarbital gr v
M. ft. cap. no. xv
Sig. One capsule t.i.d. p.r.n. asthma.

*(a)* How many grains of aminophylline would be contained in each capsule?
*(b)* What fraction of a grain of ephedrine hydrochloride would be contained in each capsule?

# 5

# Conversion

When we want to measure something, we are theoretically privileged to select any system of measure we please. But when we are required to measure a given quantity, in a formula, say, or in a prescription, the instrument at hand—the graduate or set of weights—may not happen to measure in the system specified. Consequently, a quantity called for in one system may have to be translated to its equivalent in the system of our available instrument. This translation is called *conversion*.

Conversion is frequently required in pharmacy, for the metric and common systems are sometimes jumbled together in every day experience. Pounds may not be added to grams, nor may scruples be subtracted from avoirdupois ounces, nor may a ratio be made between liters and fluidounces; and we must convert to a single system (as well as reduce to a common denomination) all miscellaneous quantities that are to be in any way compared.

Denominations in the metric system are incommensurate with those of the common systems. Hence there can be no *exact* equivalence. But the International Bureau of Standards has measured the meter in terms of inches and the kilogram in terms of pounds so precisely as to be able to express the linear equivalence with 7-figure accuracy and the weight equivalence with 9-figure accuracy. Such precision, of course, is not intended to have any ordinary practical application. From these figures the relationships of other denominations can be calculated as accurately as necessary for a given purpose.

The measurement of a denomination of one system in terms of another system is properly called a *conversion factor.* Any one conversion factor is sufficient to serve as a bridge between two systems; but in practice it is convenient to have a choice of several. We may use the equation *1 g = 15.432 gr,* for example, in converting a number of grams to grains; but in converting grains to grams, a more useful equation is *1 gr = 0.065 g*. Again, it is convenient to have one equation for converting a large denomination directly to a large denomination, and another for converting a small denomination to a small denomination.

The question just how accurate our conversion factors should be has not been satisfactorily established. According to the *United States Pharmacopeia,* when prepared dosage forms such as tablets, capsules, etc., are prescribed in the metric system, the pharmacist may dispense the corresponding *approximate* equivalent in the apothecary system, and *vice versa,* as indicated in the USP Table of Metric-Apothecary Approximate Dose Equivalents.[1] However, *"exact"* equivalents must be used for the conversion of specific quantities in converting pharmaceutical formulas. Further, the U.S.P. directs that exact equivalents rounded to three significant figures be used for prescription compounding.

Ordinary pharmaceutical procedure actually seeks something between 2- and 3-figure accuracy in final results, and the following convenient figures, although not wholly consistent, are in widespread use and are more than sufficient for all practical purposes. *These should be memorized.*

## SOME PRACTICAL EQUIVALENTS

### Conversion Equivalents of Length

| | | | |
|---|---|---|---|
| 1 m | = | 39.37 | in |
| 1 in | = | 2.54 | cm |

### Conversion Equivalents of Volume

| | | | |
|---|---|---|---|
| 1 mL | = | 16.23 | ♏ |
| 1 ♏ | = | 0.06 | mL |
| 1 fʒ | = | 3.69 | mL |
| 1 f℥ | = | 29.57 | mL |
| 1 pt | = | 473 | mL |
| 1 gal (U.S.) | = | 3785 | mL |

### Conversion Equivalents of Weight

| | | | |
|---|---|---|---|
| 1 g | = | 15.432 | gr |
| 1 kg | = | 2.20 | lb (avoir.) |
| 1 gr | = | 0.065 | g or 65 mg |
| 1 oz (avoir.) | = | 28.35 | g |
| 1 ℥ | = | 31.1 | g |
| 1 lb (avoir.) | = | 454 | g |
| 1 ℔ (apoth.) | = | 373.2 | g |

### Other Equivalents

| | | | |
|---|---|---|---|
| 1 oz (avoir.) | = | 437.5 | gr |
| 1 ℥ | = | 480 | gr |
| 1 gal (U.S.) | = | 128 | f℥ |
| 1 f℥ (water) | = | 455 | gr |

[1]Table of Metric-Apothecary Dose Equivalents, The United States Pharmacopeia XXI—The National Formulary XVI, U.S. Pharmacopeial Convention, Inc., Rockville, Md., 1985.

Note that such equivalents may be used in two ways. For example, to convert a number of fluidounces to milliliters, *multiply* by *29.57;* and to convert a number of milliliters to fluidounces, *divide* by *29.57*.

Some individuals prefer to set up a ratio of a known equivalent and solve conversion problems by proportion. For example, in determining the number of milliliters in 8 fluidounces, an equivalent relating *milliliters to fluidounces is selected* (1 f℥ = 29.57 mL) and the problem solved by proportion as follows:

$$\frac{1\ (\text{f℥})}{8\ (\text{f℥})} = \frac{29.57\ (\text{mL})}{x\ (\text{mL})}$$

$$x = 236.56 \text{ mL}, \textit{answer}.$$

In utilizing the ratio and proportion method, the equivalent which contains both the units named in the problem is the best one to use. Sometimes more than one equivalent may be appropriate. For instance, in converting grams to grains, or *vice versa,* the gram-to-grain relationship is found in the following basic equivalents, 1 g = 15.432 gr and 1 gr = 0.065 g, as well as in *derived equivalents,* as 31.1 g = 480 gr and 28.35 g = 437.5 gr. It is best to utilize the basic equivalents when converting from one system to another and to select the equivalent which provides the answer most readily.

In response to the question: *Must we round off results so as to contain no more significant figures than are contained in the conversion factor?*—the answer is *Yes.* If we desire greater accuracy, we should use a more accurate conversion factor. But to the question: *If a formula includes the 1-figure quantity 5 g, and we convert it to grains, must we round off the result to* 1 *significant figure?*—the answer is decidedly *No.* We should interpret the quantity given in a formula as expressing the precision we are expected to achieve in compounding—usually not less than 3-figure accuracy. Hence, *5 g* in a formula or prescription should be interpreted as meaning at least *5.00 g.*

## CONVERSION OF LINEAR QUANTITIES

**To convert metric lengths to common equivalents:**

We may reduce any given metric length to meters and then multiply this quantity by *39.37* (the number of inches equivalent to each meter) to get inches. But if the metric quantity is small, it may be more convenient to reduce it to centimeters and divide by *2.54* to get inches.

*Example:*

*The fiber length of a sample of purified cotton is 6.35 mm. Express the length in inches.*

6.35 mm = 0.635 cm

Solving by proportion:

$$\frac{1 \text{ (in)}}{x \text{ (in)}} = \frac{2.54 \text{ (cm)}}{0.635 \text{ (cm)}}$$

x = 0.250 in, or ¼ in, *answer.*

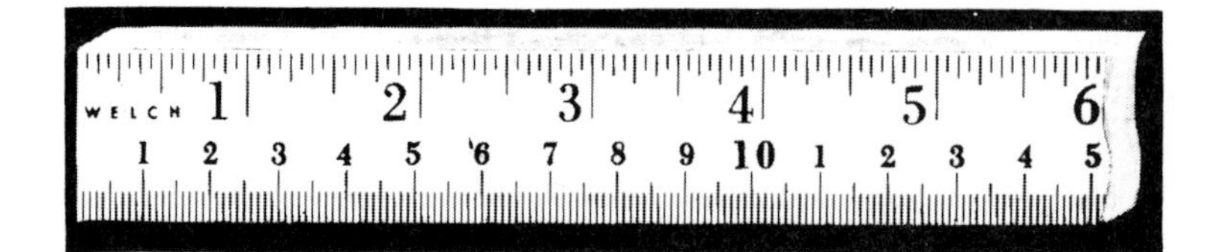


Portion of meter stick showing relation between centimeters and inches. (Courtesy of W. M. Welch Scientific Co.)

**To convert common lengths to metric equivalents:**

If given a length of a yard or more, reduce it to inches and divide by *39.37* to get meters. If given a shorter length, reduce it to inches and multiply by *2.54* to get centimeters.

*Example:*

*A medicinal plaster measures 4½ in by 6½ in. What are its dimensions in centimeters?*

Assuming 3-figure precision in the measurement,

4½ or 4.50 × 2.54 cm = 11.4 cm wide,
6½ or 6.50 × 2.54 cm = 16.5 cm long, *answers.*

## CONVERSION OF LIQUID QUANTITIES

**To convert metric volumes to apothecaries' fluid equivalents:**

For small volumes, multiply the number of milliliters by *16.23* to get minims—and reduce the result to measurable units if necessary.

For larger volumes, reduce the given volume to milliliters and divide by *29.57* to get fluidounces or by *473* to get pints.

*Examples:*

*Convert 0.4 mL to minims.*

To achieve 2-figure precision,

0.40 × 16.23 ♏ = 6.492 or 6.5 ♏, *answer.*

*Convert 2.5 L to fluidounces.*

2.5 L = 2500 mL

Solving by proportion:

$$\frac{1\ (f℥)}{x\ (f℥)} = \frac{29.57\ (mL)}{2500\ (mL)}$$

x = 84.5 f℥, *answer.*

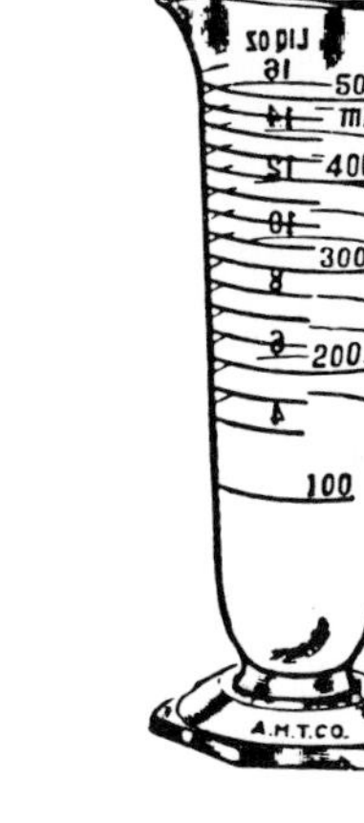


Dual scale gradulates.
(Courtesy of Corning Glass Works and Arthur H. Thomas Co.)

**To convert apothecaries' fluid volumes to metric equivalents:**

For small volumes, reduce to minims and divide by *16.23* to get milliliters.

For larger volumes, reduce to fluidounces and multiply by *29.57* to get milliliters.

*Examples:*

*Convert f℥iiss to milliliters.*

f℥iiss = 2½ × 60 ♏ = 150 ♏

Solving by proportion:

$$\frac{1\ (\text{mL})}{x\ (\text{mL})} = \frac{16.23\ (♏)}{150\ (♏)}$$

x = 9.24 mL, *answer.*

*Convert Oiiss to milliliters.*

Oiiss = 2½ × 16 f℥ = 40 f℥

40 × 29.57 mL = 1182.8 or 1180 mL, *answer.*

## CONVERSION OF WEIGHTS

**To convert metric weights to common weights:**

Reduce a given small quantity to grams and multiply by *15.432* or divide by *0.065* (whichever gives the answer more readily) to get grains, and reduce the quantity to any desired denomination.

For a larger quantity, divide the number of grams by *31.1* to get apothecaries' ounces, or by *28.35* to get avoirdupois ounces.

For a still larger quantity, divide the number of grams by *454* to get avoirdupois pounds.

*Examples:*

*Convert 12.5 g to grains.*

12.5 × 15.432 gr = 192.9 or 193 gr, *answer.*

Alternate solution (about 0.5% less accurate):

$\frac{12.5}{0.065}$ gr = 192.3 or 192 gr, *answer.*

*Convert 5 mg to grains.*

Solving by proportion:

$$\frac{1\ (\text{gr})}{x\ (\text{gr})} = \frac{65\ (\text{mg})}{5\ (\text{mg})}$$

x = $\frac{5}{65}$ gr = $\frac{1}{13}$ gr, *answer.*

*Convert 15 kg to avoirdupois pounds.*

Solving by proportion:

$$\frac{1 \text{ (kg)}}{15 \text{ (kg)}} = \frac{2.2 \text{ (lb)}}{x \text{ (lb)}}$$

x = 33.0 lb, *answer.*

**To convert common weights to metric equivalents:**

Reduce a given small quantity to grains and multiply by *65* to get milligrams; or reduce the quantity to grains and multiply by *0.065* or divide by *15.432* (whichever gives the answer more readily) to get grams. Reduce the result to any required denomination.

For larger quantities, reduce to apothecaries' ounces and multiply by *31.1*, or to avoirdupois ounces and multiply by *28.35* to get grams.

For still larger quantities, reduce to avoirdupois pounds and multiply by *454* to get grams, and then reduce, if required, to kilograms; or, more directly, reduce the given quantity to avoirdupois pounds and divide by 2.2 to get kilograms.

*Examples:*

*Convert 6.2 gr to milligrams.*

6.2 × 65 mg = 403 or 400 mg, *answer.*

*How many grams are represented by 850 grains?*

Solving by proportion:

$$\frac{1 \text{ (gr)}}{850 \text{ (gr)}} = \frac{0.065 \text{ (g)}}{x \text{ (g)}}$$

x = 55.25 or 55 g, *answer.*

*Convert 176 avoirdupois pounds to kilograms.*

$\frac{176}{2.2}$ kg = 80.0 kg, *answer.*

**Practice Problems**

1. The standard width of Type I Absorbent Gauze is 97.8 cm, and that of all other types is 91.4 cm. Express these widths in inches.

2. A mercury barometer reads 760 mm. Express this pressure in inches.

3. Convert 2 gal and 30 f℥ to liters.

4. If a mixture of powders weighing 30 g is divided into 100 dosage units, how many grains will each dosage unit weigh?

5. The inhalant dose of amyl nitrite is 0.18 mL. Express the dose in minims.

6. Ergonovine maleate ampuls each contain $\frac{1}{300}$ gr of drug. How many micrograms of ergonovine maleate are there in each ampul?

7. Adhesive tape made from film has a tensile strength, determined warpwise, of not less than 3 kg per 2.54 cm of width. Convert these quantities to common system equivalents.

8. The usual dosage range of atropine is $\frac{1}{150}$ gr to $\frac{1}{100}$ gr. Express this dosage range in milligrams.

9. The average diameter of the oil globules in an emulsion is 2.5 micrometers. What is the average size in inches?

10. The dose of a drug is $\frac{1}{10}$ gr per kg of body weight. How many milligrams should be given to a person weighing 154 lb?

11. A capsule contains $\frac{1}{8}$ gr of ephedrine sulfate, $\frac{1}{4}$ gr of theophylline and $\frac{1}{6}$ gr of phenobarbital. Convert each of these quantities to milligrams.

12. A certain elixir contains 0.325 g of potassium thiocyanate per teaspoonful (5 mL). At $15.35 per lb, what is the cost of the potassium thiocyanate required to make 1 gallon of the elixir?

13. ℞ Codeine Phosphate 30 mg
Acetaminophen 325 mg
M. ft. cap. D.T.D. no. 24
Sig. One capsule t.i.d. for pain.

How many grains each of codeine phosphate and acetaminophen should be used in compounding the prescription?

14. A prescription calls for 30 capsules, each containing $\frac{1}{200}$ gr of atropine sulfate. How many 0.4 mg tablets of atropine sulfate are needed in preparing the prescription?

15. Sustained release tablets of nitroglycerin contain the following amounts of drug: $\frac{1}{25}$ gr, $\frac{1}{10}$ gr, and $\frac{1}{50}$ gr. Express these quantities as milligrams.

16. How many $\frac{1}{4}$-gr tablets can be made from 10 g of a drug substance?

17. A hematinic tablet contains 525 mg of ferrous sulfate which is equivalent to 105 mg of elemental iron. How many grains each of ferrous sulfate and elemental iron would a patient receive from one tablet?

18. ℞ Atropine Sulfate gr $\frac{1}{200}$
Disp. xxiv tablets
Sig. One tablet t.i.d. for one week.

Assuming compliance with the prescribed dosage regimen, how many micrograms of atropine sulfate will the patient take in one week?

19. A prescription calls for 20 grains of epinephrine bitartrate. If 10 g of epinephrine bitartrate cost $9.00, what is the cost of the amount needed in the prescription?

20. The clearance between the rotor and stator of a colloid mill is set so that particles having a diameter of approximately 0.0005 in will be produced. What is the size, in micrometers, of the dispersed particles?

21. If f℥i of a cough syrup contains 10 gr of sodium citrate, how many milligrams are contained in 2.5 mL?

22. A formula for a cough syrup contains ⅛ gr of codeine phosphate per teaspoonful (fʒi). How many grams of codeine phosphate should be used in preparing one pint of the cough syrup?

23. ℞ Hydrocodone Bitartrate gr $\frac{1}{10}$
Phenacetin gr iiss
Aspirin gr v
Caffeine gr ss
M. ft. caps. D.T.D. no. xxiv
Sig. One capsule q.i.d.

*(a)* What is the weight, in milligrams, of the contents of each capsule?
*(b)* How many milligrams of hydrocodone bitartrate should be used in filling the prescription?
*(c)* How many days would the medication last if taken as directed?

24. If pentobarbital elixir contains 18.2 mg of pentobarbital per 5 mL, how many grams of pentobarbital would be used in preparing a pint of the elixir?

25. If 1000 mL of an intravenous fluid contain 2 g of an added antibiotic, how many grains of the antibiotic were administered to a patient who received 1 pint of the fluid?

26. If 15 mL of a potassium chloride solution contain 1.5 g of potassium chloride, equivalent to 20 mEq each of potassium and chloride, how many grams of potassium chloride and how many mEq each of potassium and chloride would be present in a 60-minim dose of the solution?

# 6

# Calculation of Doses

One of the prime responsibilities of the pharmacist is the checking of doses specified in prescriptions against his knowledge of the usual doses and usual dose ranges of the medicines prescribed. If he should note an unusual dose, he would be ethically bound to consult the physician, to make sure that the dosage as he reads it is correct.

For the patient, liquid dosage is almost invariably measured in "household" terms, most commonly the teaspoonful and tablespoonful. In *calculating* doses, pharmacists and physicians nowadays accept a capacity of 5 mL for the teaspoonful and 15 mL for the tablespoonful. In the past, the teaspoonful was traditionally accepted as having a capacity of 4 mL, or if the apothecaries' system was used, f℥i. It should be pointed out that household teaspoons have capacities that may vary from 3 to 7 mL. Tablespoons may vary from 15 to 22 mL in capacity.

Agreement has not been reached on a standard official teaspoon, in spite of the need for such a standard measure in connection with compounding and labeling liquid medicines. According to the *United States Pharmacopeia*, "For household purposes, an American Standard Teaspoon has been established by the American National Standards Institute as containing $4.93 \pm 0.24$ mL. In view of the almost universal practice of employing teaspoons ordinarily available in the household for the administration of medicine, the teaspoon may be regarded as representing 5 mL. Preparations intended for administration by teaspoon should be formulated on the basis of dosage in 5-mL units. Any dropper, syringe, medicine cup, special spoon, or other device used to administer liquids should deliver 5 mL wherever a teaspoon calibration is indicated." In general, pharmaceutical manufacturers use the 5-mL teaspoon and the 15-mL tablespoon as a basis for the formulation of oral liquid preparations.

Through habit and tradition, the f℥-symbol is used by many physicians in the *Signa*-portion of the prescription when indicating teaspoonful dosage. The pharmacist may interpret this symbol as a teaspoonful in dispensing prefabricated manufacturers' products called for on prescriptions and allow the patient to utilize the household teaspoon. When compounding prescriptions, the pharmacist may interpret it as a "dram spoon" and dispense a medicinal spoon having a capacity of 1 fluidrachm. Depending upon the method used, dosage calculations of the prescription are performed accordingly.

Certain factors such as viscosity and surface tension of a given liquid will influence the actual volume delivered by a teaspoon.

For calculation of dosage problems, the following Table is suggested:

## TABLE OF APPROXIMATE EQUIVALENTS

| *"Household" measure:* | | *Metric measure:* | | *Apothecaries' measure:* | |
|---|---|---|---|---|---|
| *1 teaspoonful* | = | 5 mL | = | 1⅓ fʒ | |
| *1 tablespoonful* | = | 15 mL | = | 4 fʒ | or ½f℥ |

In *judging the safety* of doses of potent substances that are prescribed in liquid form, where the liquid is to be administered in teaspoonful doses, the pharmacist should check the dosage on the basis of 6 doses per fluidounce. It should be noted that if a dramspoon is used, there will be 8 doses per fluidounce.

Frequently, the "drop" is used as a measure for medicines. It does not represent a definite quantity, since drops of different liquids vary greatly. In an attempt to standardize the drop as a unit of volume, the *United States Pharmacopeia* defines the official medicine dropper as being constricted at the delivery end to a round opening having an external diameter of about 3 mm. The dropper, when held vertically, delivers water in drops each of which weighs between 45 mg and 55 mg. Accordingly, the official dropper is calibrated to deliver 20 drops of water per mL.

However, one should keep in mind that few medicinal liquids have the same surface and flow characteristics as water, and therefore the size of drops varies materially from one liquid to another. The "drop" should not be used as a measure until the volume that it represents has been determined for each specific liquid. This is done by *calibrating* the dispensing dropper. The calibrated dropper is the only one that should be used for the measurement of medicine. Some manufacturers include a specially calibrated dropper along with their prepackaged medication for use by the patient in measuring dosage.

## CALIBRATION OF DROPPERS

A dropper may be calibrated by counting the drops of a liquid as they fall into a graduate until a measurable volume is obtained. The volume of the drop is then calculated in terms of a definite unit (mL or ♏).

## DOSAGE STATEMENTS

The monographs in the *United States Pharmacopeia Dispensing Information* (USP DI) provide *General Dosing Information* and, in addition, list under *Dosage Forms* the *usual adult dose* of a drug substance and its *usual adult prescribing limits.* In some monographs, this information is given in terms of body weight. Pediatric doses are expressed in terms of body weight or in terms of square meter of body surface area.

## "APPROXIMATE" EQUIVALENTS vs. "EXACT" EQUIVALENTS

All doses in the USP DI monographs are given in the metric system. As indicated in the preceding chapter, the *Pharmacopeia* provides a "Table of Metric-Apothecary *Approximate Dose Equivalents*" for obtaining apothecaries' equivalents for metric doses by reference. "These *approximate* dose equivalents represent the quantities usually prescribed by physicians using, respectively, the metric system and the apothecary system of weights and measures. . . . "

The pharmacist may use these *approximate* dose equivalents when dispensing prepared dosage forms.

However, the approximate dose equivalents cannot be used for the conversion of specific quantities in a prescription *which requires compounding* or in converting pharmaceutical formulas from one system of weights or measures to the other system. For such purposes *exact* equivalents must be used. For prescription compounding, these exact equivalents are to be rounded to three significant figures.

## MISCELLANEOUS DOSAGE PROBLEMS

**To calculate the number of doses in a specified amount of medicine:**

$$\text{Number of doses} = \frac{\text{Total amount}}{\text{Size of dose}}$$

The *total* amount and the *dose* must be measured in a common denomination.

*Examples:*

*If the dose of a drug is 200 milligrams, how many doses are contained in 10 grams?*

$$10 \text{ g} = 10{,}000 \text{ mg}$$

$$\text{Number of doses} = \frac{10{,}000 \text{ (mg)}}{200 \text{ (mg)}} = 50 \text{ doses, } \textit{answer.}$$

*How many 20-minim doses are contained in 40 mL of a liquid?*

$$40 \text{ ml} = 40 \times 16.23 \text{ ♏} = 649.2 \text{ ♏}$$

$$\text{Number of doses} = \frac{649.2 \text{ (♏)}}{20 \text{ (♏)}} = 32 \text{ doses, } \textit{answer.}$$

*If the dose of a medicine is ⅕ grain, how many doses are contained in ½ drachm?*

$$\tfrac{1}{2} \text{ ʒ} = \tfrac{1}{2} \times 60 \text{ gr} = 30 \text{ gr}$$

$$\text{Number of doses} = \frac{30 \text{ (gr)}}{\tfrac{1}{5} \text{ (gr)}} = 30 \times \frac{5}{1} = 150 \text{ doses, } \textit{answer.}$$

*If 1 tablespoon is prescribed as the dose of a medicine, approximately how many doses will be contained in 12 fluidounces?*

$$1 \text{ tablespoonful} = 4 \text{ fʒ}$$
$$12 \text{ f℥} = 96 \text{ fʒ}$$

$$\text{Number of doses} = \frac{96 \text{ (fʒ)}}{4 \text{ (fʒ)}} = 24 \text{ doses, } \textit{answer.}$$

*If the dose of a drug is 50 micrograms, how many doses are contained in 0.020 gram?*

$$0.020 \text{ g} = 20 \text{ mg}$$
$$50 \text{ µg} = 0.05 \text{ mg}$$
$$\text{Number of doses} = \frac{20 \text{ (mg)}}{0.05 \text{ (mg)}} = 400 \text{ doses, } \textit{answer.}$$

**To calculate the size of each dose, given a specified amount of medicine and the number of doses it contains:**

$$\text{Size of dose} = \frac{\text{Total amount}}{\text{Number of doses}}$$

The *size of the dose* will be expressed in whatever denomination is chosen for measuring the given total amount.

*Examples:*

*How many teaspoonfuls would be prescribed in each dose of an elixir if f℥vi contained 18 doses?*

f℥vi = 48 fʒ
1 teaspoonful = $1\frac{1}{3}$ fʒ
48 fʒ ÷ $1\frac{1}{3}$ fʒ = 36 teaspoonfuls

Or, 1 f℥ = 6 treaspoonfuls
6 f℥ = 36 teaspoonfuls

$$\text{Size of dose} = \frac{36 \text{ (tsp)}}{18} = 2 \text{ teaspoonfuls, } \textit{answer.}$$

*How many drops would be prescribed in each dose of a liquid medicine if 15 mL contained 60 doses? The dispensing dropper calibrates 32 drops per mL.*

15 mL = 15 × 32 drops = 480 drops

$$\text{Size of dose} = \frac{480 \text{ (drops)}}{60} = 8 \text{ drops, } \textit{answer.}$$

**To calculate the amount of a medicine, given the number of doses it contains and the size of each dose:**

Total amount = number of doses × size of dose

It is convenient first to convert the given dose to the denomination in which the total amount is to be expressed.

*Examples:*

*How many milliliters of a liquid medicine would provide a patient with 2 tablespoonfuls twice a day for 8 days?*

Number of doses = 16
Size of dose = 2 tablespoonfuls or 30 mL
Total amount = 16 × 30 ml = 480 mL, *answer.*

*How many fluidounces of a mixture would provide a patient with a teaspoonful dose to be taken 3 times a day for 16 days?*

Number of doses = 16 × 3 = 48
Size of dose = 1 teaspoonful = $1\frac{1}{3}$ fʒ
Total amount = 48 × $1\frac{1}{3}$ fʒ = 64 fʒ = 8 f℥, *answer.*

*How many milligrams of a drug will be needed to prepare 72 dosage forms if each is to contain $\frac{1}{12}$ grain?*

Number of doses = 72
Size of dose = $\frac{1}{12}$ grain = 5.4 mg
Total amount = 72 × 5.4 mg = 390 mg, *answer.*

**To calculate the quantity of an ingredient in each specified dose of a medicine, given the quantity in a total amount:**

When the number of doses in the total amount is given or can be quickly calculated, this is a convenient equation:

$$\text{Quantity in each dose} = \frac{\text{Quantity in total amount}}{\text{Number of doses}}$$

The quantity of the ingredient in the total amount should first be reduced or converted to the denomination desired in the answer.

But when the number of doses is not given, it is sometimes more convenient to use this proportion:

$$\frac{\text{Total amount}}{\text{Size of dose}} = \frac{\text{Quantity of ingredient in total}}{x}$$

$$x = \text{Quantity in each dose}$$

*Examples:*

*If 0.050 g of a substance is used in preparing 125 tablets, how many micrograms are represented in each tablet?*

$$0.050 \text{ g} = 50 \text{ mg} = 50{,}000 \text{ µg}$$

$$\frac{50{,}000 \text{ (µg)}}{125} = 400 \text{ µg, } \textit{answer.}$$

*If a preparation contains 5 g of a drug in 500 mL, how many grams are contained in each tablespoonful dose?*

$$1 \text{ tablespoonful} = 15 \text{ mL}$$

$$\frac{500 \text{ (mL)}}{15 \text{ (mL)}} = \frac{5 \text{ (g)}}{x}$$

$$x = 0.15 \text{ g, } \textit{answer.}$$

*A cough mixture contains ¾ gr of hydromorphone hydrochloride in f℥viii. How much hydromorphone hydrochloride is there in each 2-teaspoonful dose?*

2 teaspoonfuls = 2⅔ fʒ
f℥viii = 64 fʒ
64 ÷ 2⅔ = 24 doses
¾ gr ÷ 24 = 1/32 gr, *answer.*

Or, 1 ℥ = 6 teaspoonfuls
8 f℥ = 48 teaspoonfuls
48 (tsp) ÷ 2 = 24 doses

Or,

$$\frac{48 \text{ (tsp)}}{2 \text{ (tsp)}} = \frac{\frac{3}{4} \text{ (gr)}}{x \text{ (gr)}}$$

$$x = \frac{2 \times \frac{3}{4}}{48} \text{ gr} = \frac{1}{32} \text{ gr, } \textit{answer.}$$

*How many grains of codeine sulfate and of ammonium chloride will be contained in each dose of the following prescription?*

| ℞ | | |
|---|---|---|
| | Codeine Sulfate | gr vi |
| | Ammonium Chloride | ʒiss |
| | Cherry Syrup ad | f℥vi |
| | Sig. Teaspoonful for cough. | |

f℥ vi = 48 fʒ
1 teaspoonful = $1\frac{1}{3}$ fʒ
48 ÷ $1\frac{1}{3}$ = 36 doses

Or, 1 f℥ = 6 teaspoonfuls
6 f℥ = 36 teaspoonfuls
= 36 doses

6 gr ÷ 36 = $\frac{1}{6}$ gr of codeine sulfate, *and*
ʒiss or 90 gr ÷ 36 = $2\frac{1}{2}$ gr of ammonium chloride, *answers.*

Or,

$$\frac{36 \text{ (tsp)}}{1 \text{ (tsp)}} = \frac{6 \text{ (gr)}}{x \text{ (gr)}}$$

x = $\frac{1}{6}$ gr of codeine sulfate, *and*

$$\frac{36 \text{ (tsp)}}{1 \text{ (tsp)}} = \frac{90 \text{ (gr)}}{y \text{ (gr)}}$$

y = $2\frac{1}{2}$ gr of ammonium chloride, *answers.*

*How many grams of codeine phosphate and of ammonium chloride will be contained in each dose of the following prescription?*

| ℞ | | |
|---|---|---|
| | Codeine Phosphate | 0.6 g |
| | Ammonium Chloride | 6.0 g |
| | Cherry Syrup ad | 120.0 mL |
| | Sig. Teaspoonful for cough. | |

1 teaspoonful = 5 mL

120 ÷ 5 = 24 doses

0.6 g ÷ 24 = 0.025 g of codeine phosphate, *and*

6.0 g ÷ 24 = 0.25 g of ammonium chloride, *answers.*

Or,

$$\frac{120 \text{ (mL)}}{5 \text{ (mL)}} = \frac{0.6 \text{ (g)}}{x \text{ (g)}}$$

x = 0.025 g of codeine phosphate, *and*

$$\frac{120 \text{ (mL)}}{5 \text{ (mL)}} = \frac{6 \text{ (g)}}{y \text{ (g)}}$$

y = 0.25 g of ammonium chloride, *answers.*

**To calculate the quantity of an ingredient in a specified total amount of medicine, given the quantity of the ingredient in each specified dose:**

As always, we can make a sound ratio of two amounts only by measuring them in a common denomination.

Here again, when the number of doses is known or can be quickly calculated, this equation is convenient:

$$\text{Quantity in total} = \text{Quantity in dose} \times \text{Number of doses}$$

Otherwise this proportion may be used:

$$\frac{\text{Size of dose}}{\text{Total amount}} = \frac{\text{Quantity of ingredient in each dose}}{x}$$

$$x = \text{Quantity in total amount}$$

*Examples:*

*How many grams of a drug substance are required to make 120 mL of a solution each teaspoonful of which will contain 3 mg of the drug substance?*

1 teaspoonful = 5 mL

$$\frac{5 \text{ (mL)}}{120 \text{ (mL)}} = \frac{3 \text{ (mg)}}{x \text{ (mg)}}$$

x = 72 mg or 0.072 g, *answer.*

*A six-fluidounce cough mixture is to contain, in each teaspoonful, ¼ gr of codeine phosphate, ½ minim of chloroform, and 2½ gr of sodium citrate. Calculate the quantity of each ingredient to be used in filling the prescription.*

f℥vi = 48 fʒ
1 teaspoonful = $1\frac{1}{3}$ fʒ
Number of doses = 48 ÷ $1\frac{1}{3}$ = 36

Or, 1 f℥ = 6 teaspoonfuls
6 f℥ = 36 teaspoonfuls
= 36 doses

36 × ¼ gr = 9 gr of codeine phosphate,

36 × ½ ♏ = 18 ♏ of chloroform,

36 × 2½ gr = 90 gr or ʒiss of sodium citrate, *answers.*

**To calculate the dose of a drug based on body weight:**

The doses of a number of drugs for both adults and children are determined by body weight, most frequently expressed in kilograms.

*Example:*

*The usual initial dose of chlorambucil is 150 μg per kg of body weight once a day. How many milligrams should be administered to a person weighing 154 lb?*

150 μg = 0.15 mg

1 kg = 2.2 lb

$$\frac{2.2\ (\text{lb})}{154\ (\text{lb})} = \frac{0.15\ (\text{mg})}{x\ (\text{mg})}$$

x = 10.5 mg, *answer.*

## CALCULATION OF DOSES FOR CHILDREN

**To calculate the dose of a drug for children based on age:**

The age of the individual being treated is frequently a consideration in the determination of drug dosage, especially in the young or very old. Newborn infants, particularly those born prematurely, are abnormally sensitive to certain drugs because of the immature state of their hepatic and renal function by which drugs are normally inactivated and eliminated from the body. Failure to detoxify and eliminate drugs results in their accumulation in the tissues to a toxic level. Elderly individuals may also respond abnormally to the usual amount of a drug due to impaired ability to inactivate or excrete drugs or because of other concurrent pathologic conditions.

Before there was an understanding of the physiologic differences between adult and pediatric patients, the latter were treated with drugs as if they were merely miniature adults. Various rules of dosage in which the pediatric dose was a fraction of the adult dose, based on relative age, were created for youngsters (e.g., Young's Rule). Today these rules are not in general use since age alone is no longer considered to be a singularly valid criterion for use in the determination of children's dosage, especially when calculated from the *usual* adult dose which itself provides wide clinical variations in response.

*Young's Rule,* based on age:

$$\frac{\text{Age}}{\text{Age} + 12} \times \text{Adult dose} = \text{Dose for child}$$

*Examples:*

*If the usual adult dose of phenobarbital is 15 mg, what is the dose for a child 8 years old?*

$$\frac{8}{8 + 12} \times 15 \text{ mg} = \tfrac{2}{5} \times 15 \text{ mg} = 6 \text{ mg, } \textit{answer.}$$

*If the usual adult dose of an injection is 0.1 mL, what is the dose for a child 12 years old?*

$$\frac{12}{12 + 12} \times 0.1 \text{ mL} = \tfrac{1}{2} \times 0.1 \text{ mL} = 0.05 \text{ mL, } \textit{answer.}$$

Other methods based on age are:

*Cowling's Rule:*

$$\frac{\text{Age at next birthday (in years)} \times \text{Adult dose}}{24} = \text{Dose for child}$$

*Fried's Rule for Infants:*

$$\frac{\text{Age (in months)} \times \text{Adult dose}}{150} = \text{Dose for infant}$$

**To calculate the dose of a drug for children based on weight:**

The *usual doses* for drugs are considered generally suitable for 70 kg (150 pound) individuals. The ratio between the amount of drug administered and the size of the body influences the drug concentration at its site of action. Therefore, drug dosage may require adjustment from the usual adult dose for abnormally lean or obese patients. The determination of drug dosage for youngsters on the basis of body weight is considered more dependable than that based strictly on age. However, the consideration of the individual drug and patient's pathologic and physiologic state still reigns supreme and limits the clinical utility of any *general* rule of pediatric dosage. One such general rule is Clark's Rule:

*Clark's Rule,* based on weight:

$$\frac{\text{Weight (in lb)} \times \text{Adult dose}}{\text{150 (average weight of adult in lb)}} = \text{Dose for child}$$

*Example:*

*If the usual adult dose of a drug is 3 gr, what is the dose, expressed as a fraction of a grain, for a child weighing 40 lb?*

$$\frac{40 \times 3\ (\text{gr})}{150} = \tfrac{4}{15} \times 3\ (\text{gr}) = \tfrac{4}{5}\ \text{gr, } \textit{answer.}$$

The dosage of a number of drug substances is based on body weight and is frequently expressed on a *milligram* (drug) *per kilogram* (body weight) or *milligram per pound* basis.

*Example:*

*The usual dose of sulfisoxazole for infants over 2 months of age and children is 60 to 75 mg/kg of body weight. What would be the usual range for a child weighing 44 pounds?*

1 kg = 2.2 lb
20 kg = 44 lb

60 mg/kg × 20 kg = 1200 mg
75 mg/kg × 20 kg = 1500 mg

Thus, the dosage range would be 1200 to 1500 mg, *answer.*

**To calculate the dose of a drug for children based on body surface area as related to weight:**

Many physicians believe that doses for children should be based upon body surface area, since the correct dosage of drugs seems more nearly proportional to the surface area.[1]

The accompanying Table shows the approximate relation between body weight and surface area of average body dimensions. It may be used in the calculation of pediatric doses based on body surface area (BSA) as related to weight.

By reference to the Table, we find that the pediatric dose is expressed as a percent of the adult dose. This is based upon the relationship of the square meter area of a given weight and the average adult surface area of 1.73 square meters ($m^2$). Approximate doses for children may be calculated by multiplying the adult dose by this percentage.

[1]See, for instance, Shirkey, Harry C.: Drug Dosage for Infants and Children. J.A.M.A. 193:443–446, 1965.

TABLE OF THE APPROXIMATE RELATION OF SURFACE AREA AND WEIGHTS OF INDIVIDUALS OF AVERAGE BODY DIMENSION

Adapted from *Techniques of Medication* by Eric W. Martin, et al., J. B. Lippincott Co., 1969, p. 31, who adapted it from Modell's Drugs of Choice (Mosby).

| *Kilograms* | *Pounds* | *Surface Area in Square Meters* | *Per Cent of Adult Dose*[1] |
|---|---|---|---|
| 2 | 4.4 | 0.15 | 9 |
| 3 | 6.6 | 0.20 | 11.5 |
| 4 | 8.8 | 0.25 | 14 |
| 5 | 11.0 | 0.29 | 16.5 |
| 6 | 13.2 | 0.33 | 19 |
| 7 | 15.4 | 0.37 | 21 |
| 8 | 17.6 | 0.40 | 23 |
| 9 | 19.8 | 0.43 | 25 |
| 10 | 22.0 | 0.46 | 27 |
| 15 | 33.0 | 0.63 | 36 |
| 20 | 44.0 | 0.83 | 48 |
| 25 | 55.0 | 0.95 | 55 |
| 30 | 66.0 | 1.08 | 62 |
| 35 | 77.0 | 1.20 | 69 |
| 40 | 88.0 | 1.30 | 75 |
| 45 | 99.0 | 1.40 | 81 |
| 50 | 110.0 | 1.51 | 87 |
| 55 | 121.0 | 1.58 | 91 |

[1]Based on average adult surface area of 1.73 square meters.

**To calculate the dose of a drug for children based on body surface area as related to weight and height:**

For more precise calculation of pediatric doses based on body surface area, one should refer to a standard *nomogram* which includes both weight and height as factors influencing body surface area. The nomogram on page 92 may be used for determining body surface area (BSA) from weight and height. The BSA in square meters ($m^2$) is indicated where a straight line drawn to connect the height and weight of the child intersects the surface area column. In the example in the nomogram, for a child weighing 15 kg and measuring 100 cm in height, the BSA = 0.64 $m^2$. The dose is then calculated as follows:

If the adult dose is given,

$$\frac{\text{BSA of child (in m}^2\text{)}}{1.73\ \text{m}^2\ \text{(average adult BSA)}} \times \text{Adult dose} = \text{Approximate dose for child}$$

If the dose per $m^2$ is given,

$$\text{BSA of child (in m}^2\text{)} \times \text{Dose per m}^2 = \text{Approximate dose for child}$$

*Examples:*

*If the adult dose of a drug is 75 mg, what would be the dose for a child weighing 40 lb and measuring 32 in. in height? Use the body surface method.*

## BODY SURFACE AREA OF CHILDREN

Taken from Scientific Tables, 7th ed. p. 538, J. R. Geigy, S.A., Basle.

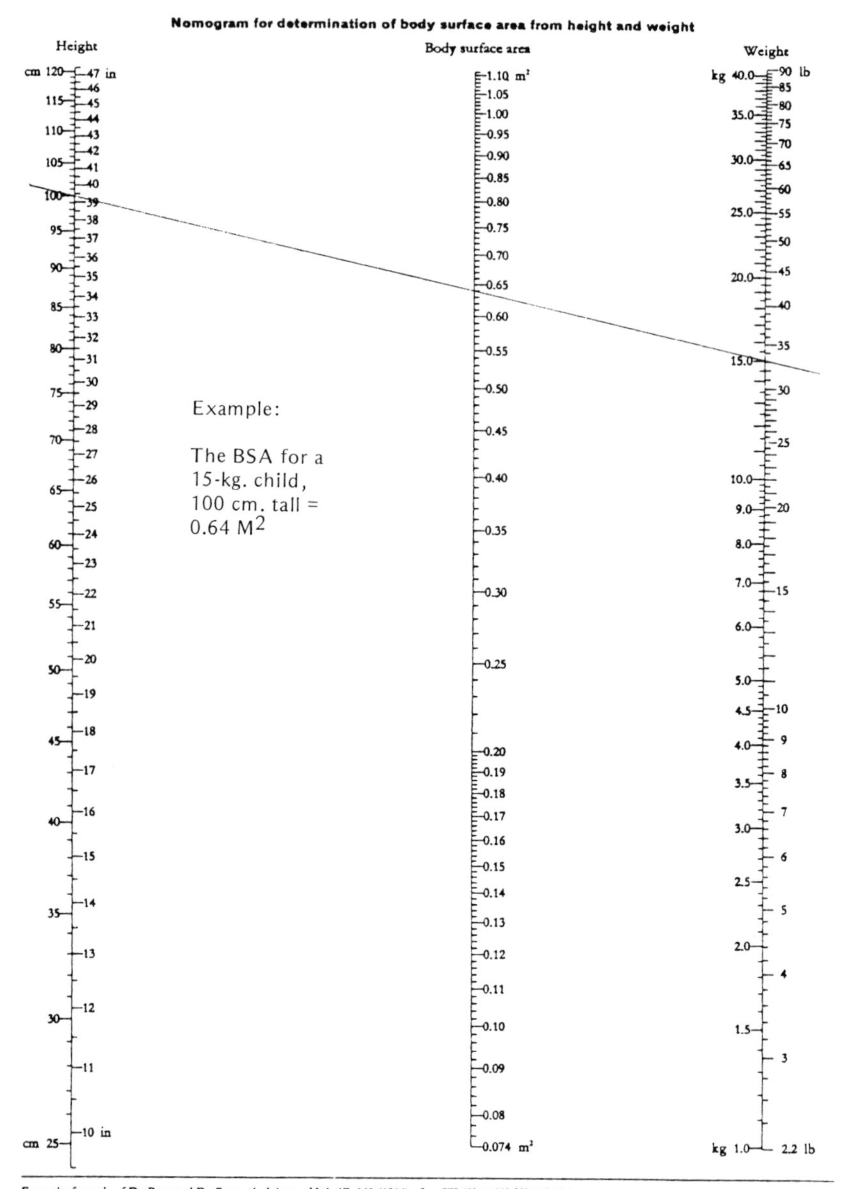


From the formula of Du Bois and Du Bois, *Arch. intern. Med.*, 17, 863 (1916): $S = W^{0.425} \times H^{0.725} \times 71.84$, or $\log S = \log W \times 0.425 + \log H \times 0.725 + 1.8564$ ($S$ = body surface in cm², $W$ = weight in kg, $H$ = height in cm)

# BODY SURFACE AREA OF ADULTS

Taken from Scientific Tables, 7th ed. p. 537, J. R. Geigy, S.A., Basle.

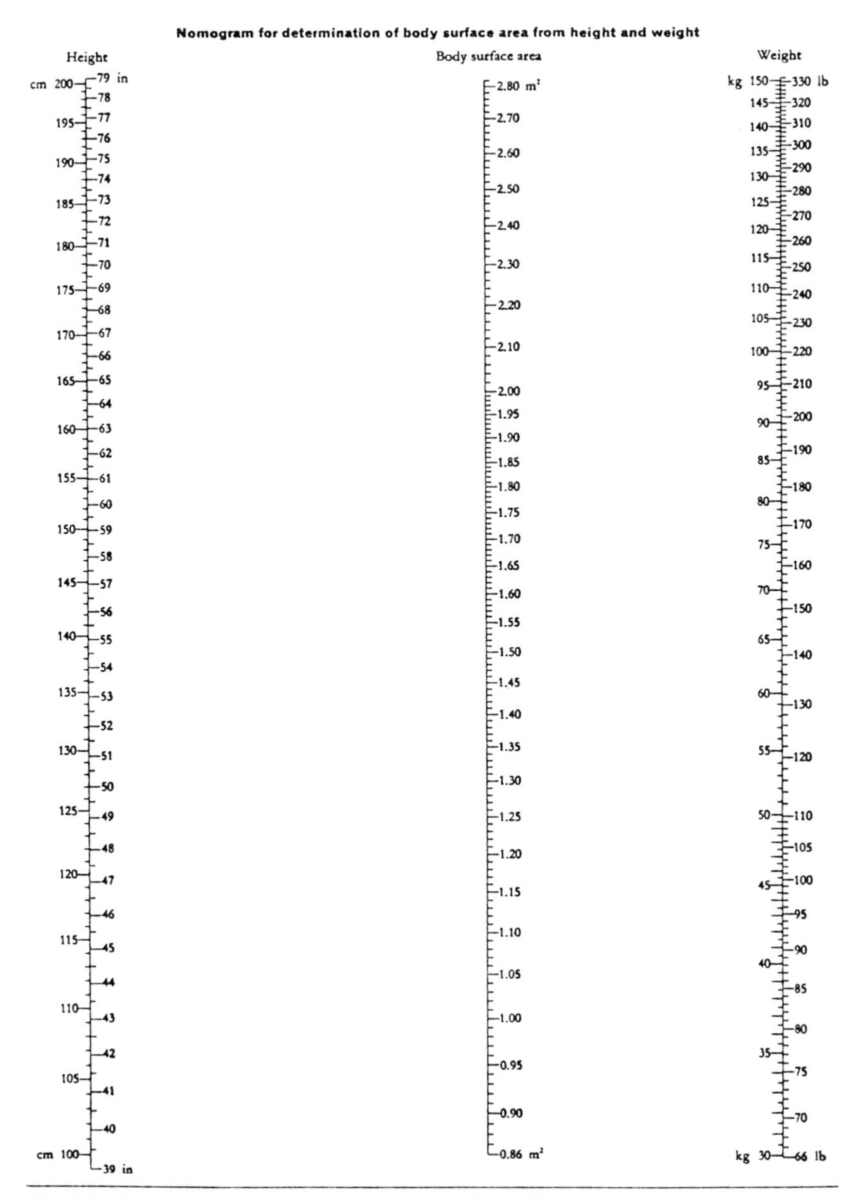


From the formula of Du Bois and Du Bois, *Arch. intern. Med.*, 17, 863 (1916): $S = W^{0.425} \times H^{0.725} \times 71.84$, or $\log S = \log W \times 0.425 + \log H \times 0.725 + 1.8564$ ($S$ = body surface in cm², $W$ = weight in kg, $H$ = height in cm)

From the nomogram, the BSA = 0.60 m²

$$\frac{0.60\ (m^2)}{1.73\ (m^2)} \times 75\ mg = 26\ mg,\ \textit{answer.}$$

*The usual pediatric dose of ephedrine sulfate is stated as 25 mg per square meter. Using the nomogram, calculate the dose for a child weighing 18 kg and measuring 82 cm in height.*

From the nomogram, the BSA = 0.60 m²

25 mg × 0.60 = 15 mg, *answer.*

Since it has been recognized that a close relationship exists between many physiological processes and the body surface area, some practitioners advocate the use of body surface area as a parameter in calculating doses for *adults* as well as for children.

The nomogram on page 93 designed specifically for determining the body surface area of *adults* may be used in the same manner as the one previously described. The adult dose is then calculated as follows:

$$\frac{\text{BSA of adult } (m^2)}{1.73\ m^2} \times \text{Usual adult dose} = \text{Dose for adult}$$

## Practice Problems

1. If the dose of a drug is 150 micrograms, how many doses are contained in 0.120 g?

2. How many 10-minim doses are contained in 60 mL of belladonna tincture?

3. If the dose of a drug is $\frac{1}{16}$ gr, how many doses are contained in ℨi?

4. If a liquid medicine is to be taken three times daily, and if 180 mL are to be taken in 4 days, how many tablespoonfuls should be prescribed for each dose?

5. If a cough syrup contains 0.24 g of codeine phosphate in 120 mL, how many milligrams are contained in each teaspoonful dose?

6. A mixture of powders contains $\frac{1}{20}$ gr of atropine sulfate. If the mixture is divided into 12 dosage forms, what fraction of a grain will each dose contain?

7. If 240 mL of a cough mixture contain $\frac{3}{4}$ gr of hydromorphinone hydrochloride, how many milligrams are contained in each teaspoonful of the mixture?

8. If f℥iv of a mixture contain 6 gr of phenobarbital, how many grains are contained in each teaspoonful dose?

9. If a solution of atropine sulfate contains 1 gr in each fluidounce, how many minims will contain $\frac{1}{120}$ gr?

10. A prescription for 250 mL of a liquid medicine contains 0.025 g of atropine sulfate and specifies a dose of 5 mL. How many micrograms of atropine sulfate are contained in each dose?

11. A physician prescribes tetracycline suspension for a patient to be taken in doses of two teaspoonfuls four times a day for 4 days, and then one teaspoonful four times a day for 2 days. How many milliliters of the suspension should be dispensed to provide the quantity for the prescribed dosage regimen?

12. Digoxin injection is available in a concentration of 0.1 mg per mL. How many milliliters of the injection will provide a dose of 75 micrograms?

13. The usual dose of digoxin for rapid digitalization is a total of 1.0 mg, divided into 2 or more portions at intervals of 6 to 8 hours. How many milliliters of digoxin elixir containing 50 μg per mL would provide this dose?

14. ℞ Dextromethorphan 15 mg/5 mL
Guaifenesin Syrup ad f℥viii
Sig. 5 mL q. 4 h. p.r.n. cough.

How many milligrams of dextromethorphan should be used in filling the prescription?

15. ℞

| | | |
|---|---|---|
| Phenobarbital | | 0.6 g |
| Belladonna Tincture | | 12.0 mL |
| Peppermint Water | ad | 120.0 mL |

Sig. 5 mL t.i.d.

How many milligrams of phenobarbital and how many milliliters of belladonna tincture will be contained in each dose?

16. What volume, in milliliters, of a solution containing 2.5 g of potassium thiocyanate per 100 mL would provide 100 mg of potassium thiocyanate three times a day for 10 days?

17. A patient has been instructed to take 15 mL of alumina and magnesium oral suspension every other hour for four doses daily. How many days will two 12-fluidounce bottles of the suspension last?

18. Kaopectate contains 90 grains of kaolin per fluidounce. How many grains of kaolin are contained in a tablespoonful dose of a mixture containing 4 f℥ of paregoric and 8 f℥ of Kaopectate?

19. One liter of Terpin Hydrate and Codeine Elixir contains 2 g of

codeine. The usual dose of the elixir is 5 mL. What is the codeine content, expressed as a fraction of a grain, of the usual dose of the elixir?

20. Amobarbital Elixir contains 4.4 g of amobarbital per liter. How many milligrams of amobarbital are contained in a teaspoonful dose of the elixir?

21. Lugol's Solution contains 5 g of iodine per 100 mL and its usual dose is 0.3 mL three times a day. How many milligrams of iodine are represented in the daily dose of the solution?

22. A patient is to receive 3¾ gr of amobarbital sodium intravenously. The drug is available in ampuls containing 500 mg of amobarbital sodium powder. Assuming that the powder is dissolved in 10 mL of sterile water, how many milliliters of the prepared solution would provide the prescribed dose?

23. A physician prescribes 1.6 million units of penicillin G potassium daily for 7 days. If 1 mg of penicillin G potassium is equal to 1595 penicillin G units, how many 250-mg tablets of penicillin G potassium should be dispensed for the prescribed dosage regimen?

24. Terpin Hydrate and Codeine Elixir contains 1 gr of codeine per fluidounce. How much additional codeine should be added to 6 f℥ of the elixir so that each teaspoonful will contain 15 mg of codeine?

25. ℞ Noscapine 0.72 g
Guaifenesin 4.80 g
Alcohol 15.0 mL
Cherry Syrup ad 120.0 mL
Sig. 5 mL t.i.d. p.r.n. cough.

How many milligrams each of noscapine and guaifenesin would be contained in each dose?

26. ℞ Lincocin 1.2 g
Propylene Glycol 4.0 mL
Isopropyl Alcohol 70%
Purified Water aa ad 60 mL
Sig. Apply b.i.d. for acne.

*(a)* If the source of lincocin is an injection containing the equivalent of 300 mg of lincocin per mL, how many milliliters of the injection should be used in filling the prescription?

*(b)* How many milliliters each of 70% isopropyl alcohol and purified water would be required in filling the prescription?

27. How many milliliters of an injection containing 20 mg of gentamicin in each 2 mL should be used in filling a medication order calling for 2.5 mg of gentamicin to be administered intramuscularly?

28. A physician ordered 1.5 milligrams of theophylline to be administered orally to a baby. How many milliliters of theophylline elixir containing 80 mg of theophylline per 15 mL should be used in filling the medication order?

29. How many milliliters of aminophylline injection containing 250 mg of aminophylline in each 10 mL should be used in filling a medication order calling for 15 mg of aminophylline?

30. A physician ordered 20 mg of Demerol and 0.3 mg of atropine sulfate to be administered preoperatively to a patient. Demerol is available in a syringe containing 25 mg per mL and atropine sulfate is in an ampul containing 0.4 mg per 0.5 mL. How many milliliters of each should be used in filling the medication order?

31. A solution contains 660 mg of sodium fluoride per 120 mL and has a dose of 10 drops. If the dispensing dropper calibrates 25 drops per mL, how many milligrams of sodium fluoride are contained in each dose?

32. ℞ Acetaminophen Drops
Disp. 15 mL
Sig. 0.6 mL t.i.d.

*(a)* If acetaminophen drops contain 25 gr of acetaminophen per 15-mL container, how many milligrams are there in each prescribed dose?

*(b)* If the dropper calibrates 20 drops per mL, how many drops should be administered per dose?

33. ℞ Potassium Thiocyanate
Aromatic Elixir aa qs
Make a solution to contain 0.2 g/tsp
Disp. 180 mL
Sig. 5 mL in water daily.

How many grams of potassium thiocyanate should be used in compounding the prescription?

34. ℞ Dihydrocodeinone gr $\frac{1}{12}$/tsp
Hydriodic Acid Syrup
Cherry Syrup aa f℥iii
Sig. Tsp. every 2 hr. for cough.

How many grains of dihydrocodeinone should be used in compounding the prescription?

35. The dose of a drug is 500 μg per kg of body weight. How many milligrams should be given to a child weighing 55 lb?

36. The usual dosage range of dimercaprol is 2.5 to 5 mg per kg of body weight. What would be the dosage range, in grams, for a person weighing 165 lb?

37. ℞ Erythromycin Estolate 400 mg/5 mL
Disp. 100 mL
Sig. ______tsp. q.i.d. until all medication is taken.

If the dose of erythromycin estolate is given as 40 mg per kg per day, *(a)* what would be the proper dose of the medication in the *Signa* if the prescription is for a 44 lb child, and *(b)* how many days will the medication last?

38. An intravenous infusion contains 1 g of carbenicillin in each 20 mL. How many milliliters of the infusion should be administered daily to a 154 lb patient if the dose of carbenicillin is 200 mg per kg per day?

39. The adult dose of a liquid medication is 0.1 mL per kg of body weight to be administered as a single dose. How many teaspoonfuls should be administered to a person weighing 220 lb?

40. A physician orders 2 mg of ampicillin to be added to each milliliter of a 250-mL bottle of 5% dextrose in water ($D_5W$) for intravenous infusion. *(a)* How many mg of ampicillin should be added? *(b)* If the 250 mL of solution represents a single dose and if the dose of ampicillin is 25 mg per kg of body weight, how many pounds does the patient weigh?

41. ℞ Piperazine Syrup 500 mg/5 mL
Disp. ______mL
Sig. Parents: Take ______teaspoonfuls daily for 2 days.
Child: Take ______teaspoonfuls daily for 2 days.

The dose of piperazine for adults is 3.5 g as a single daily dose for two consecutive days. For children, the dose is 75 mg per kg of body weight per day for two consecutive days. If both parents and a 66 lb child are to take the medication as directed, *(a)* how many milliliters of piperazine syrup should be dispensed, and *(b)* how many teaspoonfuls each should the parents and the child take daily?

42. A physician desires a dose of 40 μg per kg of digoxin for an eight-pound newborn child. How many milliliters of an injection containing 0.25 mg of digoxin per mL should be given?

43. The dose of gentamicin sulfate is 1.7 mg per kg of body weight. How many milliliters of an injectable solution containing the equivalent of 40 mg of gentamicin per mL should be administered to a person weighing 198 lb?

44. The usual intramuscular dose of kanamycin sulfate is the equivalent of 7.5 mg of kanamycin per kg of body weight. How many milliliters

of kanamycin sulfate injection containing the equivalent of 250 mg of kanamycin per mL should be given to a person weighing 176 lb?

45. The dose of pyrvinium pamoate is 5 mg per kg of body weight as a single dose. How many tablets, each containing 50 mg of pyrvinium pamoate, should be dispensed for a person weighing 110 lb to provide an initial dose and a second dose in 2 weeks?

46. How many chloramphenicol capsules, each containing 250 mg of chloramphenicol, are needed to provide 25 mg per kg of body weight per day for 1 week for a person weighing 154 lb?

47. A child weighing 25 lb is to receive 4 mg of phenytoin per kg of body weight daily as an anticonvulsant. How many milliliters of pediatric phenytoin suspension containing 30 mg per 5 mL should the child receive?

48. If the usual dose of a drug is 325 mg, what is the dose, in milligrams, for a child 6 years old? Use Young's Rule to calculate the dose.

49. If the usual adult dose of paregoric is 5 mL, what is the dose, in milliliters, for a child 4 years old. Use Young's Rule to calculate the dose.

50. The usual adult dose of atropine sulfate is 0.5 mg. Using Young's Rule calculate the dose, in micrograms, for a child 8 years old.

51. The usual adult dose of scopolamine hydrobromide is 0.6 mg. Using Clark's Rule calculate the dose, in micrograms, for a child weighing 45 lb.

52. What is the body surface area (BSA) for a child weighing 20 kg and measuring 80 cm in height?

53. What is the body surface area for an adult measuring 5′10″ in height and weighing 176 lb?

54. If the adult dose of a drug is 100 mg, what would be the dose for a child with a body surface area of 0.70 square meters?

55. If the adult dose of a drug is 25 mg, what would be the dose for a child weighing 40 lb and measuring 32 in. in height? Use the body surface area method.

56. The daily dose of diphenhydramine hydrochloride for a child may be determined on the basis of 5 mg per kg of body weight or on the basis of 150 mg per $m^2$. Calculate the dose on each basis for a child weighing 55 lb and measuring 40 in. in height?

57. If the dose of a drug is 10 mg per $m^2$ per day, what would be the daily dose, in milligrams, for a child weighing 30 lb and measuring 26 in. in height?

58. The dose of mitocin injection is 20 mg per $m^2$ per day. Using the nomogram on p. 93, determine the daily dose for a patient who weighs 144 lb and measures 68 in. in height.

59. The usual pediatric dose of a drug is 300 mg per square meter. Using the nomogram, calculate the dose for a child weighing 20 kg and measuring 90 cm in height.

60. A medication order calls for tobramycin sulfate, 1 mg per kg of body weight, to be administered by IM injection to a patient weighing 220 pounds. Tobramycin sulfate is available in a vial containing 80 mg per 2 mL. How many milliliters of the injection should the patient receive?

61. The usual pediatric dose of cefazolin sodium is 25 mg/kg/day divided equally into three doses. What would be the single dose, in milligrams, for a child weighing 33 pounds?

62. A medication order calls for 6 μg/kg of body weight of pentagastrin to be administered subcutaneously to a patient weighing 154 pounds. The source of the drug is an ampul containing 0.5 mg in each 2 mL of the solution. How many milliliters of the solution should be injected?

63. If the loading dose of kanamycin is 7 mg/kg of body weight, how many grams should be administered to a patient weighing 165 lb?

64. How many grams of fluorouracil will a 154-lb patient receive in five (5) successive days at a dosage rate of 12 mg/kg/day?

65. A beclomethasone diproprionate inhaler contains 10 mg of active ingredient and delivers 200 doses. How many micrograms of beclomethasone diproprionate are delivered per dose?

# 7

# Reducing and Enlarging Formulas

Pharmacists may have to reduce or enlarge formulas for pharmaceutical preparations in the course of their professional practice or manufacturing activities. Official formulas and most other formulas for manufacturing are based on the preparation of 1000 mL or 1000 g of product. The pharmacist may be called upon to make either a smaller or greater quantity and thus must reduce or enlarge the formula while maintaining the correct proportion of each ingredient.

When a formula specifies a *total amount,* we may determine how much of each ingredient is needed to obtain a desired total amount by this proportion:

$$\frac{\text{Total amount specified in formula}}{\text{Total amount desired}} = \frac{\text{Quantity of each ingredient in formula}}{x}$$

$x$ = Quantity of each ingredient in amount desired

Although all problems specifying a total amount may be solved by this proportion, it is usually more convenient—particularly if the quantities are given in the metric system—to solve them by the use of short cuts. Thus, given a formula for 1000 mL or 1000 g, we may divide or multiply the quantity of each ingredient by a power of 10 simply by moving the decimal point to the left or right the required number of places. Or, given a formula for the same amounts, we may reduce or enlarge it by using factors. For example, if we wish to prepare 1 gallon (3785 mL) of a formula whose specified total amount is 1000 mL, we would multiply the quantity of each ingredient by the factor 3.785. And, if we were to prepare 50 g of a formula whose specified total amount is 1000 g, we would multiply the quantity of each ingredient by $\frac{1}{20}$ (since 50 g is $\frac{1}{20}$ of 1000 g).

Some formulas, however, do not specify a total amount, instead indicating relative quantities of ingredients or *proportional parts* to be used in obtaining any desired total amount. Such problems may be solved by this proportion:

$$\frac{\text{Total number of parts in formula}}{\text{Number of parts of each ingredient}} = \frac{\text{Total amount desired}}{x}$$

x = Quantity of each ingredient in amount desired

In solving problems that involve reducing and enlarging formulas, these facts should be noted:

(1) To make a valid ratio, the total amounts compared must be expressed in a common denomination, whether in grams, fluidounces, pounds, or anything else. Consequently, if they are unlike to start with, one or the other must be reduced or converted. If, for example, the formula is given in the metric system and the required quantity is in the common system, it is generally best to convert the required quantity into the metric system. The answers may then be converted into weighable or measurable denominations in the common system or, if this is not indicated, the results may be left in the metric system.

(2) Since the quantity of each ingredient is calculated separately, it does not matter if the formula includes an assortment of terms (pounds and fluidounces, grams and milliliters, and so on).

## FORMULAS THAT SPECIFY AMOUNTS OF INGREDIENTS

**To calculate the quantities of ingredients to be used when reducing or enlarging a formula for a specified total amount:**

*Examples:*

*From the following formula, calculate the quantity of each ingredient required to make 240 mL of Calamine Lotion.*

| | |
|---|---|
| Calamine | 80 g |
| Zinc Oxide | 80 g |
| Glycerin | 20 mL |
| Bentonite Magma | 250 mL |
| Calcium Hydroxide Topical Solution, to make | 1000 mL |

Using the factor 0.24 (since 240 mL is 0.24 × 1000 mL), the quantity of each ingredient is calculated as follows:

| | | |
|---|---|---|
| Calamine | = 80 × 0.24 = | 19.2 g |
| Zinc Oxide | = 80 × 0.24 = | 19.2 g |
| Glycerin | = 20 × 0.24 = | 4.8 mL |
| Bentonite Magma | = 250 × 0.24 = | 60 mL |
| Calcium Hydroxide Topical Solution, to make | | 240 mL, *answers.* |

If, in this problem, the required amount were *60 mL*, we should *move the decimal point one place to the left and multiply by 0.6*. Or, if the required amount were *50 mL*, we would either *divide by 20* or *move the decimal point one place to the left and divide by 2*. And, if the required amount were *125 mL*, we should *multiply by the fraction* ⅛ (since 125 mL is ⅛ of 1000 mL).

*From the following formula, calculate the quantity of each ingredient required to make 1 gallon of Compound Benzoin Tincture.*

| | |
|---|---|
| Benzoin | 100 g |
| Aloe | 20 g |
| Storax | 80 g |
| Tolu Balsam | 40 g |
| Alcohol, to make | 1000 mL |

Using the factor 3.785, the quantity of each ingredient is calculated as follows:

| | | |
|---|---|---|
| Benzoin | = 100 × 3.785 = | 378.5 g |
| Aloe | = 20 × 3.785 = | 75.7 g |
| Storax | = 80 × 3.785 = | 302.8 g |
| Tolu Balsam | = 40 × 3.785 = | 151.4 g |
| Alcohol, to make | | 3785 mL or 1 gal, *answers.* |

*From the following formula, calculate the quantity of each ingredient required to make 1 lb (avoir.) of the ointment.*

| | |
|---|---|
| Coal Tar | 50 g |
| Starch | 250 g |
| Zinc Oxide | 150 g |
| Petrolatum | 550 g |

Since the formula is for 1000 g, and using the factor 0.454, the quantity of each ingredient is calculated as follows:

| | | | | |
|---|---|---|---|---|
| Coal Tar | = | 50 × 0.454 | = | 22.7 g |
| Starch | = | 250 × 0.454 | = | 113.5 g |
| Zinc Oxide | = | 150 × 0.454 | = | 68.1 g |
| Petrolatum | = | 550 × 0.454 | = | 249.7 g |
| | | | | 454.0 g |
| | | | | or 1 lb, *answers.* |

*From the following formula for 100 capsules, calculate the quantity of each ingredient required to make 24 capsules.*

| | |
|---|---|
| Belladonna Extract | 1.0 g |
| Ephedrine Sulfate | 1.6 g |
| Phenobarbital | 2.0 g |
| Aspirin | 32.0 g |

Using the factor 0.24 (since 24 capsules are represented by 0.24 × 100), the quantity of each ingredient is calculated as follows:

| | | | | |
|---|---|---|---|---|
| Belladonna Extract | = | 1.0 × 0.24 | = | 0.24 g |
| Ephedrine Sulfate | = | 1.6 × 0.24 | = | 0.384 g |
| Phenobarbital | = | 2.0 × 0.24 | = | 0.48 g |
| Aspirin | = | 32.0 × 0.24 | = | 7.68 g, |
| | | | | *answers.* |

## FORMULAS THAT SPECIFY PROPORTIONAL PARTS

**To calculate the quantities of ingredients required to prepare a desired amount of a formula when it specifies proportional parts:**

If a formula gives us quantities in terms of *proportional parts,* these facts should be noted:

(1) When parts by weight are specified, we can convert only to weights and not to volumes, whereas when parts by volume are specified, we can convert only to volumes.

(2) Just as the formula measures all quantities in a common denomination (namely, in terms of parts), so will our calculations result in a single denomination, and this will be the denomination we select at the outset for measuring the desired total amount.

*Examples:*

*From the following formula, calculate the quantity of each ingredient required to make 1000 g of the ointment.*

| | |
|---|---|
| Coal Tar | 5 parts |
| Zinc Oxide | 10 parts |
| Hydrophilic Ointment | 50 parts |

Total number of parts (by weight) = 65

1000 g will contain 65 parts

$$\frac{65\ \text{(parts)}}{5\ \text{(parts)}} = \frac{1000\ \text{(g)}}{x\ \text{(g)}}$$

x = 76.92 g of Coal Tar,

and

$$\frac{65\ \text{(parts)}}{10\ \text{(parts)}} = \frac{1000\ \text{(g)}}{y\ \text{(g)}}$$

y = 153.85 g of Zinc Oxide,

and

$$\frac{65\ \text{(parts)}}{50\ \text{(parts)}} = \frac{1000\ \text{(g)}}{z\ \text{(g)}}$$

z = 769.23 g of Hydrophilic Ointment, *answers.*

(Check total: 1000 g)

*From the same formula, calculate the quantity of each ingredient required to make ℥i of the ointment.*

Total number of parts (by weight) = 65

℥i or 480 grains will contain 65 parts

$$\frac{65\ \text{(parts)}}{5\ \text{(parts)}} = \frac{480\ \text{(gr)}}{x\ \text{(gr)}}$$

x = 36.9 gr of Coal Tar,

and

$$\frac{65\ \text{(parts)}}{10\ \text{(parts)}} = \frac{480\ \text{(gr)}}{y\ \text{(gr)}}$$

y = 73.9 gr of Zinc Oxide,

and

$$\frac{65\text{ (parts)}}{50\text{ (parts)}} = \frac{480\text{ (gr)}}{z\text{ (gr)}}$$

$z = 369.2$ gr of Hydrophilic Ointment, *answers.*

(Check total: 480 gr or ℥i)

*From the following formula, calculate the quantity of each ingredient required to make 5 lb (avoir.) of the powder.*

| | |
|---|---|
| Bismuth Subcarbonate | 8 parts |
| Kaolin | 15 parts |
| Magnesium Oxide | 2 parts |

Total number of parts (by weight) = 25 parts

5 lb (454 g × 5) or 2270 g will contain 25 parts

$$\frac{25\text{ (parts)}}{8\text{ (parts)}} = \frac{2270\text{ (g)}}{x\text{ (g)}}$$

$x = 726.4$ g of Bismuth Subcarbonate,

and

$$\frac{25\text{ (parts)}}{15\text{ (parts)}} = \frac{2270\text{ (g)}}{y\text{ (g)}}$$

$y = 1362$ g of Kaolin,

and

$$\frac{25\text{ (parts)}}{2\text{ (parts)}} = \frac{2270\text{ (g)}}{z\text{ (g)}}$$

$z = 181.6$ g of Magnesium Oxide, *answers.*

(Check total: 2270 g)

**To calculate the quantities of ingredients in a desired amount when proportional parts may be reckoned from the formula:**

If the ingredients are all measured by weight, or all by volume, we may consider the sum of the weights (or volumes) when expressed in a common denomination as specifying a total number of parts.

*Example:*

*From the following formula, calculate the quantity of each ingredient required to make 500 g of the powder.*

| | |
|---|---|
| Boric Acid | 5 g |
| Starch | 20 g |
| Talc | 50 g |

Total number of parts (by weight) = 75

500 g will contain 75 parts

$$\frac{75 \text{ (parts)}}{5 \text{ (parts)}} = \frac{500 \text{ (g)}}{x \text{ (g)}}$$

x = 33.3 g of Boric Acid,

and

$$\frac{75 \text{ (parts)}}{20 \text{ (parts)}} = \frac{500 \text{ (g)}}{y \text{ (g)}}$$

y = 133.3 g of Starch,

and

$$\frac{75 \text{ (parts)}}{50 \text{ (parts)}} = \frac{500 \text{ (g)}}{z \text{ (g)}}$$

z = 333.3 g of Talc, *answers.*

(Check total: 500 g)

### Practice Problems

1. From the following formula, calculate the quantities required to make 180 mL of benzyl benzoate lotion.

| | |
|---|---|
| Benzyl Benzoate | 250 mL |
| Triethanolamine | 5 g |
| Oleic Acid | 20 g |
| Purified Water, to make | 1000 mL |

2. From the following formula, calculate the quantities required to make 5 gallons of a phenobarbital elixir.

| | | |
|---|---|---|
| Phenobarbital | 4 | g |
| Orange Oil | 0.25 | mL |
| Certified Red Color | | q.s. |
| Alcohol | 200 | mL |
| Propylene Glycol | 100 | mL |
| Sorbitol Solution | 600 | mL |
| Water, to make | 1000 | mL |

3. From the following formula, calculate the quantities required to make 5 lb (avoir.) of hydrophilic ointment.

| | | |
|---|---|---|
| Methylparaben | 0.25 | g |
| Propylparaben | 0.15 | g |
| Sodium Lauryl Sulfate | 10 | g |
| Propylene Glycol | 120 | g |
| Stearyl Alcohol | 250 | g |
| White Petrolatum | 250 | g |
| Purified Water, to make | 1000 | g |

4. From the following formula, calculate the quantities required to prepare 1 gallon of an antihistamine elixir.

| | | |
|---|---|---|
| Chlorpheniramine Maleate | 0.4 | g |
| Benzaldehyde | 0.1 | mL |
| Vanillin | 0.2 | g |
| Certified Red Color | | q.s. |
| Alcohol | 100 | mL |
| Sorbitol Solution | 450 | mL |
| Water, to make | 1000 | mL |

5. From the following formula, calculate the amount, in grams, of each ingredient required to make 1 lb (avoir.) of cold cream.

| | | |
|---|---|---|
| Cetyl Esters Wax | 12.5 | parts |
| White Wax | 12.0 | parts |
| Mineral Oil | 56.0 | parts |
| Sodium Borate | 0.5 | parts |
| Water | 19.0 | parts |

6. From the following formula for 100 capsules, calculate the quantity of each ingredient required to prepare 36 capsules.

| | | |
|---|---|---|
| Codeine Phosphate | 1.6 | g |
| Acetophenetidin | 4.0 | g |
| Acetylsalicylic Acid | 16.0 | g |
| Atropine Sulfate | 0.025 | g |

7. From the following formula, calculate the quantity of each ingredient present in 8 f℥ of the antacid suspension.

| | | |
|---|---|---|
| Aluminum Hydroxide Compressed Gel | 362.8 | g |
| Sorbitol Solution | 282 | mL |
| Syrup | 93 | mL |
| Glycerin | 25 | mL |
| Methylparaben | 0.9 | g |
| Propylparaben | 0.3 | g |
| Flavor | | q.s. |
| Water, to make | 1000 | mL |

8. From the following formula, calculate the quantity of each ingredient required to make 1500 g of the powder.

| | |
|---|---|
| Calcium Carbonate | 5 parts |
| Magnesium Oxide | 1 part |
| Sodium Bicarbonate | 4 parts |
| Bismuth Subcarbonate | 3 parts |

9. From the following formula, calculate the number of grams of each ingredient required to make 1000 g of the ointment.

| | |
|---|---|
| Salicylic Acid | 0.5 part |
| Precipitated Sulfur | 4.5 parts |
| Hydrophilic Ointment | 35.0 parts |

10. From the following formula, calculate the quantity of each ingredient required to make 1 lb (avoir.) of the ointment.

| | | |
|---|---|---|
| Vioform Powder | | 0.2 g |
| Hydrocortisone Powder | | 0.6 g |
| Cold Cream | ad | 20. g |

11. From the following formula, calculate the quantity of each ingredient required to make 4 liters of the lotion.

| | |
|---|---|
| Witch Hazel | 4 parts (by volume) |
| Glycerin | 1 part " " |
| Boric Acid Solution | 15 parts " " |

12. From the following formula, calculate the quantity of each ingredient required to prepare 5 lb (avoir.) of the ointment.

| | |
|---|---|
| Benzoic Acid | 6 parts |
| Salicylic Acid | 3 parts |
| Polyethylene Glycol Ointment | 91 parts |

13. From the following formula, calculate the quantity of each ingredient required to make 1 pint of the hematinic syrup.

| | |
|---|---|
| Cyanocobalamin | 400 μg |
| Ascorbic Acid | 20 g |
| Ferrous Gluconate | 17 g |
| Sodium Citrate | 100 g |
| Flavor | q.s. |
| Sorbitol Solution, to make | 1000 mL |

14. From the following formula, calculate the quantity of each ingredient required to prepare 1 gallon of the lotion.

| | | |
|---|---|---|
| Calamine | | 8 g |
| Starch | | 20 g |
| Glycerin | | 10 mL |
| Isopropyl Alcohol 70% | | 30 mL |
| Purified Water | ad | 100 mL |

15. From the following formula, calculate the quantity of each ingredient required to prepare 5 pints of the solution.

| | |
|---|---|
| Resorcinol Monoacetate | 50 mL |
| Castor Oil | 25 mL |
| Chloral Hydrate | 75 g |
| Isopropyl Alcohol, to make | 1000 mL |

16. From the following formula, calculate the quantity of each ingredient required to prepare 1 lb (avoir.) of the ointment base.

| | |
|---|---|
| Cetyl Alcohol | 225 g |
| White Wax | 15 g |
| Glycerin | 150 g |
| Sodium Lauryl Sulfate | 30 g |
| Water | 1080 g |

17. From the following U.S.P. formula for Cherry Syrup, calculate the quantity of each ingredient needed to prepare 120 mL of the syrup.

| | |
|---|---|
| Cherry Juice | 475 mL |
| Sucrose | 800 g |
| Alcohol | 20 mL |
| Purified Water, to make | 1000 mL |

18. How much of each ingredient is required to prepare one thousand APC Capsules each containing the following?

| | |
|---|---|
| Acetylsalicylic Acid | 250 mg |
| Phenacetin | 120 mg |
| Caffeine | 30 mg |

19. From the following formula for a corn removal product, calculate the quantity of each ingredient in a pint of the product.

| | |
|---|---|
| Salicylic Acid | 2.0 g |
| Alcohol | 3.0 mL |
| Ether, to make | 15.0 mL |

20. From the following formula, calculate the quantity of each ingredient required to prepare 10 pints of the lotion.

| | |
|---|---|
| Hexachlorophene | 0.1 g |
| Cetyl Alcohol | 0.5 g |
| Isopropyl Alcohol | 70.0 g |
| Purified Water, to make | 100.0 mL |

21. An antihypertensive tablet contains the following medicinal agents. How many grams of each ingredient are required to prepare 5000 tablets?

| | |
|---|---|
| Reserpine | 100 μg |
| Hydralazine Hydrochloride | 25 mg |
| Hydrochlorothiazide | 15 mg |

22. A formula for 30 suppositories contains the following:

| | |
|---|---|
| Bismuth Subgallate | 6.0 g |
| Peruvian Balsam | 2.5 g |
| Zinc Oxide | 4.5 g |
| Cocoa Butter | 50.0 g |

How much of each ingredient should be used to prepare 144 suppositories?

23. From the following formula for an antacid tablet, calculate the quantity of each ingredient required to prepare a batch of 5 M tablets.

| | |
|---|---|
| Magnesium Trisilicate | 500 mg |
| Aluminum Hydroxide Dried Gel | 250 mg |
| Mannitol | 300 mg |
| Magnesium Stearate | 10 mg |
| Starch | 10 mg |
| Flavor | q.s. |

24. From the following formula, calculate the quantity of each ingredient required to prepare two 5-lb (avoir.) containers of Zinc Gelatin.

| | |
|---|---|
| Zinc Oxide | 100 g |
| Gelatin | 150 g |
| Glycerin | 400 g |
| Purified Water | 350 mL |

25. From the following formula, calculate the quantity of each ingredient required to prepare five 1-pint containers of acetaminophen syrup.

| | |
|---|---|
| Acetaminophen | 24 g |
| Benzoic Acid | 1 g |
| Disodium Calcium EDTA | 1 g |
| Propylene Glycol | 150 mL |
| Alcohol | 150 mL |
| Soluble Saccharin | 1.8 g |
| Water | 200 mL |
| Flavor | q.s. |
| Sorbitol Solution, to make | 1000 mL |

26. Each 5 mL of a pediatric cough syrup is to contain the following amounts of medication. Calculate the amount of each ingredient needed to prepare a pint of the syrup.

| | |
|---|---|
| Dextromethorphan Hydrobromide | 7.5 mg |
| Phenylpropanolamine Hydrochloride | 9.0 mg |
| Guaifenesin | 100.0 mg |
| Flavored Syrup, to make | 5.0 mL |

27. A nasal inhaler contains 250 mg of propylhexedrine and 12.5 mg of menthol. How much of each ingredient would be used in preparing 5,000 inhalers?

28. From the following formula for a typical chewable antacid tablet, calculate the amount of each ingredient needed to manufacture 50,000 tablets.

| | |
|---|---|
| Aluminum Hydroxide | 325 mg |
| Mannitol | 812 mg |
| Sodium Saccharin | 0.4 mg |
| Sorbitol (10% solution) | 32.5 mg |
| Magnesium Stearate | 35 mg |
| Mint Flavor Concentrate | 4 mg |

# 8

# Density, Specific Gravity, and Specific Volume

The relative weights of equal volumes of substances are shown by their densities and their specific gravities.

## DENSITY

*Density* is mass per unit volume of a substance, *e.g.*, the number of grams per cubic centimeter or milliliter, or the number of grains per fluidounce, or the number of pounds per gallon, and so on. It is *usually* expressed as *g per cc*. Since the *gram* is defined as the mass of 1 cc of water at 4°C, the density of water is *1 g per cc*. Since the *Pharmacopeia* states that 1 mL may be used as the equivalent of 1 cc, for our purposes the density of water may be expressed as *1 g per mL*. One (1) mL of mercury, on the other hand, weighs 13.6 g, hence its density is *13.6 g per mL*.

Density may be calculated by dividing mass by volume. Thus, if 10 mL of sulfuric acid weigh 18 g, its density is:

$$\frac{18\ (\text{g})}{10\ (\text{mL})} = 1.8\ g\ per\ mL$$

## SPECIFIC GRAVITY

*Specific gravity* is a ratio, *expressed decimally*, of the weight of a substance to the weight of an equal volume of a substance chosen as a standard, both substances having the same temperature or the temperature of each being definitely known. Water is used as the standard for the specific gravities of liquids and solids; the most useful standard for gases—which have little or no pharmaceutical significance—is hydrogen (although sometimes air is used).

Specific gravity may be calculated by dividing the weight of a given substance by the weight of an equal volume of water. Thus, if 10 mL of sulfuric acid weigh 18 g, and 10 mL of water, under similar conditions, weigh 10 g, the specific gravity of the acid is

$$\frac{\text{Weight of 10 mL of sulfuric acid}}{\text{Weight of 10 mL of water}} = \frac{18\ (g)}{10\ (g)} = 1.8$$

Specific gravities can be expressed decimally to as many places as the accuracy of their determination warrants. In pharmaceutical work this may be two, three, or four decimal places. Since substances expand or contract at different rates when their temperatures change, variations in the specific gravity of a substance must be carefully allowed for in accurate work. In the *United States Pharmacopeia* the standard temperature for specific gravities is 25°C, except for that of alcohol, which is 15.56°C by government regulation.

## DENSITY VS. SPECIFIC GRAVITY

The density of a substance is a concrete number (*1.8 g per mL* in the example), while specific gravity, being a ratio between like quantities, is an abstract number (*1.8* in the example). Whereas density must vary with the table of measure, specific gravity has no dimension and is, therefore, a constant value for each substance (when measured under controlled conditions). Thus, the density of water may be variously expressed as *1 g per mL*, or *455 gr per f℥*, or *62½ lb per cu ft*; but the specific gravity of water is always 1.

The specific gravity of a substance and its density in the metric system are numerically equal (as a result of the definition of the gram), but they are quite different when the density is expressed in the common system.

The factor *455* (rounded off from 454.57 or 454.6 gr, the weight of 1 f℥ of water at 25°C) is useful for calculating the approximate weight of a small volume of water measured in the apothecaries' system. But if *455* is used, the result should be expressed in no more than three significant figures. When quantities greater than a pint are involved, it is usually more convenient to convert them to their metric equivalent before calculating. For a discussion of the derivation of the factor *455*, refer to page 131 under "Percentage Preparations."

## SPECIFIC GRAVITY OF LIQUIDS

**To calculate the specific gravity of a liquid when its weight and volume are known:**

*Examples:*

*If 54.96 mL of an oil weigh 52.78 g, what is the specific gravity of the oil?*

54.96 mL of water weigh 54.96 g

$$\text{Specific gravity of oil} = \frac{52.78 \text{ (g)}}{54.96 \text{ (g)}} = 0.9603, \textit{ answer.}$$

*If a pint of a certain liquid weighs 9250 grains, what is the specific gravity of the liquid?*

1 pint = 16 f℥

16 f℥ of water weigh 7280 grains

$$\text{Specific gravity of liquid} = \frac{9250 \text{ (gr)}}{7280 \text{ (gr)}} = 1.27, \textit{ answer.}$$

**To calculate the specific gravity of a liquid, determined with a specific gravity bottle:**

In the determination of the specific gravity of a liquid by means of a *specific gravity bottle,*[1] the container is filled and weighed first with water and then with the liquid. By subtracting the weight of the empty container from the two weights, we have the *weights of equal volumes*—even though we may not know exactly what the volumes are.

*Example:*

*A specific gravity bottle weighs 23.66 g. When filled with water it weighs 72.95 g; when filled with another liquid it weighs 73.56 g. What is the specific gravity of the liquid?*

73.56 g − 23.66 g = 49.90 g of liquid
72.95 g − 23.66 g = 49.29 g of water

$$\text{Specific gravity of liquid} = \frac{49.90 \text{ (g)}}{49.29 \text{ (g)}} = 1.012, \textit{ answer.}$$

**To calculate the specific gravity of a liquid determined by the displacement or plummet method:**

The basis for the determination of the specific gravity of a liquid by this method is *Archimedes' principle,* which states that a body immersed in a liquid displaces an amount of the liquid equal to its own volume and suffers an apparent loss in weight equal to the weight of the displaced liquid. Thus, we can weigh a plummet when suspended in water and when suspended in a liquid whose specific gravity is to be determined, and by subtracting these weights from the weight of the plummet

[1]A container intended to be used as a specific gravity bottle, with a known capacity (commonly 10, 25, or 100 mL) so that the weight of water it will contain is already known, is called a *pycnometer.*

in air, we get the *weights of equal volumes of the liquids* needed in our calculation.

*Example:*

*A glass plummet weighs 12.64 g in air, 8.57 g when immersed in water, and 9.12 g when immersed in an oil. Calculate the specific gravity of the oil.*

$$12.64 \text{ g} - 9.12 \text{ g} = 3.52 \text{ g of displaced oil}$$
$$12.64 \text{ g} - 8.57 \text{ g} = 4.07 \text{ g of displaced water}$$

$$\text{Specific gravity of oil} = \frac{3.52 \text{ (g)}}{4.07 \text{ (g)}} = 0.865, \textit{ answer.}$$

## SPECIFIC GRAVITY OF SOLIDS

**To calculate the specific gravity of a solid heavier than and insoluble in water:**

The specific gravity of a solid *heavier than* and *insoluble in water* may be calculated simply by dividing the weight of the solid in air by the weight of water that it displaces when immersed in it. The weight of water displaced (apparent loss of weight in water) is equal to the *weight of an equal volume of water.*

*Example:*

*A piece of glass weighs 38.525 g in air and 23.525 g when immersed in water. What is its specific gravity?*

$$38.525 \text{ g} - 23.525 \text{ g} = 15.000 \text{ g of displaced water}$$
*(weight of an equal volume of water)*

$$\text{Specific gravity of glass} = \frac{38.525 \text{ (g)}}{15.000 \text{ (g)}} = 2.568, \textit{ answer.}$$

**To calculate the specific gravity of a solid heavier than and soluble in water:**

*The weights of equal volumes of any two substances are proportional to their specific gravities.* Therefore, given a solid heavier than and soluble in water, we may use the method just discussed, but *substituting some liquid of known specific gravity* in which the solid is insoluble.

*Example:*

*A crystal of a chemical salt weighs 6.423 g in air and 2.873 g when immersed in an oil having a specific gravity of 0.858. What is the specific gravity of the salt?*

$$6.423 \text{ g} - 2.873 \text{ g} = 3.550 \text{ g of displaced oil}$$

$$\frac{3.550 \text{ (g of oil)}}{6.423 \text{ (g of salt)}} = \frac{0.858 \text{ (sp. gr. of oil)}}{x \text{ (sp. gr. of salt)}}$$

$x = 1.55$, *answer.*

**To calculate the specific gravity of a solid lighter than and insoluble in water:**

The determination of the specific gravity of a solid *lighter than* and *insoluble in water* involves the use of a sinker which is attached to the solid in order to prevent it from floating (and therefore, having no apparent weight at all). The weight of the sinker in air is of no interest to us here, but its weight when immersed in water alone must be known so that the combined weight of the solid in air and the sinker in water may be calculated. By subtracting from this weight the weight of solid and sinker when immersed in water, the weight of the water displaced by the solid (and therefore the *weight of an equal volume of water*) is calculated.

*Example:*

*A piece of wax weighs 16.35 g in air, and a sinker weighs 32.84 g immersed in water. When they are fastened together and immersed in water, their combined weight is 29.68 g. Calculate the specific gravity of the wax.*

$32.84 \text{ g} + 16.35 \text{ g} = 49.19 \text{ g}$, combined weight of sinker in water and of wax in air

$49.19 \text{ g} - 29.68 \text{ g} = 19.51 \text{ g}$, weight of water displaced by wax *(weight of equal volume of water)*

$$\text{Specific gravity of wax} = \frac{16.35 \text{ (g)}}{19.51 \text{ (g)}} = 0.838, \textit{ answer.}$$

**To calculate the specific gravity of granulated solids heavier than and insoluble in water:**

A specific gravity bottle can be used with crystals, powders, and other forms of solids whose volume cannot be directly measured. If such a substance is *insoluble in water,* we may weigh a portion of it, introduce this amount into the bottle, fill up the bottle with water, and weigh the mixture. The solid will displace a *volume of water equal to its own volume,* and the weight of this displaced water can be calculated.

*Example:*

*A bottle weighs 50.0 g when empty and 96.8 g when filled with water. If 28.8 g of a granulated metal are placed in the bottle and the bottle is filled with water, the total weight is 118.4 g. What is the specific gravity of the metal?*

96.8 g − 50.0 g = 46.8 g, weight of water filling the bottle

46.8 g + 28.8 g = 75.6 g, combined weight of water and metal

118.4 g − 50.0 g = 68.4 g, combined weight of water and metal in bottle

75.6 g − 68.4 g = 7.2 g, weight of water displaced by metal *(weight of equal volume of water)*

$$\text{Specific gravity of metal} = \frac{28.8\ (\text{g})}{7.2\ (\text{g})} = 4.0, \textit{ answer.}$$

## SPECIFIC VOLUME

The volume of a unit weight of a substance may be expressed in any convenient denominations, such as so-many *cubic feet per lb* or *gallons per lb,* but more frequently as *mL per g.*

*Specific volume,* in pharmaceutical practice, is usually defined as an abstract number representing the ratio, *expressed decimally,* of the volume of a substance to the volume of an equal weight of another substance taken as a standard, both having the same temperature. Water is the standard for liquids and solids.

Whereas specific gravity is a comparison of weights of equal volumes, specific volume is a comparison of volumes of equal weights. Because of this relationship, specific gravity and specific volume are *reciprocals* of each other—that is, if they are multiplied together the product is 1. Specific volume tells us how much greater (or smaller) in volume a mass is than the same weight of water. It may be calculated by dividing the volume of a given mass by the volume of an equal weight of water. Thus, if 25 g of glycerin measure 20 mL and 25 g of water measure 25 mL under the same conditions, the specific volume of the glycerin is

$$\frac{\text{Volume of 25 g of glycerin}}{\text{Volume of 25 g of water}} = \frac{20\ (\text{mL})}{25\ (\text{mL})} = 0.8$$

**To calculate the specific volume of a liquid, given the volume of a specified weight:**

*Example:*

*Calculate the specific volume of a syrup, 91.0 mL of which weigh 107.16 g.*

107.16 g of water measure 107.16 mL

$$\text{Specific volume of syrup} = \frac{91.0\ (\text{mL})}{107.16\ (\text{mL})} = 0.849, \textit{ answer.}$$

**To calculate the specific volume of a liquid, given its specific gravity, and to calculate its specific gravity given its specific volume:**

Since specific gravity and specific volume are reciprocals of each other, a substance that is heavier than water will have a higher specific gravity and a lower specific volume, whereas a substance that is lighter than water will have a lower specific gravity and a higher specific volume. It follows, therefore, that we may determine the specific volume of a substance by dividing 1 by its specific gravity; and we may determine the specific gravity of a substance by dividing 1 by its specific volume.

*Examples:*

*What is the specific volume of phosphoric acid having a specific gravity of 1.71?*

$$\frac{1}{1.71} = 0.585, \textit{ answer.}$$

*If a liquid has a specific volume of 1.396, what is its specific gravity?*

$$\frac{1}{1.396} = 0.716, \textit{ answer.}$$

### Practice Problems

1. If 250 mL of alcohol weight 203 g, what is its density?

2. A piece of copper metal weighs 53.6 g, and has a volume of 6 mL. Calculate its density.

3. A 30-mL sample of sulfuric acid weighs 55 g. Calculate its density.

4. If 150 mL of polyethylene glycol 400 weigh 170 g, what is its specific gravity?

5. If a liter of sorbitol solution weighs 1285 g, what is its specific gravity?

6. If 500 mL of ferric chloride solution weigh 650 g, what is its specific gravity?

7. If 380 g of cottonseed oil measure 415 mL, what is its specific gravity?

8. If 2 f℥ of glycerin weigh 1140 grains, what is its specific gravity?

9. Five pints of hydrochloric acid weigh 2.79 kg. Calculate its specific gravity.

10. A pycnometer weighs 50.0 g. When filled with water, it weighs 100.0 g; when filled with an oil, it weighs 94.0 g. Calculate the specific gravity of the oil.

11. A pycnometer weighs 21.62 g. Filled with water it weighs 46.71 g; filled with another liquid it weighs 43.28 g. Calculate the specific gravity of the liquid.

12. A glass stopper weighs 39.625 g in air, 24.625 g in water, and 28.375 g in ether. What is the specific gravity of the ether?

13. A glass plummet weighs 14.35 g in air, 11.40 g when immersed in water, and 8.95 g when immersed in sulfuric acid. Calculate the specific gravity of the acid.

14. A piece of metal weighs 8.624 g in air and 5.615 g when immersed in water. What is its specific gravity?

15. If a solid weighs 84.62 g in air and 58.48 g when immersed in water, what is its specific gravity?

16. A chemical crystal weighs 3.630 g in air and 1.820 g when immersed in an oil. If the specific gravity of the oil is 0.837, what is the specific gravity of the chemical?

17. A piece of wax weighs 42.65 g in air, and a sinker weighs 38.42 g in water. Together they weigh 33.18 g in water. Calculate the specific gravity of the wax.

18. An insoluble powder weighs 12 g. A specific gravity bottle, weighing 21 g when empty, weighs 121 g when filled with water. When the powder is introduced into the bottle and the bottle is filled with water, the three together weigh 130 g. What is the specific gravity of the powder?

19. If 73.42 g of a liquid measure 81.5 mL, what is its specific volume?

20. If 120 g of acetone measure 150 mL, what is its specific volume?

21. If olive oil has a specific gravity of 0.912, what is its specific volume?

22. The specific gravity of alcohol is 0.815. What is its specific volume?

23. What is the specific volume of sulfuric acid having a specific gravity of 1.826?

24. If chloroform has a specific gravity of 1.476, what is its specific volume?

25. What is the specific gravity of a liquid having a specific volume of 0.825?

# 9

# Weights and Volumes of Liquids

The weights of equal volumes and the volumes of equal weights of liquids are proportional to their specific gravities. To calculate, therefore, the *weight of a given volume* or the *volume of a given weight* of a liquid, its specific gravity must be known.

When *specific gravity is used as a factor in a calculation, the result should contain no more significant figures than the number in the factor.*

Because of the simple relationship between the units in the metric system, such problems are simply and easily solved when only metric quantities are involved, but they become more complex when units of the common systems are used.

## CALCULATIONS OF WEIGHT

**To calculate the weight of a liquid when given its volume and specific gravity:**

The *weight of any given volume* of a liquid of known specific gravity can be calculated by this proportion:

$$\frac{\text{Specific gravity of water}}{\text{Specific gravity of liquid}} = \frac{\text{Weight of equal volume of water}}{x}$$

$$x = \text{Weight of liquid}$$

And from this we may derive a useful equation:

$$\text{Weight of liquid} = \text{Weight of equal volume of water} \times \text{Specific gravity of liquid}$$

*Examples:*

*What is the weight of 3620 mL of alcohol having a specific gravity of 0.820?*

3620 mL of water weigh 3620 g

3620 g × 0.820 = 2968 g, *answer.*

*What is the weight of 4 f℥ of paraldehyde having a specific gravity of 0.990?*

4 f℥ of water weigh 455 gr × 4 or 1820 gr

1820 gr × 0.990 = 1802 gr, or (retaining only significant figures) 1800 gr, *answer.*

*What is the weight, in grams, of 2 f℥ of a liquid having a specific gravity of 1.118?*

In this type of problem it is generally best to convert the given volume to its metric equivalent first and then to solve the problem in the metric system.

2 × 29.57 mL = 59.14 mL

59.14 mL of water weigh 59.14 g

59.14 g × 1.118 = 66.12 g, *answer.*

*What is the weight, in grains, of 50 mL of ether having a specific gravity of 0.715?*

In problems of this type it is generally best to solve the problem in the metric system and then to convert the weight to the common system.

50 mL of water weigh 50 g

50 g × 0.715 = 35.75 g = 551 gr, *answer.*

## CALCULATIONS OF VOLUME

**To calculate the volume of a liquid when given its weight and specific gravity:**

The *volume of any given weight* of a liquid of known specific gravity can be calculated by this proportion:

$$\frac{\text{Specific gravity of liquid}}{\text{Specific gravity of water}} = \frac{\text{Volume of equal weight of water}}{x}$$

$x$ = Volume of liquid

And the derived equation will be:

$$\text{Volume of liquid} = \frac{\text{Volume of equal weight of water}}{\text{Specific gravity of liquid}}$$

*Examples:*

*What is the volume of 492 g of nitric acid with a specific gravity of 1.40?*

492 g of water measure 492 mL

$$\frac{492 \text{ mL}}{1.40} = 351 \text{ mL, } \textit{answer.}$$

*What is the volume, in minims, of 1 oz of a perfume oil having a specific gravity of 0.850?*

1 oz = 437.5 gr

437.5 gr of water measure $\frac{437.5}{455}$ f℥ or 462 ♏

$$\frac{462 \text{ ♏}}{0.850} = 544 \text{ or } 540 \text{ ♏, } \textit{answer.}$$

Or:

1 oz = 28.35 g

28.35 g of water measure 28.35 mL

$$\frac{28.35 \text{ mL}}{0.850} = 33.25 \text{ mL} = 541 \text{ or } 540 \text{ ♏, } \textit{answer.}$$

*What is the volume, in f℥, of 1 lb of methyl salicylate with a specific gravity of 1.185?*

1 lb = 454 g

454 g of water measure 454 mL

$$\frac{454 \text{ mL}}{1.185} = 383.1 \text{ mL} = 12.96 \text{ f℥, or (with 3-figure accuracy),}$$

13.0 f℥, *answer.*

*What is the volume, in pints, of 50 lb of glycerin having a specific gravity of 1.25?*

50 lb = 454 × 50 = 22700 g

22700 g of water measure 22700 mL

$$\frac{22700 \text{ mL}}{1.25} = 18160 \text{ mL} = 38.4 \text{ pints, } \textit{answer.}$$

**To calculate the cost of a given volume of a liquid bought by weight:**

*Examples:*

*What is the cost of 1000 mL of glycerin, specific gravity 1.25, bought at $2.00 per lb?*

1000 mL of water weigh 1000 g

Weight of 1000 mL of glycerin = 1000 g × 1.25 = 1250 g

1 lb = 454 g

$$\frac{454 \text{ (g)}}{1250 \text{ (g)}} = \frac{(\$)\ 2.00}{(\$)\ x}$$

x = $5.50, *answer.*

*What is the cost of 2 f℥ of cinnamon oil, specific gravity 1.055, bought at $27.00 per ¼ lb?*

2 f℥ = 59.14 mL

59.14 mL of water weigh 59.14 g

Weight of 59.14 mL of oil = 59.14 g × 1.055 = 62.39 g

¼ lb = 113.5 g

$$\frac{113.5 \text{ (g)}}{62.39 \text{ (g)}} = \frac{(\$)\ 27.00}{(\$)\ x}$$

x = $14.84, *answer.*

*What is the cost of 1 pint of chloroform, specific gravity 1.475, bought at $6.25 per lb?*

1 pint = 473 mL

473 mL of water weigh 473 g

Weight of 473 mL of chloroform = 473 g × 1.475 = 697.7 g

1 lb = 454 g

$$\frac{454\ (g)}{697.7\ (g)} = \frac{(\$)\ 6.25}{(\$)\ x}$$

x = $9.60, *answer.*

**Practice Problems**

1. What is the weight of 100 mL of hydrochloric acid having a specific gravity of 1.16?

2. What is the weight of 300 mL of glycerin having a specific gravity of 1.25?

3. What is the weight, in grams, of 14 mL of mercury having a specific gravity of 13.6?

4. What is the weight, in grams, of 225 mL of sulfuric acid having a specific gravity of 1.83?

5. What is the weight, in kilograms, of 5 liters of sulfuric acid with a specific gravity of 1.84?

6. What is the weight of 650 mL of chloroform having a specific gravity of 1.475?

7. If the specific gravity of alcohol is 0.812, what is the weight, in kilograms, of 10 liters?

8. What is the weight, in grains, of 4 f℥ of glycerin having a specific gravity of 1.25?

9. What is the weight, in pounds, of 5 pints of nitric acid having a specific gravity of 1.42?

10. What is the weight, in grams, of 1 pint of chloroform having a specific gravity of 1.475?

11. What is the weight, in grams, of 4 f℥ of orange oil with a specific gravity of 0.844?

12. Calculate the weight, in grams, of 10 pints of hydrochloric acid having a specific gravity of 1.155.

13. What is the weight, in kilograms, of 1 gallon of sorbitol solution having a specific gravity of 1.285?

14. What is the weight, in grams, of 1 pint of a mixture of equal parts of alcohol (specific gravity 0.812) and glycerin (specific gravity 1.25)?

15. What is the weight, in pounds, of 1 gallon of a medicated syrup with a specific gravity of 1.27?

16. What is the weight, in pounds, of 1 liter of glycerin having a specific gravity of 1.25?

17. What is the volume, in milliliters, of 100 g of phosphoric acid having a specific gravity of 1.71?

18. What is the volume, in milliliters, of 1 lb of benzyl benzoate having a specific gravity of 1.120?

19. What is the volume, in milliliters, of 1 kg of sulfuric acid with a specific gravity of 1.83?

20. What is the volume of 1000 g of mercury having a specific gravity of 13.6?

21. A formula calls for 425 g of hydrochloric acid with a specific gravity of 1.155. How many milliliters of the acid should be used?

22. What is the volume of 650 g of ferric chloride solution with a specific gravity of 1.30?

23. A formula for 1000 mL of a preparation calls for 800 g of cottonseed oil with a specific gravity of 0.920. How many milliliters of cottonseed oil should be used in preparing 5 liters of the formula?

24. A formula for a vanishing cream contains 750 g of glycerin. How many milliliters of glycerin (specific gravity 1.25) should be used?

25. What is the volume, in milliliters, of 1 kilogram of peppermint oil with a specific gravity of 0.908?

26. What is the volume, in milliliters, of a liniment containing 1 lb of chloroform (specific gravity 1.475) and 5 lb of methyl salicylate (specific gravity 1.180)?

27. What is the volume, in pints, of 9 lb of sulfuric acid having a specific gravity of 1.83?

28. Calculate the volume, in fluidounces, of 1 lb of an oil with a specific gravity of 0.904?

29. What is the volume, in pints, of 40 lb of a liquid with a specific gravity of 1.32?

30. What is the volume, in pints, of 10 lb of peppermint oil having a specific gravity of 0.904?

31. What is the cost of 10 liters of a liquid (specific gravity 1.20) bought at $4.40 per lb?

32. What is the cost of 3 liters of chloroform (specific gravity 1.475) bought at $6.25 per lb?

33. What will 10 lb of glycerin (specific gravity 1.25) cost at $2.50 per pt?

34. A formula for a mouth rinse contains 1.6 mL of cinnamon oil per 1000 mL. If the cinnamon oil (specific gravity 1.050) is bought at $27.00 per ¼ lb, calculate the cost of the oil required to prepare 5 gallons of the mouth rinse.

35. A perfume oil has a specific gravity of 0.960 and costs $28.75 per kg. What is the cost of 4 f℥?

36. A prescription calls for 0.3 g of phosphoric acid (specific gravity 1.71). How many milliliters should be used in compounding the prescription?

37. A formula for 1000 g of a soft soap contains 380 g of a vegetable oil. If the oil has a specific gravity of 0.890, how many milliliters should be used in preparing 10 lb of the soft soap?

38. A cosmetic formula calls for 500 g of peach kernel oil (specific gravity 0.910) per 1000 g of finished product. How many milliliters of the oil should be used in preparing 5000 g of the formula?

39. A sunscreen lotion contains 5 g of menthyl salicylate (specific gravity 1.045) per 100 mL. How many milliliters of menthyl salicylate should be used in preparing 1 gallon of the lotion?

40. The formula for 1000 g of Polyethylene Glycol Ointment, N.F., calls for 600 g of polyethylene glycol 400. At $3.55 per pint, what is the cost of the polyethylene glycol 400, specific gravity 1.140, needed to prepare 4000 g of the ointment?

41.

| | |
|---|---|
| Stearic Acid | 14.0 g |
| Triethanolamine | 0.7 g |
| Cetyl Alcohol | 3.0 g |
| Sodium Lauryl Sulfate | 0.5 g |
| Propylene Glycol | 5.0 g |
| Distilled Water | 76.8 g |

How many milliliters of triethanolamine (specific gravity 1.125) and how many milliliters of propylene glycol (specific gravity 1.035) should be used in preparing 2500 g of the above formula?

# 10

# Percentage Preparations

## PERCENTAGE

The term *percent* and its corresponding sign (%) mean "by the hundred" or "in a hundred," and *percentage* means "rate per hundred"; so *50 percent* (or 50%) and *a percentage of 50* are equivalent expressions. A percent may also be expressed as a *ratio,* represented as a common or decimal fraction. For example, *50%* means *50 parts in 100* of the same kind, and may be expressed as $\frac{50}{100}$ or *0.50.* Percent, therefore, is simply another fraction of such frequent and familiar use that its numerator is expressed, but its denominator is left understood. It should be noted that percent is always an abstract quantity, and that, as such, it may be applied to anything.

For the purposes of computation, percents are usually changed to equivalent decimal fractions. This is done by dropping the % sign and dividing the expressed numerator by *100.* Thus, *12.5%* $= \frac{12.5}{100}$, or *0.125;* and *0.05%* $= \frac{0.05}{100}$, or *0.0005.* We must not forget that in the reverse process (changing a decimal to a percent) the decimal is multiplied by *100* and the % sign is affixed.

Percentage is an essential part of pharmaceutical calculations. The pharmacist encounters it frequently and uses it as a convenient means of expressing the concentration of a solute in a solution, of the amount of active material in a drug or preparation, or of the quantity of an ingredient in a mixture.

## PERCENTAGE PREPARATIONS

Percentage, as it applies to solutions and liquid preparations (mixtures, lotions, suspensions), expresses *parts per 100 parts.* Obviously, then, in a *true percentage solution* or *liquid preparation* the *parts* of the percentage would represent the *grams* of solute or constituent in *100 g* of solution or liquid preparation. In general practice, however, the pharmacist most frequently encounters a different kind of percentage solution or liquid preparation, one in which the *parts* of the percentage represent *grams* of a solute or constituent in *100 mL* of solution or liquid preparation.

In order to avoid the possibility of any misinterpretation of the meaning of the term "percentage solution or liquid preparation," percentage concentrations are expressed as follows:

*Percent weight-in-volume*—(w/v) expresses the number of *g* of a constituent in *100 mL* of solution or liquid preparation, and is used regardless of whether water or another liquid is the solvent or vehicle.

*Percent volume-in-volume*—(v/v) expresses the number of *mL* of a constituent in *100 mL* of solution or liquid preparation.

*Percent weight-in-weight*—(w/w) expresses the number of *g* of a constituent in *100 g* of solution or mixture.

The term *percent* used without qualification means, for mixtures of solids and semisolids, percent weight-in-weight; for solutions or suspensions of solids in liquids, percent weight-in-volume; for solutions of liquids in liquids, percent volume-in-volume; and for solutions of gases in liquids, percent weight-in-volume. For example, a 1 percent solution is prepared by dissolving 1 g of a solid or 1 mL of a liquid in sufficient of the solvent to make 100 mL of the solution. In the dispensing of prescription medications, slight changes in volume owing to variations in room temperature may be disregarded.

The term *milligrams percent* (mg%) expresses the number of milligrams of a substance in 100 mL of liquid. It is used frequently to denote the concentration of a drug or natural substance in a biological fluid, as in the blood. Thus, the statement that the concentration of nonprotein nitrogen in the blood is 30 mg% means that each 100 mL of blood contains 30 milligrams of nonprotein nitrogen.

For very dilute solutions, it is convenient to express concentrations in terms of *parts per million* (ppm). The term is commonly used in designating test limits, as in the example, the limit of arsenic in zinc oxide is 6 parts per million (6 ppm) or 0.0006%.

## PERCENTAGE WEIGHT-IN-VOLUME

One way of making all weight-in-volume solutions conform to the definition would be to convert all common and apothecaries' weights to grams and all volumes to milliliters before expressing percentage strength. But such a procedure is not required.

For, if 1 gram in 100 milliliters of solution is taken as the only "correct" strength of a 1% (w/v) solution, this means that 1 gram of solute is contained in a volume of solution *that would weigh 100 grams if, like water, the solution had a specific gravity of 1*—if, in other words, each milliliter of solution weighed *1 gram*. Hence, to make a solution of the same strength by any system of measure, we have only to dissolve *1* weight unit of solute in sufficient solvent to make a volume that would weigh *100* of those weight units if the solution were pure water.

A solution so compounded, then, would contain not only *1 g* in every *100 mL* (the volume of *100 g* of water) but likewise approximately *4.55* grains[1] in every fluidounce (the volume of *455 grains* of water at 25°C). Therefore, we may look upon a *weight-in-volume* solution as a kind of *weight-in-weight* solution in disguise: the percentage strength being based after all upon a comparison of parts by weight, but the weight of the solution being arbitrarily calculated from its designated volume as if it has a specific gravity of *1.00*.

**To calculate the weight of the active ingredient in a specified volume of solution or liquid preparation, given its percentage weight-in-volume:**

Taking water to represent any solvent or vehicle, we may prepare weight-in-volume percentage solutions or liquid preparations which are

---

[1]"Disregarding the difference between cubic centimeter and milliliter, which is so small that it does not affect the equivalents used, this quantity was derived as follows:

1 cubic centimeter of water at 4°C. weighs 1 gram
1 fluidounce = 29.573 cubic centimeters
1 gram = 15.4324 grains

Using these equivalents

100 cc. : 29.573 cc. = 1 Gm. : x
x = 0.29573 Gm.
1 Gm. : 0.29573 Gm. = 15.4324 gr. : y
y = 4.5638 grains

"This would be the number of grains of a solid in 1 fluidounce of a 1 percent solution if the liquid were measured at 4°C., but percentage solutions are generally prepared at or near the official temperature of 25°C., and any volume of a liquid weighs slightly less at 25°C. than it does at 4°C. The effect of this is that a theoretical 1% solution, containing 4.5638 grains of a chemical in 1 fluidounce at 4°C., will contain less than this weight in 1 fluidounce if it were prepared at 4°C. and the fluidounce is measured at 25°C. The quantities are approximately proportional to the quantities of water in fluidounces measured at each of the respective temperatures. The correction of this slight difference can be made by the following methods:

1 fluidounce of water weighs 456.38 grains in vacuum at 4°C.
1 fluidounce of water weighs 454.57 grains in air at 25°C.
Using these numbers, we have this proportion:
456.38 : 454.57 = 4.5638 : z
z = 4.5457 grains in 1 fluidounce of a 1 percent solution at 25°C.

In this correction, water is taken to represent any solvent, and the small amount of solvent displaced by the solid is disregarded. This can be done without introducing an appreciable error for any ordinary percentage solution, because the total difference is so small.

The number of grains in one fluidounce of a 1 percent weight-in-volume solution may be rounded off to 4.5, 4.55, or 4.546, to attain different degrees of accuracy in preparing such solutions."

(Quoted from "The Calculation of Percentage Solutions in the U.S.P. XI" by Dr. Theodore J. Bradley, *American Druggist*, July, 1936.)

equivalent in strength when calculated by either the metric or the apothecaries' system if we use the following rules:

*Rule 1.* In the metric system, multiply the required number of milliliters by the percentage strength, expressed as a decimal, to obtain the number of grams of solute or constituent in the solution or liquid preparation. *The volume in milliliters represents the weight in grams of the solution or liquid preparation as if it were pure water.*

Vol. in mL (representing grams) × % (expressed as a decimal) = g of solute or constituent

*Rule 2.* In the apothecaries' system, multiply the *weight* of a fluidounce of water (455 grains) by the required number of fluidounces and by the percentage strength, expressed as a decimal, to obtain the number of grains of solute or constituent in the solution or liquid preparation. *The volume in fluidounces times 455 grains represents the weight in grains of the solution or liquid preparation as if it were pure water.*

Vol. in f℥ × 455 gr × % (expressed as a decimal) = gr of solute or constituent

*Examples:*

*How many grams of dextrose are required to prepare 4000 mL of a 5% solution?*

4000 mL represent 4000 g of solution

5% = 0.05
4000 g × 0.05 = 200 g, *answer.*

*How many grams of potassium permanganate should be used in compounding the following prescription?*

| ℞ | Potassium Permanganate | | 0.02% |
|---|---|---|---|
| | Distilled Water | ad | 250.0 |
| | Sig. As directed. | | |

250 mL represent 250 g of solution

0.02% = 0.0002
250 g × 0.0002 = 0.05 g, *answer.*

*How many grains of aminobenzoic acid should be used in preparing 8 f℥ of a 5% solution in 70% alcohol?*

8 f℥ represent 8 × 455 gr of solution

5% = 0.05
8 × 455 gr × 0.05 = 182 gr, *answer.*

*How many grains of atropine sulfate should be used in compounding the following prescription?*

℞ Atropine Sulfate 2%
Distilled Water q.s. ad ℥iv
Sig. Use in the eye.

$$℥iv = \frac{1}{2}\ f℥$$

$\frac{1}{2}$ f℥ represents $\frac{1}{2} \times 455$ gr of solution

$$2\ \% = 0.02$$

$$\frac{1}{2} \times 455\ \text{gr} \times 0.02 = 4.55\ \text{gr}, \textit{answer}.$$

**To calculate the percentage weight-in-volume of a solution or liquid preparation, given the weight of the solute or constituent and the volume of the solution or liquid preparation:**

It should be remembered that the volume, in milliliters, of the solution represents the weight, in grams, of the solution or liquid preparation as if it were pure water.

*Examples:*

*What is the percentage strength (w/v) of a solution of urea, if 80 mL contain 12 g?*

80 mL of water weigh 80 g

$$\frac{80\ (\text{g})}{12\ (\text{g})} = \frac{100\ (\%)}{x\ (\%)}$$

$x = 15\%$, *answer.*

*What is the percentage strength (w/v) of a solution of boric acid if 45.5 grains are dissolved in enough water to make 8 f℥?*

8 f℥ of water weigh 3640 gr

$$\frac{3640\ (\text{gr})}{45.4\ (\text{gr})} = \frac{100\ (\%)}{x\ (\%)}$$

$x = 1.25\%$, *answer.*

**To calculate the volume of a solution or liquid preparation, given its percentage strength weight-in-volume and the weight of the solute or constituent:**

*Examples:*

*How many milliliters of a 3% solution can be made from 27 g of ephedrine sulfate?*

$$\frac{3\ (\%)}{100\ (\%)} = \frac{27\ (\text{g})}{\text{x}\ (\text{g})}$$

x = 900 g, weight of the solution if it were water

Volume in mL = 900 mL, *answer.*

*How many fluidounces of a 10% solution can be made from 182 grains of silver nitrate?*

$$\frac{10\ (\%)}{100\ (\%)} = \frac{182\ (\text{gr})}{\text{x}\ (\text{gr})}$$

x = 1820 gr, weight of solution if it were water

Volume in f℥ = $^{1820}/_{455}$ f℥ = 4 f℥, *answer.*

## PERCENTAGE VOLUME-IN-VOLUME

Liquids are usually measured by volume, and the percentage strength indicates the number of parts by volume of the active ingredient that are contained in the total volume of the solution or liquid preparation considered as 100 parts by volume. If there is any possibility of misinterpretation, this kind of percentage should be specified: *e.g., 10% (v/v).*

**To calculate the volume of the active ingredient in a specified volume of a solution or liquid preparation, given its percentage strength volume-in-volume:**

*Examples:*

*How many milliliters of liquefied phenol should be used in compounding the following prescription?*

| ℞ | | | |
|---|---|---|---|
| ℞ | Liquefied Phenol | | 2.5% |
| | Calamine Lotion | ad | 240.0 mL |
| | Sig. For external use. | | |

Volume in mL × % (expressed as a decimal) = mL of active ingredient

240 mL × 0.025 = 6 mL, *answer.*

*How many minims of methyl salicylate should be used in compounding the following prescription?*

| | | | |
|---|---|---|---|
| ℞ | Methyl Salicylate | | 5% |
| | Isopropyl Alcohol | ad | f℥iv |
| | Sig. Apply. | | |

Vol. in ♏ × % (expressed as a decimal) = vol. in ♏ of active ingredient

480 ♏ × 4 × 0.05 = 96 ♏, *answer.*

**To calculate the percentage volume-in-volume of a solution or liquid preparation, given the volume of active ingredient and the volume of the solution or liquid preparation:**

The required volumes may have to be calculated from given weights and specific gravities.

*Examples:*

*In preparing 250 mL of a certain lotion, a pharmacist used 4 mL of liquefied phenol. What was the percentage (v/v) of liquefied phenol in the lotion?*

$$\frac{250\ (\text{mL})}{4\ (\text{mL})} = \frac{100\ (\%)}{x\ (\%)}$$

x = 1.6%, *answer.*

*A formula for 8 f℥ of a mouth rinse contains 10 ♏ of a flavoring oil. What is the percentage (v/v) of the oil in the mouth rinse?*

8 f℥ = 3840 ♏

$$\frac{3840\ (♏)}{10\ (♏)} = \frac{100\ (\%)}{x\ (\%)}$$

x = 0.26%, *answer.*

*What is the percentage strength (v/v) of a solution of 800 g of a liquid with a specific gravity of 0.800 in enough water to make 4000 mL?*

800 g of water measure 800 mL

800 mL ÷ 0.800 = 1000 mL of active ingredient

$$\frac{4000\ (\text{mL})}{1000\ (\text{mL})} = \frac{100\ (\%)}{x\ (\%)}$$

x = 25%, *answer.*

**To calculate the volume of a solution or liquid preparation, given the volume of the active ingredient and its percentage strength (v/v):**

The volume of the active ingredient may have to be first calculated from its weight and specific gravity.

*Examples:*

*Peppermint spirit contains 10% (v/v) of peppermint oil. What volume of the spirit will contain 75 mL of peppermint oil?*

$$\frac{10\ (\%)}{100\ (\%)} = \frac{75\ (\text{mL})}{x\ (\text{mL})}$$

x = 750 mL, *answer.*

*Chloroform liniment contains 30% (v/v) of chloroform. How many milliliters of chloroform liniment can be prepared from 1 lb of chloroform (sp. gr. 1.475)?*

1 lb = 454 g

454 g of water measure 454 mL

454 mL ÷ 1.475 = 308 mL of chloroform

$$\frac{30\ (\%)}{100\ (\%)} = \frac{308\ (\text{mL})}{x\ (\text{mL})}$$

x = 1027 or 1030 mL, *answer.*

## PERCENTAGE WEIGHT-IN-WEIGHT

Percentage weight-in-weight (*true percentage* or *percentage by weight)* indicates the number of parts by weight of active ingredient that are contained in the total weight of the solution or mixture considered as 100 parts by weight.

Liquids are not customarily measured by weight, and therefore, a weight-in-weight solution or liquid preparation of a solid or a liquid in a liquid should be so designated: *e.g., 10% (w/w).*

**To calculate the weight of the active ingredient in a specified weight of the solution or liquid preparation, given its weight-in-weight percentage strength:**

*Examples:*

*How many grams of phenol should be used to prepare 240 g of a 5% (w/w) solution in water?*

Weight of solution in g × % (expressed as a decimal) = g of solute

240 g × 0.05 = 12 g, *answer.*

*How many g of a drug substance are required to make 120 mL of a 20% (w/w) solution having a specific gravity of 1.15?*

120 mL of water weigh 120 g

120 g × 1.15 = 138 g, weight of 120 mL of solution

138 g × 0.20 = 27.6 g plus enough water to make 120 mL, *answer.*

**To calculate the weight of either active ingredient or diluent, given the weight of the other and the percentage strength (w/w) of the solution or liquid preparation:**

The weights of active ingredient and diluent are proportional to their percentages.

*Examples:*

*How many grams of a drug substance should be dissolved in 240 mL of water to make a 4% (w/w) solution?*

100% − 4% = 96% (by weight) of water

240 mL of water weigh 240 g

$$\frac{96\ (\%)}{4\ (\%)} = \frac{240\ (g)}{x\ (g)}$$

x = 10 g, *answer.*

It is usually impossible to prepare a specified *volume* of a solution or liquid preparation of given weight-in-weight percentage strength, since the volume displaced by the active ingredient cannot be known in advance. If an excess is not undesirable, we may make a volume somewhat more than that specified by taking the given volume to refer to the solvent or vehicle and from this quantity calculating the weight of the solvent or vehicle (the specific gravity of the solvent or vehicle must be known). Using this weight, we may follow the method above to calculate the corresponding weight of the active ingredient needed.

*Example:*

*How should you prepare 100 mL of a 2% (w/w) solution of a drug substance in a solvent having a specific gravity of 1.25?*

100 mL of water weigh 100 g

100 g × 1.25 = 125 g, weight of 100 mL of solvent

100% − 2% = 98% (by weight) of solvent

$$\frac{98\ (\%)}{2\ (\%)} = \frac{125\ (g)}{x\ (g)}$$

x = 2.55 g

Therefore, dissolve 2.55 g of drug substance in 125 g (or 100 mL) of solvent, *answer.*

**To calculate the percentage strength (w/w) of a solution of liquid preparation, given the weight of the active ingredient and the weight of the solution or liquid preparation:**

If the weight of the finished solution or liquid preparation is not given, other data must be supplied from which it may be calculated: the weights of both ingredients, for instance, or the volume and the specific gravity of the solution or liquid preparation.

*Examples:*

*If 1500 g of a solution contain 75 g of a drug substance, what is the percentage strength (w/w) of the solution?*

$$\frac{1500\ (g)}{75\ (g)} = \frac{100\ (\%)}{x\ (\%)}$$

x = 5%, *answer.*

*If 5 g of boric acid are dissolved in 100 mL of water, what is the percentage strength (w/w) of the solution?*

100 mL of water weigh 100 g

100 g + 5 g = 105 g, weight of solution

$$\frac{105\ (g)}{5\ (g)} = \frac{100\ (\%)}{x\ (\%)}$$

x = 4.76%, *answer.*

*If 1000 mL of syrup with a specific gravity of 1.313 contain 850 g of sucrose, what is its percentage strength (w/w)?*

1000 mL of water weigh 1000 g

1000 g × 1.313 = 1313 g, weight of 1000 mL of syrup

$$\frac{1313\ (g)}{850\ (g)} = \frac{100\ (\%)}{x\ (\%)}$$

x = 64.7%, *answer.*

**To calculate the weight of a solution or liquid preparation, given the weight of its active ingredient and its percentage strength (w/w):**

*Example:*

*What weight of a 5% (w/w) solution can be prepared from 2 g of active ingredient?*

$$\frac{5\ (\%)}{100\ (\%)} = \frac{2\ (g)}{x\ (g)}$$

x = 40 g, *answer.*

### Weight-in-Weight Mixtures of Solids

Solids are usually measured by weight, and the percentage strength of a mixture of solids indicates the number of parts by weight of the active ingredient that are contained in the total weight of the mixture considered as *100 parts* by weight.

**To calculate the amount of active ingredient in a specified weight of a mixture of solids, given its percentage strength (w/w):**

*Examples:*

*How many milligrams of hydrocortisone should be used in compounding the following prescription?*

| ℞ | | | |
|---|---|---|---|
| ℞ | Hydrocortisone | | ⅛% |
| | Hydrophilic Ointment | ad | 10.0 g |
| | Sig. Apply. | | |

⅛% = 0.125%

10 g × 0.00125 = 0.0125 g or 12.5 mg, *answer.*

*How many grains of hexachlorophene should be used in compounding the following prescription?*

| ℞ | | | |
|---|---|---|---|
| ℞ | Hexachlorophene | | 0.5% |
| | Coal Tar Solution | | ʒii |
| | Hydrophilic Base | ad | ℥i |
| | Sig. Apply to affected areas. | | |

℥i = 480 gr

480 gr × 0.005 = 2.4 gr, *answer.*

*How many grams of benzocaine should be used in compounding the following prescription?*

| ℞ | | | |
|---|---|---|---|
| ℞ | Benzocaine | | 2% |
| | Polyethylene Glycol Base | ad | 2.0 |
| | Make 24 such suppositories | | |
| | Sig. Insert one as directed. | | |

2 g × 24 = 48 g, total weight of mixture

48 g × 0.02 = 0.96 g, *answer.*

*How many grains of calcium undecylenate should be used in compounding the following prescription?*

| ℞ | | | |
|---|---|---|---|
| ℞ | Calcium Undecylenate | | 10% |
| | Talc | ad | ℥iv |
| | Sig. Apply locally. | | |

℥iv = 1920 gr

1920 gr × 0.10 = 192 gr, *answer.*

## RATIO STRENGTH

The concentration of weak solutions or liquid preparations is frequently expressed in terms of ratio strength. Since all percentages are a ratio of parts per hundred, ratio strength is merely another way of expressing the percentage strength of solutions or liquid preparations (and, less frequently, of mixtures of solids). For example, *5%* means *5 parts per 100* or *5:100*. Although *5 parts per 100* designates a ratio strength, it is customary to translate this designation into a ratio the first figure of which is *1*; thus, *5:100 = 1:20*.

When a ratio strength, for example, *1:1000*, is used to designate a concentration, it is to be interpreted as follows:

*For solids in liquids*—*1 gram* of solute or constituent in *1000 milliliters* of solution or liquid preparation, or *1 grain* of solute or constituent in a volume of solution or liquid preparation represented by that of *1000 grains* of water.

*For liquids in liquids*—*1 milliliter* of constituent in *1000 milliliters* of solution or liquid preparation, or *1 minim* of active ingredient in *1000 minims* of solution or liquid preparation.

*For solids in solids*—*1 gram* of constituent in *1000 grams* of mixture or *1 grain* of active ingredient in *1000 grains* of mixture.

The ratio and percentage strengths of any solution or mixture of solids are proportional, and either is easily converted to the other by the use of proportion.

**To calculate ratio strength, given the percentage strength:**

*Example:*

*Express 0.02% as a ratio strength.*

$$\frac{0.02\ (\%)}{100\ (\%)} = \frac{1\ (\text{part})}{x\ (\text{parts})}$$

$$x = 5000$$

Ratio strength = 1:5000, *answer.*

**To calculate percentage strength, given the ratio strength:**

*Example:*

*Express 1:4000 as a percentage strength.*

$$\frac{4000\ (\text{parts})}{1\ (\text{part})} = \frac{100\ (\%)}{x\ (\%)}$$

$x = 0.025\%$, *answer.*

**To calculate the ratio strength of a solution or liquid preparation, given the weight of solute or constituent in a specified volume of solution or liquid preparation:**

*Examples:*

*A certain injectable contains 2 mg of a drug per mL of solution. What is the ratio strength (w/v) of the solution?*

$$2 \text{ mg} = 0.002 \text{ g}$$

$$\frac{0.002 \text{ (g)}}{1 \text{ (g)}} = \frac{1 \text{ (mL)}}{x \text{ (mL)}}$$

$$x = 500 \text{ mL}$$

Ratio strength = 1:500, *answer.*

*What is the ratio strength (w/v) of a solution made by dissolving five tablets, each containing 2.25 g of sodium chloride, in enough water to make 1800 mL?*

$$2.25 \text{ g} \times 5 = 11.25 \text{ g of sodium chloride}$$

$$\frac{11.25 \text{ (g)}}{1 \text{ (g)}} = \frac{1800 \text{ (mL)}}{x \text{ (mL)}}$$

$$x = 160 \text{ mL}$$

Ratio strength = 1:160, *answer.*

**To solve problems involving ratio strength:**

In solving problems in which the calculations are based on ratio strength, it is sometimes convenient to translate the problem into one based on percentage strength and to solve it according to the rules and methods discussed under percentage preparations.

*Examples:*

*How many grams of potassium permanganate should be used in preparing 500 mL of a 1:2500 solution?*

$$1:2500 = 0.04\%$$

$$500 \text{ (g)} \times 0.0004 = 0.2 \text{ g}, \textit{answer.}$$

Or,

1:2500 means 1 g in 2500 mL of solution

$$\frac{2500 \text{ (mL)}}{500 \text{ (mL)}} = \frac{1 \text{ (g)}}{x \text{ (g)}}$$

$$x = 0.2 \text{ g}, \textit{answer.}$$

*How many milligrams of gentian violet should be used in preparing the following solution?*

| ℞ | Gentian Violet Solution 1:10,000 | 500 mL |
|---|---|---|
| | Sig. Instill as directed. | |

1:10,000 = 0.01%

500 (g) × 0.0001 = 0.050 g or 50 mg, *answer.*

Or,

1:10,000 means 1 g of 10,000 mL of solution

$$\frac{10{,}000\ (\text{mL})}{500\ (\text{mL})} = \frac{1\ (\text{g})}{x\ (\text{g})}$$

x = 0.050 g or 50 mg, *answer.*

*How many grains of benzethonium chloride are required to prepare f℥viii of a 1:4000 solution?*

1:4000 = 0.025%

455 (gr) × 0.00025 × 8 = 0.91, or 0.9 gr, *answer.*

Or,

1:4000 means 1 gr in a volume of solution represented by that of 4000 gr of water

8 f℥ of water weigh 3640 gr

$$\frac{4000\ (\text{gr})}{3640\ (\text{gr})} = \frac{1\ (\text{gr})}{x\ (\text{gr})}$$

x = 0.91 or 0.9 gr, *answer.*

*How many milligrams of hexachlorophene should be used in compounding the following prescription?*

| ℞ | Hexachlorophene | | 1:400 |
|---|---|---|---|
| | Hydrophilic Ointment | ad | 10 g |
| | Sig. Apply. | | |

1:400 = 0.25%

10 (g) × 0.0025 = 0.025 g or 25 mg, *answer.*

Or,

1:400 means 1 g in 400 g of ointment

$$\frac{400\ (g)}{10\ (g)} = \frac{1\ (g)}{x\ (g)}$$

x = 0.025 g or 25 mg, *answer.*

*How many grains of tetracaine should be used in compounding the following prescription?*

| ℞ Tetracaine | | 1:200 |
|---|---|---|
| White Petrolatum | ad | ℨii |
| Sig. Apply to eye. | | |

1:200 = 0.5%

ℨii = 120 gr

120 gr × 0.005 = 0.6 gr, *answer.*

Or,

1:200 means 1 gr in 200 gr of ointment

$$\frac{200\ (gr)}{120\ (gr)} = \frac{1\ (gr)}{x\ (gr)}$$

x = 0.6 gr, *answer.*

## SIMPLE CONVERSIONS OF CONCENTRATIONS TO "mg/mL"

Occasionally, pharmacists, particularly those practicing in patient-care settings, need to *convert rapidly* product concentrations expressed as percentage strength, ratio strength or as grams per liter (as in I.V. infusions) *to* mg/mL. These conversions may be made quickly by simple techniques. Here are some suggestions:

**To convert product percentage strengths to mg/mL:**

Multiply the percentage strength, expressed as a whole number, by 10 to obtain mg/mL.

*Example:*

*Convert 4% (w/v) to mg/mL.*

4 × 10 = 40 mg/mL, *answer.*

Proof: 4% (w/v) = 4 g/100 mL = 4000 mg/100 mL = 40 mg/mL

**To convert product ratio strengths to mg/mL:**

Divide the ratio strength by 1000 to obtain mg/mL.

*Example:*

*Convert 1:10000 (w/v) to mg/mL.*

10000 ÷ 1000 = 1 mg/10 mL, *answer.*

Proof: 1:10000 (w/v) = 1 g/10000 mL = 1000 mg/10000 mL = 1 mg/10 mL

**To convert product strengths expressed as grams/liter to mg/mL:**

Convert the numerator to milligrams and divide by the number of milliliters in the denominator to obtain mg/mL.

*Example:*

*Convert a product concentration of 1 g per 250 mL to mg/mL.*

1000 ÷ 250 = 4 mg/mL, *answer.*

Proof: 1 g/250 mL = 1000 mg/250 mL = 4 mg/mL

**Practice Problems**

1. ℞ Antipyrine 5%
Glycerin ad 60.0
Sig. Five drops in right ear.

How many grams of antipyrine should be used in compounding the prescription?

2. ℞ Sol. Ephedrine Sulfate
½% 30 mL
Sig. For the nose.

How many milligrams of ephedrine sulfate should be used in compounding the prescription?

3. ℞ Resin of Podophyllum 25%
Compound Benzoin Tincture ad 30.0
Sig. Apply to papillomas t.i.d.

How many grams of resin of podophyllum should be used in compounding the prescription?

4. How many milligrams of a certified red color should be used in preparing 5 liters of a 0.01% solution?

5. ℞ Potassium Iodide Solution (10%)
Ephedrine Sulfate Solution (3%) aa 15.0 mL
Sig. Five drops in water as directed.

How many grams each of potassium iodide and ephedrine sulfate should be used in compounding the prescription?

6. ℞ Cocaine 2%
Mineral Oil ad f℥i
Sig. Nasal spray.

How many grains of cocaine should be used in compounding the prescription?

7. ℞ Sol. Potassium Iodide
100% f℥i
Sig. Ten drops in water a.c.

How many grains of potassium iodide should be used in compounding the prescription?

8. ℞ Iodine 1%
Potassium Iodide 2%
Glycerin ad f℥ii
Sig. Use as a swab.

How many grains each of iodine and potassium iodide should be used in compounding the prescription?

9. A formula for a mouth rinse contains $\frac{1}{10}$% (w/v) of zinc chloride. How many grams of zinc chloride should be used in preparing 25 liters of the mouth rinse?

10. ℞ Pilocarpine Nitrate 4%
Phosphate Buffer Solution ad f3ii
Sig. For the eye.

How many grains of pilocarpine nitrate should be used in compounding the prescription?

11. An injection contains 50 mg of pentobarbital sodium in each mL of solution. What is the percentage strength (w/v) of the solution?

12. If 425 g of sucrose are dissolved in enough water to make 500 mL, what is the percentage strength (w/v) of the solution?

13. An ear drop formula contains 54 mg of antipyrine and 14 mg of benzocaine in each mL of solution. Calculate the percentage strength (w/v) of each ingredient in the formula.

14. How many liters of 2% (w/v) iodine tincture can be made from 123 g of iodine?

15. How many milliliters of 0.9% (w/v) sodium chloride solution can be made from 1 lb (avoir.) of sodium chloride?

16. How many milliliters of a 0.9% (w/v) solution of sodium chloride can be prepared from 50 tablets, each containing 2.25 g of sodium chloride?

17. If an intravenous injection contains 20% (w/v) of mannitol, how many milliliters of the injection should be administered to provide a patient with 100 g of mannitol?

18. An inhalant aerosol contains 0.25% (w/v) of isoproterenol hydrochloride. If each depression of the aerosol valve delivers 0.12 mg of the drug, how many doses are contained in a 15-mL aerosol package?

19. The intravenous dose of mannitol is 1.5 g per kg of body weight, administered as a 15% (w/v) solution. How many milliliters of the solution should be administered to a 150-lb patient?

20. If a physician orders a 25 mg "test dose" of sodium thiopental for a patient prior to anesthesia, how many milliliters of a 2.5% (w/v) solution of sodium thiopental should be used?

21. How many milliliters of resorcinol monoacetate should be used to prepare 1 pint of a 15% (v/v) lotion?

22. A sunscreen lotion contains 5% (v/v) of menthyl salicylate. How many milliliters of menthyl salicylate should be used in preparing 5 pt of the lotion?

23. Peppermint Spirit contains 10% (v/v) of peppermint oil. How many milliliters of peppermint oil should be used in preparing 1 gallon of the spirit?

24. ℞ Coal Tar Solution 10%
Green Soap Tincture ad f℥viii
Sig. Shampoo weekly.

How many fluidrachms of coal tar solution should be used in compounding the prescription?

25. ℞ Salicylic Acid 0.1%
Resorcinol Monoacetate 3.0%
Isopropyl Alcohol ad 250 mL
Sig. For the scalp.

How many milligrams of salicylic acid and how many milliliters of resorcinol monoacetate should be used in compounding the prescription?

26. ℞ Hydrocortisone powder 1.0%
Menthol 0.25%
Phenol 0.25%
Lubriderm Lotion ad 250 mL
Sig. Apply to rash several times a day.

How many grams of hydrocortisone powder and how many milligrams each of menthol and phenol should be used in compounding the prescription?

27. A lotion vehicle contains 15% (v/v) of glycerin. How many liters of glycerin should be used in preparing 5 gallons of the lotion?

28. ℞ Liquefied Phenol 0.5%
Zinc Oxide 5.0%
Lime Water ad f℥viii
Sig. Apply.

How many minims of liquefied phenol and how many grains of zinc oxide should be used in compounding the prescription?

29. One gallon of a certain lotion contains 946 mL of benzyl benzoate. Calculate the percentage (v/v) of benzyl benzoate in the lotion.

30. The formula for 1 liter of an elixir contains 0.25 mL of a flavoring oil. What is the percentage (v/v) of the flavoring oil in the elixir?

31. Paregoric contains the equivalent of 0.4% of opium. How many milligrams of opium are represented in a tablespoonful dose of a mixture of equal parts of paregoric and Kaopectate?

32. Belladonna leaf contains 0.3% of alkaloids. If 10 g of leaf are used to prepare 100 mL of belladonna tincture, how many milligrams of alkaloids are contained in this volume of the tincture?

33. ℞ Phenobarbital 1.0 g
Belladonna Tincture 30.0 mL
Peppermint Water ad 250.0 mL
Sig. One teaspoonful a.c.

If belladonna tincture contains 0.03% of alkaloids, how many micrograms of alkaloids are represented in each dose of the prescription?

34. A liniment contains 15% (v/v) of methyl salicylate. How many milliliters of the liniment can be made from 1 pt of methyl salicylate?

35. How many grams of sucrose must be dissolved in 475 mL of water to make a 65% (w/w) solution?

36. How many grams of tannic acid must be dissolved in 320 mL of glycerin having a specific gravity of 1.25 to make a 20% (w/w) solution?

37. How many grams of a drug substance should be dissolved in 1800 mL of water to make a 10% (w/w) solution?

38. What is the percentage strength (w/w) of a solution made by dissolving 62.5 g of potassium chloride in 187.5 mL of water?

39. If 198 g of dextrose are dissolved in 1000 mL of water, what is the percentage strength (w/w) of the solution?

40. One (1) lb of a fungicidal ointment contains 9.08 g of undecylenic acid. Calculate the percentage (w/w) of undecylenic acid in the ointment.

41. One (1) liter of purified water is mixed with 5 lb (avoir.) of wool fat. Calculate the percentage (w/w) of purified water in the finished product.

42. How many grams each of resorcinol and hexachlorophene should be used in preparing 5 lb (avoir.) of an acne ointment which is to contain 2% of resorcinol and 0.25% of hexachlorophene?

43. ℞ Gentian Violet 0.5%
Hydrophilic Ointment ad ℥i
Sig. Apply to affected area.

How many grains of gentian violet should be used in compounding the prescription?

44. ℞ Vioform Powder 2.0%
Hydrocortisone Powder 1.5%
Cold Cream ad ʒiv
Sig. Apply.

How many grains each of vioform powder and hydrocortisone powder should be used in compounding the prescription?

45. ℞ Iodochlorhydroxyquin 0.9 g
Hydrocortisone 0.15 g
Cream Base ad 30.0 g
Sig. Apply.

What is the percentage strength (w/w) each of iodochlorhydroxyquin and hydrocortisone in the prescription?

46. ℞ Salicylic Acid 2%
Menthol ¼%
Talc ad 60 g
Sig. Dust on.

How many grams of salicylic acid and how many milligrams of menthol should be used in compounding the prescription?

47. How many milligrams of procaine hydrochloride should be used in preparing 120 suppositories each weighing 2 g and containing ¼% of procaine hydrochloride?

48. If a topical cream contains 1.8% (w/w) of hydrocortisone, how many milligrams of hydrocortisone should be used in preparing 15 g of the cream?

49. A topical cream contains 0.2% (w/w) of nitrofurazone. How many grams of nitrofurazone are there in 4 oz (avoir.) of the cream?

50. You are directed to mix ℥i of Whitfield's Ointment (containing 6% of salicylic acid) and ℥ii of Lassar's Paste with Salicylic Acid (containing 2% of salicylic acid) with enough white petrolatum to make ℥iv. What is the percentage (w/w) of salicylic acid in the finished product?

51. ℞ Salicylic Acid ʒss
Boric Acid Ointment
Zinc Oxide Ointment aa ℥ss
Sig. Apply.

Calculate the percentage (w/w) of salicylic acid in the prescription.

52. A pharmacist incorporates 6 g of coal tar into 120 g of a 5% coal tar ointment. Calculate the percentage (w/w) of coal tar in the finished product.

53. From the following formula calculate the quantity, in grams, each of benzocaine, ephedrine sulfate, zinc oxide and camphor required to prepare 250 suppositories.

| | | |
|---|---|---|
| Benzocaine | | 0.8% |
| Ephedrine Sulfate | | 0.2% |
| Zinc Oxide | | 4.0% |
| Camphor | | 2.1% |
| Cocoa Butter | ad | 2.0 g |
| M. ft. suppos. no. i | | |

54. ℞ Phenobarbital Elixir 60 mL
Aludrox Suspension 180 mL
Sig. Two teaspoonfuls t.i.d.

If phenobarbital elixir contains 0.4% of phenobarbital, how many milligrams of phenobarbital would be contained in each dose of the prescription?

55. Plasma protein fraction (PPF) is available as a 5% (w/v) solution.

If the dose of the solution for a child is given as 5 mL per lb, how many grams of PPF would be administered to a child weighing 20 kg?

56. Express each of the following as a percentage strength:

(a) 1:1500 (d) 1:400
(b) 1:10,000 (e) 1:3300
(c) 1:250 (f) 1:4000

57. Express each of the following as a ratio strength:

(a) 0.125% (d) 0.6%
(b) 2.5% (e) $\frac{1}{3}$%
(c) 0.80% (f) $\frac{1}{20}$%

58. Express each of the following concentrations as a ratio strength:

(a) 2 mg of active ingredient in 2 mL of solution
(b) 0.275 mg of active ingredient in 5 mL of solution
(c) 2 g of active ingredient in 250 mL of solution
(d) 1 mg of active ingredient in 0.5 mL of solution

59. Echothiophate iodide solution is available in four strengths: 1.5 mg/mL; 3.0 mg/5 mL; 6.25 mg/5 mL and 12.5 mg/5 mL. Express each concentration as a percentage strength (w/v).

60. Triamcinolone acetonide ointment is available in three strengths: 0.025%, 0.1% and 0.5%. Express these concentrations in terms of mg of triamcinolone acetonide per g of ointment.

61. What is the percent concentration of cholesterol in a patient's blood serum if the cholesterol level is determined to be 200 mg%?

62. A patient is determined to have 0.8 mg of glucose in each mL of blood. Express the concentration of glucose in the blood as mg%.

63. Purified water contains not more than 10 ppm of total solids. Express this concentration as a percentage.

64. A vaginal foam contains 0.01% (w/v) of dienestrol. Express this concentration as a ratio strength.

65. A tetracycline syrup is preserved with 0.08% (w/v) of methylparaben, 0.02% (w/v) of propylparaben and 0.10% (w/v) of sodium metabisulfite. Express these concentrations as ratio strengths.

66. An ophthalmic solution of naphazoline hydrochloride is stabilized with 0.0006% (w/v) of sodium carbonate and preserved with 0.002% (w/v) of phenylmercuric nitrate. Express these concentrations as ratio strengths.

67. An injection contains 0.50% (w/v) of lidocaine hydrochloride and

1:200,000 (w/v) of epinephrine. Express the concentration of lidocaine hydrochloride as a ratio strength and that of epinephrine as percentage.

68. A sample of white petrolatum contains 10 mg of tocopherol per kg as a preservative. Express the amount of tocopherol as a ratio strength.

69. Calcium Hydroxide Topical Solution contains 170 mg of calcium hydroxide per 100 mL at 15°C. Express this concentration as a ratio strength.

70. Dibucaine hydrochloride solution is used for spinal anesthesia in a concentration of 1:1500 (w/v). How many milligrams of dibucaine hydrochloride are contained in a 20-mL vial of the solution?

71. ℞ Potassium Permanganate Tablets 0.2 g
Disp. #100
Sig. Two tablets in 4 pt of water
and use as directed.

Express the concentration, as a ratio strength, of the solution prepared according to the directions given in the prescription.

72. How many grams of sodium fluoride should be added to 100,000 liters of drinking water containing 0.8 ppm of sodium fluoride to provide a recommended concentration of 1.75 ppm?

73. How many grams of benzalkonium chloride should be used in preparing 5 gallons of a 1:5000 (w/v) solution?

74. ℞ Epinephrine Solution 1:1000 7.5 mL
Simple Syrup ad 60.0 mL
Sig. Teaspoonful as directed.

What is the concentration of epinephrine in the compounded prescription?

75. ℞ Phenacaine Hydrochloride 1:100
Mercury Bichloride 1:4000
Ophthalmic Base ad 10 g
Sig. Apply to right eye.

How many milligrams of phenacaine hydrochloride and of mercury bichloride should be used in compounding the prescription?

76. ℞ Atropine Base 1:200
Castor Oil ad 5 g
Sig. Apply topically to eye.

How many milligrams of atropine base should be used in compounding the prescription?

77. ℞ Menthol 1:500
Hexachlorophene 1:800
Hydrophilic Ointment Base ad 30 g
Sig. Apply to hands.

How many milligrams each of menthol and hexachlorophene should be used in compounding the prescription?

78. How many milligrams of isoflurophate are contained in 15 g of a 1:10,000 ophthalmic solution of isoflurophate in peanut oil?

79. If a dry powder mixture of the antibiotic amoxicillin is diluted with water to 80 mL by a pharmacist in order to prepare a prescription containing 125 mg of amoxicillin per 5 mL, (a) how many grams of amoxicillin are there in the dry mixture, and (b) what is the percentage strength of amoxicillin in the filled prescription?

80. A prefilled syringe of lidocaine hydrochloride contains 100 mg per 5 mL of the injection. Express the concentration of lidocaine hydrochloride as percentage (w/v).

81. If 10 mL of a nitroglycerin injection (5 mg of nitroglycerin per mL) is added to make a liter of intravenous fluid, what is the percentage strength (w/v) of nitroglycerin in the final product?

82. A cupric chloride injection (0.4 mg of copper per mL) is used as an additive to intravenous solutions for total parenteral nutrition (TPN). What is the final ratio strength of copper in the TPN solution if 2.5 mL of the cupric chloride injection is added to enough of the intravenous solution to prepare 500 mL?

83. Nitro-Bid Ointment contains 2% (w/w) of nitroglycerin. According to the manufacturer, each inch of the ointment squeezed from the tube contains 15 mg of nitroglycerin. How many grams would each inch of ointment weigh?

# 11

# Dilution and Concentration

In the previous chapter we have considered problems arising from the quantitative relationship, in given solutions or mixtures, between the active ingredients and the total amounts of solution or mixture, or between the ingredients themselves.

Problems of a slightly different character arise when given solutions or mixtures are *diluted* (by the addition of diluent, or by admixture with solutions or mixtures of lower strength) or are *concentrated* (by the addition of active ingredient, or by admixture with solutions or mixtures of greater strength, or by evaporation of the diluent).

Such problems sometimes seem complicated and difficult. But the complication proves to be nothing more than a series of steps required in the calculation, and the difficulty usually vanishes as each step, in itself, proves to be a simple matter.

Often a problem can be solved in several ways. The best way is not necessarily the shortest: the best way is the one that clearly is grasped and that leads to the correct answer.

These two rules, wherever they may be applied, will greatly simplify the calculations:

*(1) When ratio strengths are given, convert them to percentage strengths before setting up a proportion.* It is much more troublesome to calculate with a ratio like $\frac{1}{10}:\frac{1}{500}$ than with the equivalent *10 (%):0.2 (%).*

*(2) Whenever proportional parts enter into a calculation, reduce them to lowest terms.* Instead of calculating with a ratio like 75 *(parts):25 (parts),* simplify it to *3 (parts):1 (part).*

## RELATIONSHIP BETWEEN STRENGTH AND TOTAL QUANTITY

If a mixture of a given percentage or ratio strength is diluted to twice its original quantity, its active ingredient will be contained in twice as many parts of the whole, and its strength therefore will be reduced by one-half. Contrariwise, if a mixture is concentrated by evaporation to one-half its original quantity, the active ingredient (assuming that none was lost by evaporation) will be contained in one-half as many parts of the whole, and the strength will be doubled. So, if 50 mL of a solution containing 10 g of active ingredient with a strength of 20% or 1:5 (w/v) are diluted to 100 mL, the original volume is doubled, but the original strength is now reduced by one-half to 10% or 1:10 (w/v). And if by evaporation of the solvent the volume of the solution is reduced to 25 mL or one-half the original quantity, the 10 g of the active ingredient now indicate a strength of 40% or 1:2.5 (w/v).

It turns out, then, that *if the amount of active ingredient remains constant, any change in the quantity of a solution or mixture of solids is inversely proportional to the percentage or ratio strength;* that is, the percentage or ratio strength decreases as the quantity increases, and conversely.

This relationship is generally true for all mixtures except volume-in-volume and weight-in-volume solutions containing components that contract when mixed together.

Problems in this section generally may be solved by (1) inverse proportion, (2) the equation, (quantity) × (concentration) = (quantity) × (concentration), or (3) determining the quantity of active constituent (solute) needed and then calculating the quantity of the available solution (usually concentrated or stock solution) which will provide the needed amount of constituent.

## DILUTION AND CONCENTRATION OF LIQUIDS

**To calculate the percentage or ratio strength of a solution made by diluting or concentrating (by evaporation) a solution of given quantity and strength:**

*Examples:*

*If 500 mL of a 15% (v/v) solution of methyl salicylate in alcohol are diluted to 1500 mL, what will be the percentage strength (v/v)?*

$$\frac{1500\ (\text{mL})}{500\ (\text{mL})} = \frac{15\ (\%)}{x\ (\%)}$$

x = 5%, *answer.*

Or,

$$\begin{aligned}(\text{quantity}) \times (\text{concentration}) &= (\text{quantity}) \times (\text{concentration})\\ 500\ (\text{mL}) \times 15\ (\%) &= 1500\ (\text{mL}) \times x\ (\%)\\ x &= 5\%,\ \textit{answer.}\end{aligned}$$

Or,

500 mL of 15% (v/v) solution contain 75 mL of methyl salicylate (active ingredient)

$$\frac{1500\ (\text{mL})}{75\ (\text{mL})} = \frac{100\ (\%)}{x\ (\%)}$$

x = 5%, *answer.*

*If 50 mL of a 1:20 (w/v) solution of aluminum acetate are diluted to 1000 mL, what is the ratio strength (w/v)?*

1:20 = 5%

$$\frac{1000\ (\text{mL})}{50\ (\text{mL})} = \frac{5\ (\%)}{x\ (\%)}$$

x = 0.25% = 1:400, *answer.*

Or,

$$\frac{1000\ (\text{mL})}{50\ (\text{mL})} = \frac{1/20}{x}$$

$$x = \frac{1}{400} = 1{:}400,\ \textit{answer.}$$

Or,

50 (mL) × 5 (%) = 1000 (mL) × x (%)

x = 0.25% = 1:400, *answer.*

Or,

50 mL of a 1:20 solution contain 2.5 g of aluminum acetate

$$\frac{2.5\ (\text{g})}{1\ (\text{g})} = \frac{1000\ (\text{mL})}{x\ (\text{mL})}$$

x = 400 mL

Ratio strength = 1:400, *answer.*

*If 4 f℥ of a 1:2000 (w/v) solution of cetylpyridinium chloride are diluted to 1 pint, what will be the ratio strength (w/v) of the dilution?*

1 pint = 16 f℥

1:2000 = 0.05%

$$\frac{16\ (\text{f℥})}{4\ (\text{f℥})} = \frac{0.05\ (\%)}{x\ (\%)}$$

x = 0.0125% = 1:8000, *answer.*

Or,

$$4\ (\text{f}℥) \times 0.05\ (\%) = 16\ (\text{f}℥) \times x\ (\%)$$

$$x = 0.125\% = 1{:}8000, \textit{answer.}$$

Or,

$$\frac{16\ (\text{f}℥)}{4\ (\text{f}℥)} = \frac{1/2000}{x}$$

$$x = \frac{1}{8000} = 1{:}8000, \textit{answer.}$$

*If a syrup containing 65% (w/v) of sugar is evaporated to 85% of its volume, what percent (w/v) of sugar will it contain?*

Any convenient amount of the syrup—say, 100 mL—may be used in the calculation. If we evaporate 100 mL of the syrup to 85% of its volume, we shall have 85 mL.

$$\frac{85\ (\text{mL})}{100\ (\text{mL})} = \frac{65\ (\%)}{x\ (\%)}$$

$$x = 76.47\% \text{ or } 76\%, \textit{answer.}$$

**To calculate the amount of solution of desired strength that can be made by diluting or concentrating (by evaporation) a specified quantity of a solution of given strength:**

*Examples:*

*How many grams of 10% (w/w) ammonia water can be made from 1800 g of 28% (w/w) ammonia water?*

$$\frac{10\ (\%)}{28\ (\%)} = \frac{1800\ (\text{g})}{x\ (\text{g})}$$

$$x = 5040\ \text{g}, \textit{answer.}$$

Or,

$$1800\ (\text{g}) \times 28\ (\%) = x\ (\text{g}) \times 10\%$$

$$x = 5040\ \text{g}, \textit{answer.}$$

Or,

1800 g of 28% ammonia water contain 504 g of ammonia (100%)

$$\frac{10\ (\%)}{100\ (\%)} = \frac{504\ (g)}{x\ (g)}$$

x = 5040 g, *answer.*

*How many milliliters of a 1:5000 (w/v) solution of phenylmercuric acetate can be made from 125 mL of a 0.2% solution?*

1:5000 = 0.02%

$$\frac{0.02\ (\%)}{0.2\ (\%)} = \frac{125\ (mL)}{x\ (mL)}$$

x = 1250 mL, *answer.*

Or,

0.2% = 1:500

$$\frac{1/5000}{1/500} = \frac{125\ (mL)}{x\ (mL)}$$

x = 1250 mL, *answer.*

Or,

125 mL of a 0.2% solution contain 0.25 g of phenylmercuric acetate

$$\frac{1\ (g)}{0.25\ (g)} = \frac{5000\ (mL)}{x\ (mL)}$$

x = 1250 mL, *answer.*

Or,

$$125\ (mL) \times 0.2\ (\%) = x\ (mL) \times 0.02\ (\%)$$

x = 1250 mL, *answer.*

*If 1 gallon of a 30% (w/v) solution is to be evaporated so that the solution will have a strength of 50% (w/v), what will be its volume in fluidounces?*

1 gallon = 128 f℥

$$\frac{50\ (\%)}{30\ (\%)} = \frac{128\ (f℥)}{x\ (f℥)}$$

x = 76.8 f℥, *answer.*

## STOCK SOLUTIONS

Stock solutions are solutions of known concentration that are frequently prepared by the pharmacist for convenience in dispensing. They are usually strong solutions from which weaker ones may be conveniently made; and, when correctly prepared, they enable the pharmacist to obtain small quantities of medicinal substances that are to be dispensed in solution.

Stock solutions are invariably prepared on a weight-in-volume basis, and their concentration is expressed as a ratio strength or, less frequently, as a percentage strength.

**To calculate the amount of a solution of given strength that must be used to prepare a solution of desired amount and strength:**

*Examples:*

*How many milliliters of a 1:400 (w/v) stock solution should be used to make 4 liters of a 1:2000 (w/v) solution?*

4 liters = 4000 mL

1:400 = 0.25% 1:2000 = 0.05%

$$\frac{0.25\ (\%)}{0.05\ (\%)} = \frac{4000\ (\text{mL})}{x\ (\text{mL})}$$

x = 800 mL, *answer.*

Or,

$$\frac{1/400}{1/2000} = \frac{4000\ (\text{mL})}{x\ (\text{mL})}$$

x = 800 mL, *answer.*

Or,

4000 mL of a 1:2000 (w/v) solution require 2 g of active constituent (solute), thus:

$$\frac{1\ (\text{g})}{2\ (\text{g})} = \frac{400\ (\text{mL})}{x\ (\text{mL})}$$

x = 800 mL, *answer.*

*How many fluidounces of a 1:400 (w/v) stock solution should be used in preparing 1 gallon of a 1:2000 (w/v) solution?*

1 gallon = 128 f℥

1:400 = 0.25% 1:2000 = 0.05%

$$\frac{0.25\ (\%)}{0.05\ (\%)} = \frac{128\ (f℥)}{x\ (f℥)}$$

x = 25⅗ f℥, *answer.*

Or,

1 gallon of a 1:2000 (w/v) solution requires 1.89 g of active constituent, thus:

$$\frac{1.89\ (g)}{1\ (g)} = \frac{x\ (mL)}{400\ (mL)}$$

x = 756 mL = 25.6 or 25⅗ f℥, *answer.*

*How many milliliters of a 1% stock solution of a certified red dye should be used in preparing 4000 mL of a mouth wash which is to contain 1:20,000 (w/v) of the certified red dye as a coloring agent?*

1:20,000 = 0.005%

$$\frac{1\ (\%)}{0.005\ (\%)} = \frac{4000\ (mL)}{x\ (mL)}$$

x = 20 mL, *answer.*

Check:

1% stock solution contains 20 (mL) × 0.01 → 0.2 g certified red dye ← 1:20,000 solution contains 4000 (mL) × 0.00005

Or,

4000 mL of a 1:20,000 (w/v) solution require 0.2 g of certified red dye, thus:

$$\frac{1\ (g)}{0.2\ (g)} = \frac{100\ (mL)}{x\ (mL)}$$

x = 20 mL, *answer.*

*How many milliliters of a 1:16 solution of sodium hypochlorite should be used in preparing 5000 mL of a 0.5% solution of sodium hypochlorite for irrigation?*

$1{:}16 = 6.25\%$

$$\frac{6.25\ (\%)}{0.5\ (\%)} = \frac{5000\ (\text{mL})}{x\ (\text{mL})}$$

x = 400 mL, *answer.*

Or,

5000 mL of a 0.5% (w/v) solution require 25 g of sodium hypochlorite, thus:

$$\frac{25\ (\text{g})}{1\ (\text{g})} = \frac{x\ (\text{mL})}{16\ (\text{mL})}$$

x = 400 mL, *answer.*

*How many milliliters of a 1:50 stock solution of ephedrine sulfate should be used in compounding the following prescription?*

| ℞ Ephedrine Sulfate | | 0.25% |
|---|---|---|
| Rose Water | ad | 30.0 mL |
| Sig. For the nose. | | |

$1{:}50 = 2\%$

$$\frac{2\ (\%)}{0.25\ (\%)} = \frac{30\ (\text{mL})}{x\ (\text{mL})}$$

x = 3.75 mL, *answer.*

Or,

30 (g) × 0.0025 = 0.075 g of ephedrine sulfate needed

1:50 means 1 g in 50 mL of stock solution.

$$\frac{1\ (\text{g})}{0.075\ (\text{g})} = \frac{50\ (\text{mL})}{x\ (\text{mL})}$$

x = 3.75 mL, *answer.*

**To calculate the quantity of active ingredient in any specified amount of solution when given the strength of a diluted portion of the solution:**

From the strength of the diluted portion we may calculate the *quantity* of *active ingredient* that the undiluted portion must have contained, and then by proportion we may calculate how much active ingredient must be present in any other amount of the stock solution.

*Examples:*

*How much silver nitrate should be used in preparing 50 mL of a solution such that 5 mL diluted to 500 mL will yield a 1:1000 solution?*

1:1000 means 1 g of silver nitrate in 1000 mL of solution

$$\frac{1000 \text{ (mL)}}{500 \text{ (mL)}} = \frac{1 \text{ (g)}}{x \text{ (g)}}$$

x = 0.5 g of silver nitrate in 500 mL of *diluted* solution (1:1000) which is also the amount in 5 mL of the *stronger* (stock) solution,

and,

$$\frac{5 \text{ (mL)}}{50 \text{ (mL)}} = \frac{0.5 \text{ (g)}}{y \text{ (g)}}$$

y = 5 g, *answer.*

The accompanying diagrammatic sketch should prove helpful in solving the problem.

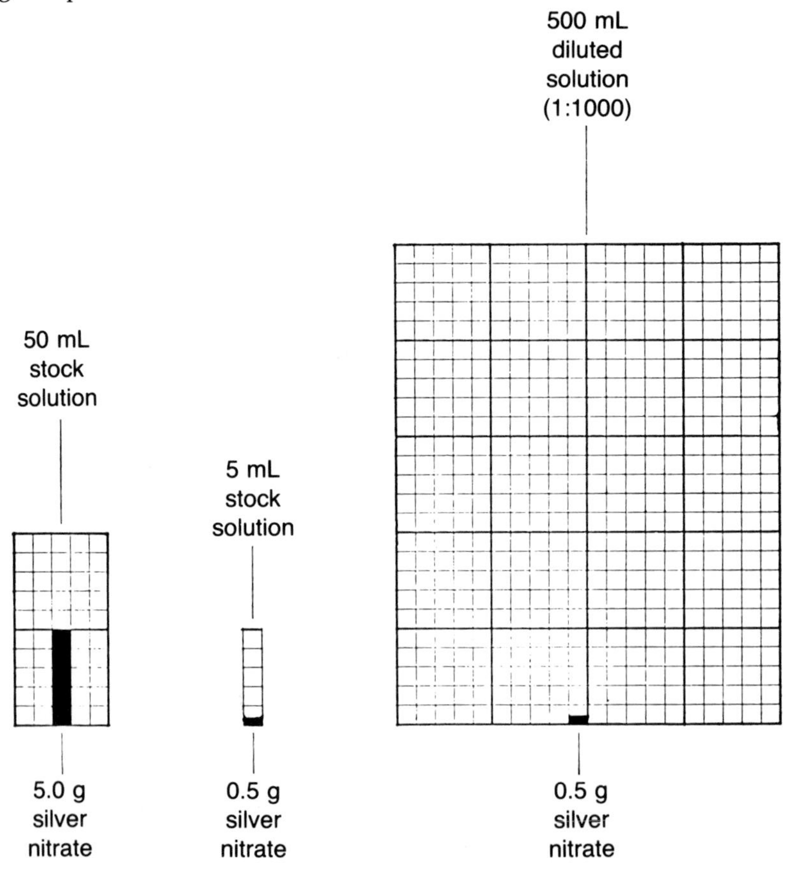

*How many grams of sodium chloride should be used in preparing 500 mL of a stock solution such that 50 mL diluted to 1000 mL will yield a "⅓ normal saline" (0.3% w/v) for irrigation?*

1000 (mL) × 0.003 = 3 g of sodium chloride in 1000 mL of "⅓ normal saline" (0.3% w/v) which is *also* the amount in 50 mL of the *stronger* (stock) solution to be prepared.

and,

$$\frac{50\ (\text{mL})}{500\ (\text{mL})} = \frac{3\ (\text{g})}{x\ (\text{g})}$$

x = 30 g, *answer.*

*How many milliliters of a 17% (w/v) concentrate of benzalkonium chloride should be used in preparing 300 mL of a stock solution such that 15 mL diluted to a liter will yield a 1:5000 solution?*

1 liter = 1000 mL

1:5000 means 1 g of benzalkonium chloride in 5000 mL of solution

$$\frac{5000\ (\text{mL})}{1000\ (\text{mL})} = \frac{1\ (\text{g})}{x\ (\text{g})}$$

x = 0.2 g of benzalkonium chloride in 1000 mL of *diluted* solution (1:5000) which is *also* the amount in 15 mL of the *stronger* (stock) solution to be prepared.

and,

$$\frac{15\ (\text{mL})}{300\ (\text{mL})} = \frac{0.2\ (\text{g})}{y\ (\text{g})}$$

y = 4 g of benzalkonium chloride needed

Since a 17% (w/v) concentrate contains 17 g per 100 mL

then,

$$\frac{17\ (\text{g})}{4\ (\text{g})} = \frac{100\ (\text{mL})}{z\ (\text{mL})}$$

z = 23.5 mL, *answer.*

**To calculate the amount of diluent that should be added to a solution of given strength and quantity to make a solution of specified lower strength:**

When given the quantity and strength of a solution, we may easily determine how much diluent should be added to reduce its strength as desired by first calculating the quantity of weaker solution that can be made and then subtracting from this the original quantity.

*Examples:*

*How many milliliters of water should be added to 300 mL of a 1:750 (w/v) solution of benzalkonium chloride to make a 1:2500 (w/v) solution?*

1:750 = 0.133% 1:2500 = 0.04%

$$\frac{0.04\ (\%)}{0.133\ (\%)} = \frac{300\ (\text{mL})}{\text{x}\ (\text{mL})}$$

x = 997.5 or 1000 mL of 0.04% (w/v) solution to be prepared

The difference between the volume of *diluted* (weaker) solution prepared and the volume of *stronger* solution used represents the volume of water (diluent) to be used.

1000 mL − 300 mL = 700 mL, *answer.*

*How many fluidounces of water should be added to a pint of a 5% (w/v) solution of boric acid to make a 2% (w/v) solution?*

1 pint = 16 f℥

$$\frac{2\ (\%)}{5\ (\%)} = \frac{16\ (\text{f℥})}{\text{x}\ (\text{f℥})}$$

x = 40 f℥

and,

40 f℥ − 16 f℥ = 24 f℥, *answer.*

If we are not given the strength of the original solution, but the quantity of active ingredient it contains, the simplest procedure is to calculate directly what must be the amount of solution of the strength desired if it contains this quantity of active ingredient; then by subtraction of the given original amount, as above, we may determine the required amount of diluent.

*Example:*

*How many milliliters of water should be added to 375 mL of a solution containing 0.5 g of benzalkonium chloride to make a 1:5000 solution?*

1:5000 means 1 g in 5000 mL of solution

$$\frac{1\ (\text{g})}{0.5\ (\text{g})} = \frac{5000\ (\text{mL})}{\text{x}\ (\text{mL})}$$

x = 2500 mL of 1:5000 (w/v) solution containing 0.5 g of benzalkonium chloride and,

2500 mL − 375 mL = 2125 mL, *answer.*

## DILUTION OF ALCOHOL

Since there is a noticeable contraction in volume when alcohol and water are mixed, we cannot calculate the volume of water needed to dilute alcohol to a desired *volume-in-volume* strength. But this contraction does not affect the *weights* of the components, and hence the *weight of water* (and from this, the *volume)* needed to dilute alcohol to a desired *weight-in-weight* strength may be calculated.

**To solve miscellaneous problems involving dilution of alcohol:**

*Examples:*

*How much water should be mixed with 5000 mL of 85% (v/v) alcohol to make 50% (v/v) alcohol?*

$$\frac{50\ (\%)}{85\ (\%)} = \frac{5000\ (\text{mL})}{x\ (\text{mL})}$$

$$x = 8500\ \text{mL}$$

Therefore, use 5000 mL of 85% (v/v) alcohol and enough water to make 8500 mL, *answer.*

*How many milliliters of 95% (v/v) alcohol and how much water should be used in compounding the following prescription?*

℞ Boric Acid 1.0 g
Alcohol 70% 30.0 mL
Sig. Ear drops.

$$\frac{95\ (\%)}{70\ (\%)} = \frac{30\ (\text{mL})}{x\ (\text{mL})}$$

$$x = 22\ \text{mL}$$

Therefore, use 22 mL of 95% (v/v) alcohol and enough water to make 30 mL, *answer.*

*How much water should be added to 4000 g of 90% (w/w) alcohol to make 40% (w/w) alcohol?*

$$\frac{40\ (\%)}{90\ (\%)} = \frac{4000\ (g)}{x\ (g)}$$

x = 9000 g, weight of 40% (w/w) alcohol equivalent to 4000 g of 90% (w/w) alcohol

9000 g − 4000 g = 5000 g or 5000 mL, *answer.*

## DILUTION OF ACIDS

The strength of an official undiluted *(concentrated)* acid is expressed as percentage weight-in-weight. For example, Phosphoric Acid contains not less than 85.0% and not more than 88.0%, by weight, of $H_3PO_4$. But the strength of an official *diluted* acid is expressed as percentage weight-in-volume. For example, Diluted Phosphoric Acid contains, in each 100 mL, not less than 9.5 g and not more than 10.5 g of $H_3PO_4$.

It is necessary, therefore, to consider the specific gravity of concentrated acids in calculating the volume to be used in preparing a desired quantity of a diluted acid.

**To calculate the volume of a concentrated acid required to prepare a desired quantity of a diluted acid:**

*Examples:*

*How many milliliters of 96% (w/w) sulfuric acid having a specific gravity of 1.84 are required to make 1000 mL of diluted sulfuric acid 10% (w/v)?*

1000 g × 0.10 = 100 g of $H_2SO_4$ (100%) in 1000 mL of 10% (w/v) acid

$$\frac{96\ (\%)}{100\ (\%)} = \frac{100\ (g)}{x\ (g)}$$

x = 104 g of 96% acid

104 g of water measure 104 mL

104 (mL) ÷ 1.84 = 56.5 mL, *answer.*

*How many milliliters of 85% (w/w) phosphoric acid having a specific gravity of 1.71 should be used in preparing 1 gallon of ¼% (w/v) phosphoric acid solution which is to be used for bladder irrigation?*

1 gallon = 3785 mL

3785 (g) × 0.0025 = 9.46 g of $H_3PO_4$ (100%) in 3785 mL (1 gallon) of ¼% (w/v) solution

$$\frac{85\ (\%)}{100\ (\%)} = \frac{9.46\ (g)}{x\ (g)}$$

x = 11.13 g of 85% phosphoric acid

11.13 g of water measure 11.13 mL

11.13 (mL) ÷ 1.71 = 6.5 mL, *answer.*

## DILUTION AND CONCENTRATION OF SOLIDS

**To solve miscellaneous problems involving dilution and concentration of solids:**

*Examples:*

*How many grams of opium containing 15% (w/w) of morphine and how many grams of lactose should be used to prepare 150 g of opium containing 10% (w/w) of morphine?*

$$\frac{15\ (\%)}{10\ (\%)} = \frac{150\ (g)}{x\ (g)}$$

x = 100 g of 15% opium, *and*

150 g − 100 g = 50 g of lactose, *answers.*

*If some moist crude drug contains 7.2% (w/w) of active ingredient and 21.6% of water, what will be the percentage (w/w) of active ingredient after the drug is dried?*

100 g of moist drug would contain 21.6 g of water and would therefore weigh 78.4 g after drying.

$$\frac{78.4\ (g)}{100\ (g)} = \frac{7.2\ (\%)}{x\ (\%)}$$

x = 9.2%, *answer.*

*How many grams of 20% benzocaine ointment and how many grams of ointment base (diluent) should be used in preparing 5 lb (avoir.) of 2.5% benzocaine ointment?*

5 lb = 454 g × 5 = 2270 g

$$\frac{20\ (\%)}{2.5\ (\%)} = \frac{2270\ (g)}{x\ (g)}$$

x = 283.75 or 284 g of 20% ointment, *and*

2270 g − 284 g = 1986 g of ointment base, *answers.*

*How many grains of 20% zinc oxide ointment and how many grains of ophthalmic base should be used in compounding the following prescription?*

℞ Ophthalmic Zinc Oxide Ointment 3% ʒii
Sig. Apply to lids.

ʒii = 120 gr

$$\frac{20\ (\%)}{3\ (\%)} = \frac{120\ (gr)}{x\ (gr)}$$

x = 18 gr of 20% ointment, *and*

120 gr − 18 gr = 102 gr of ophthalmic base, *answers.*

*How many grams of coal tar should be added to 3200 g of 5% coal tar ointment to prepare an ointment containing 20% of coal tar?*

3200 g × 0.05 = 160 g of coal tar in 3200 g of 5% ointment

3200 g − 160 g = 3040 g of base (diluent) in 3200 g of 5% ointment

In the 20% ointment the diluent will represent 80% of the total weight.

$$\frac{80\ (\%)}{20\ (\%)} = \frac{3040\ (g)}{x\ (g)}$$

x = 760 g of coal tar in the 20% ointment

But since the 5% ointment already contains 160 g of coal tar, 760 g − 160 g = 600 g, *answer.*

A much simpler method of solving the problem above can be used if we mentally translate it to read:

*How many grams of coal tar should be added to 3200 g of coal tar ointment containing 95% diluent to prepare an ointment containing 80% diluent?*

$$\frac{80\ (\%)}{95\ (\%)} = \frac{3200\ (g)}{x\ (g)}$$

x = 3800 g of ointment containing 80% diluent and 20% coal tar

3800 g − 3200 g = 600 g, *answer.*

NOTE: For another simple method, using alligation alternate, see page 178.

*How many milliliters of water should be added to 150 g of wool fat to prepare hydrous wool fat containing 25% of water?*

100% − 25% = 75% wool fat in hydrous wool fat

$$\frac{75\ (\%)}{100\ (\%)} = \frac{150\ (g)}{x\ (g)}$$

x = 200 g of hydrous wool fat

200 g − 150 g = 50 g or mL of water, *answer.*

A more direct solution:

$$\frac{75\ (\%)}{25\ (\%)} = \frac{150\ (g)}{x\ (g)}$$

x = 50 g or mL of water, *answer.*

## TRITURATIONS

Triturations are dilutions of potent medicinal substances. They were at one time official and were prepared by *diluting one part by weight of the finely powdered medicinal substance with nine parts by weight of finely powdered lactose.* They are, therefore, *10%* or *1:10 (w/w)* mixtures.

These dilutions offer a means of obtaining conveniently and accurately small quantities of potent drugs for compounding purposes.

**To calculate the quantity of a trituration required to obtain a given amount of a medicinal substance:**

*Examples:*

*How many grams of a 1:10 trituration of atropine sulfate are required to obtain 25 mg of atropine sulfate?*

10 g of trituration contain 1 g of atropine sulfate

25 mg = 0.025 g

$$\frac{1 \text{ (g)}}{0.025 \text{ (g)}} = \frac{10 \text{ (g)}}{x \text{ (g)}}$$

x = 0.25 g, *answer.*

*How many grains of a 1:10 trituration of colchicine are needed to obtain the amount needed for 100 capsules each containing $\frac{1}{120}$ gr of colchicine and 5 gr of aspirin?*

$\frac{1}{120}$ gr × 100 = $\frac{100}{120}$ gr or $\frac{5}{6}$ gr of colchicine needed

10 gr of trituration contain 1 gr of colchicine

$$\frac{1 \text{ (gr)}}{\frac{5}{6} \text{ (gr)}} = \frac{10 \text{ (gr)}}{x \text{ (gr)}}$$

x = $8\frac{1}{3}$ gr, *answer.*

*How many milligrams of a 10% trituration of atropine sulfate should be used in preparing 500 mL of a solution of atropine sulfate which is to contain $\frac{1}{400}$ gr of atropine sulfate per teaspoonful?*

1 teaspoonful = 5 mL

500 ÷ 5 = 100 doses

$\frac{1}{400}$ gr × 100 = $\frac{100}{400}$ or $\frac{1}{4}$ gr of atropine sulfate needed

10% trituration contains 1 gr of atropine sulfate in 10 gr

$$\frac{1 \text{ (gr)}}{\frac{1}{4} \text{ (gr)}} = \frac{10 \text{ (gr)}}{x \text{ (gr)}}$$

x = $2\frac{1}{2}$ gr, *answer.*

## ALLIGATION

Alligation is an arithmetical method of solving problems that involve the mixing of solutions or mixtures of solids possessing different percentage strengths.

## ALLIGATION MEDIAL

*Alligation medial* is a method by which the "weighted average" percentage strength of a mixture of two or more substances whose quantities and concentrations are known may be quickly calculated. The percentage strength, expressed as a whole number, of each component of the mixture is multiplied by its corresponding quantity, and the sum of the products is divided by the sum of the quantities to give the percentage strength of the mixture—provided, of course, that the quantities have been expressed in a common denomination, whether of weight or of volume.

**To calculate the percentage strength of a mixture that has been made by mixing two or more components of given percentage strengths:**

*Examples:*

*What is the percentage (v/v) of alcohol in a mixture of 3000 mL of 40% (v/v) alcohol, 1000 mL of 60% (v/v) alcohol, and 1000 mL of 70% (v/v) alcohol?*

$$\begin{array}{rcrcr} 40 & \times & 3000 & = & 120000 \\ 60 & \times & 1000 & = & 60000 \\ 70 & \times & \underline{1000} & = & \underline{70000} \\ \text{Totals:} & & 5000 & & 250000 \end{array}$$

250000 ÷ 5000 = 50%, *answer.*

*What is the percentage of zinc oxide in an ointment prepared by mixing 200 g of 10% ointment, 50 g of 20% ointment, and 100 g of 5% ointment?*

$$\begin{array}{rcrcr} 10 & \times & 200 & = & 2000 \\ 20 & \times & 50 & = & 1000 \\ 5 & \times & \underline{100} & = & \underline{500} \\ \text{Totals:} & & 350 & & 3500 \end{array}$$

3500 ÷ 350 = 10%, *answer.*

In some problems the addition of a solvent or vehicle must be considered. It is generally best to consider the diluent as of zero percentage strength as in the following problem.

*Example:*

*What is the percentage (v/v) of alcohol in a cough mixture containing 500 mL of terpin hydrate elixir, 100 mL of chloroform spirit, and enough hydriodic acid syrup to make 1000 mL? Terpin hydrate elixir contains 40% (v/v) of alcohol, and chloroform spirit contains 90% (v/v) of alcohol.*

| | | | |
|---|---|---|---|
| 40 × | 500 | = | 20000 |
| 90 × | 100 | = | 9000 |
| 0 × | 400 | = | 0 |
| Totals: | 1000 | | 29000 |

29000 ÷ 1000 = 29%, *answer.*

## ALLIGATION ALTERNATE

*Alligation alternate* is a method by which we may calculate the number of parts of two or more components of a given strength when they are to be mixed to prepare a mixture of desired strength. A final proportion permits us to translate relative parts to any specific denomination.

The strength of a mixture must lie somewhere between the strengths of its components—that is, the mixture must be somewhat stronger than its weakest component and somewhat weaker than its strongest; and, as already indicated, the strength of the mixture is always a "weighted" average: it lies nearer to that of its weaker or stronger components depending upon the relative amounts involved.

This "weighted" average can be found by means of an extremely simple scheme, as illustrated in the diagram below.

**To find the relative amounts of solutions or other substances of different strengths that should be used to make a mixture of required strength:**

*Example:*

*In what proportion should alcohols of 95% and 50% strengths be mixed to make 70% alcohol?*

Note that the difference between the *strength of the stronger component* (95%) and the *desired strength* (70%) indicates the *number of parts of the weaker* to be used (25 parts); and the difference between the *desired strength* (70%) and the *strength of the weaker component* (50%) indicates the *number of parts of the stronger* to be used (20 parts).

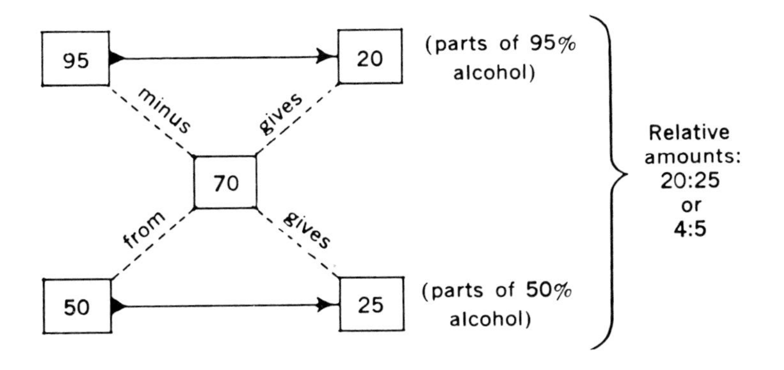


The mathematical validity of this relationship can be demonstrated.

| *Percent given* | *Percent desired* | *Proportional parts required* |
|---|---|---|
| a | | x |
| | c | |
| b | | y |

Given these data, the ratio of x to y may be derived algebraically as follows:

$$ax + by = c(x + y)$$
$$ax + by = cx + cy$$
$$ax - cx = cy - by$$
$$x(a - c) = y(c - b)$$

$$\frac{x}{y} = \frac{c - b}{a - c}$$

And given a = 95%, b = 50%, and c = 70%, we may therefore solve the problem as follows:

$$.95\ x + .50\ y = .70\ (x + y)$$

$$\text{Or, } 95\ x + 50\ y = 70\ x + 70\ y$$

$$95\ x - 70\ x = 70\ y - 50\ y$$

$$x(95 - 70) = y\ (70 - 50)$$

$$\frac{x}{y} = \frac{70 - 50}{95 - 70} = \frac{20}{25} = \frac{4\ \text{(parts)}}{5\ \text{(parts)}},\ \textit{answer.}$$

The result can be shown to be correct by *alligation medial:*

$$95 \times 4 = 380$$
$$50 \times 5 = 250$$
$$\text{Totals: } 9 \quad 630$$

$$630 \div 9 = 70\%$$

The customary layout of *alligation alternate,* used in the examples below, is a convenient simplification of the diagram above.

*Examples:*

*In what proportion should 20% benzocaine ointment be mixed with an ointment base to produce a 2.5% benzocaine ointment?*

| | | |
|---|---|---|
| 20% | | 2.5 parts of 20% |
| | 2.5% | |
| 0% | | 17.5 parts of ointment base |

Relative amounts: 2.5:17.5, or 1:7, *answer.*

$$\text{Check: } 20 \times 1 = 20$$
$$0 \times 7 = 0$$
$$\text{Totals: } 8 \quad 20$$

$$20 \div 8 = 2.5\%$$

*A hospital pharmacist wants to use three lots of ichthammol ointment containing respectively 50%, 20%, and 5% of ichthammol. In what proportion should they be mixed to prepare a 10% ichthammol ointment?*

Here the two lots containing *more* (50% and 20%) than the desired percentage may be separately linked to the lot containing *less* (5%) than the desired percentage:

| | | |
|---|---|---|
| 50% | | 5 parts of 50% ointment |
| 20% | 10% | 5 parts of 20% ointment |
| 5% | | 10 + 40 = 50 parts of 5% ointment |

Relative amounts: 5:5:50, or 1:1:10, *answer.*

Check: $50 \times 1 = 50$
$20 \times 1 = 20$
$5 \times 10 = 50$
Totals: 12   120

$120 \div 12 = 10\%$

There are, of course, other answers, for the two stronger lots may be mixed first in any proportions desired, yielding a mixture that may then be mixed with the weakest lot in a proportion giving the desired strength.

*In what proportions may a manufacturing pharmacist mix 20%, 15%, 5%, and 3% zinc oxide ointments to produce a 10% ointment?*

Each of the weaker lots is paired with one of the stronger to give the desired strength; and since we may pair them in two ways, we may get two sets of correct answers.

| | | |
|---|---|---|
| 20% | | 7 parts of 20% ointment |
| 15% | 10% | 5 parts of 15% ointment |
| 5% | | 5 parts of 5% ointment |
| 3% | | 10 parts of 3% ointment |

Relative amounts: 7:5:5:10, *answer.*

Check: $20 \times 7 = 140$
$15 \times 5 = 75$
$5 \times 5 = 25$
$3 \times 10 = 30$
Totals: 27   270

$270 \div 27 = 10\%$

Or,

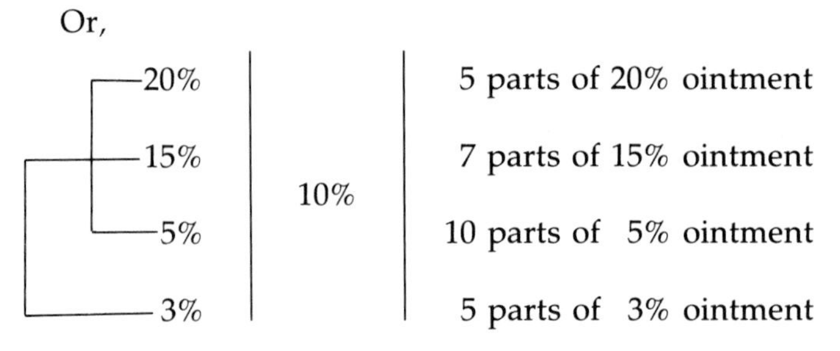


Relative amounts: 5:7:10:5, *answer.*

Check:

| | | | |
|---|---|---|---|
| 20 × | 5 | = | 100 |
| 15 × | 7 | = | 105 |
| 5 × | 10 | = | 50 |
| 3 × | 5 | = | 15 |
| Totals: | 27 | | 270 |

$270 \div 27 = 10\%$

*How many milliliters of 50% (w/v) dextrose solution and how many milliliters of 5% (w/v) dextrose solution are required to prepare 4500 mL of a 10% (w/v) solution?*

| | | |
|---|---|---|
| 50% | | 5 parts of 50% solution |
| | 10% | |
| 5% | | 40 parts of 5% solution |

Relative amounts 5:40, or 1:8, with a total of 9 parts

$$\frac{9 \text{ (parts)}}{1 \text{ (part)}} = \frac{4500 \text{ (mL)}}{x \text{ (mL)}}$$

x = 500 mL of 50% solution, *and*

$$\frac{9 \text{ (parts)}}{8 \text{ (parts)}} = \frac{4500 \text{ (mL)}}{y \text{ (mL)}}$$

y = 4000 mL of 5% solution, *answers.*

*How many milliliters each of 2% iodine tincture and 7% stronger iodine tincture should be used in preparing 1 gallon of a tincture containing 3.5% of iodine?*

1 gallon = 3785 mL

| | | |
|---|---|---|
| 2% | | 3.5 parts of 2% tincture |
| | 3.5% | |
| 7% | | 1.5 parts of 7% tincture |

Relative amounts: 3.5:1.5, or 7:3, with a total of 10 parts

$$\frac{10 \text{ (parts)}}{7 \text{ (parts)}} = \frac{3785 \text{ (mL)}}{x \text{ (mL)}}$$

x = 2650 mL of 2% iodine tincture, *and*

$$\frac{10 \text{ (parts)}}{3 \text{ (parts)}} = \frac{3785 \text{ (mL)}}{y \text{ (mL)}}$$

y = 1135 mL of 7% stronger iodine tincture, *answers.*

**To calculate the quantity of a solution or mixture of given strength that should be mixed with a specified quantity of another solution or mixture of given strength to make a solution or mixture of desired strength:**

*Examples:*

*How many grams of 2.5% hydrocortisone cream should be mixed with 360 g of 0.25% cream to make a 1% hydrocortisone cream?*

| | | |
|---|---|---|
| 2.5% | | 0.75 part of 2.5% cream |
| | 1% | |
| 0.25% | | 1.5 parts of 0.25% cream |

Relative amounts: 0.75:1.5, or 1:2

$$\frac{2 \text{ (parts)}}{1 \text{ (part)}} = \frac{360 \text{ (g)}}{x \text{ (g)}}$$

x = 180 g, *answer.*

*Alternate (algebraic) solution of the same problem:*

$$\begin{aligned} 2.5(x) + 0.25(360) &= 1(360 + x) \\ 2.5x + 90 &= 360 + x \\ 1.5x &= 270 \\ x &= 180 \text{ g, } \textit{answer.} \end{aligned}$$

*How many grams of white petrolatum should be mixed with 250 g of 5% and 750 g of 15% sulfur ointments to prepare a 10% ointment?*

$$\begin{aligned} 5 \times 250 &= 1250 \\ 15 \times 750 &= 11250 \\ \text{Totals: } 1000 &\quad 12500 \end{aligned}$$

12500 ÷ 1000 = 12.5% of sulfur in 1000 g of a mixture of 5% and 15% ointments

| | | |
|---|---|---|
| 12.5% | | 10 parts of 12.5% mixture |
| | 10% | |
| 0% | | 2.5 parts of white petrolatum |

Relative amounts: 10:2.5, or 4:1

$$\frac{4 \text{ (parts)}}{1 \text{ (part)}} = \frac{1000 \text{ (g)}}{x \text{ (g)}}$$

x = 250 g, *answer.*

$$\begin{aligned} \text{Check: } 12.5 \times 1000 &= 12500 \\ 0 \times 250 &= 0 \\ \text{Totals: } 1250 \quad &\quad 12500 \end{aligned}$$

$$12500 \div 1250 = 10\%$$

**To calculate the amount of active ingredient that must be added to increase the strength of a mixture of given amount and strength:**

*Example:*

*How many grams of coal tar should be added to 3200 g of 5% coal tar ointment to prepare an ointment containing 20% of coal tar?*

Coal tar (active ingredient) = 100%

| | | |
|---|---|---|
| 100% | | 15 parts of 100% coal tar |
| | 20% | |
| 5% | | 80 parts of 5% ointment |

Relative amounts: 15:80, or 3:16

$$\frac{16 \text{ (parts)}}{3 \text{ (parts)}} = \frac{3200 \text{ (g)}}{x \text{ (g)}}$$

x = 600 g, *answer.*

$$\begin{aligned} \text{Check: } 100 \times 600 &= 60000 \\ 5 \times 3200 &= 16000 \\ \text{Totals: } 3800 \quad &\quad 76000 \end{aligned}$$

$$76000 \div 3800 = 20\%$$

Compare the solution of this problem by use of alligation alternate with other methods on page 169.

## SPECIFIC GRAVITY OF MIXTURES

The methods of alligation medial and alligation alternate may be used in solving problems involving the specific gravities of different quantities of liquids of known specific gravities—provided that there is no change in volume when the liquids are mixed, and that they are measured in a common denomination of *volume*.

**To calculate the specific gravity of a mixture given the specific gravities of its ingredients:**

*Example:*

*What is the specific gravity of a mixture of 1000 mL of syrup with a specific gravity of 1.300, 400 mL of glycerin with a specific gravity of 1.250, and 1000 mL of an elixir with a specific gravity of 0.950?*

$$\begin{aligned} 1.300 \times 1000 &= 1300 \\ 1.250 \times 400 &= 500 \\ 0.950 \times \underline{1000} &= \underline{950} \\ \text{Totals: } 2400 & \quad 2750 \end{aligned}$$

$2750 \div 2400 = 1.146$, *answer.*

**To calculate the relative or specific amounts of ingredients of given specific gravities required to make a mixture of desired specific gravity:**

*Examples:*

*In what proportion must glycerin with a specific gravity of 1.25 and water be mixed to give a liquid having a specific gravity of 1.10?*

| | | |
|---|---|---|
| 1.25 | | 0.10 parts of glycerin |
| | 1.10 | |
| 1.00 | | 0.15 parts of water |

Relative amounts: 0.10:0.15, or 2:3, *answer.*

*How many milliliters of each of two liquids with specific gravities of 0.950 and 0.875 should be used to prepare 1500 mL of a liquid having a specific gravity of 0.925?*

| | | |
|---|---|---|
| 0.950 | | 0.050, or 50 parts of liquid with specific gravity of 0.950 |
| | 0.925 | |
| 0.875 | | 0.025, or 25 parts of liquid with specific gravity of 0.875 |

Relative amounts: 50:25, or 2:1, with a total of 3 parts

$$\frac{3 \text{ (parts)}}{2 \text{ (parts)}} = \frac{1500 \text{ (mL)}}{x \text{ (mL)}}$$

x = 1000 mL of liquid with specific gravity of 0.950, *and*

$$\frac{3 \text{ (parts)}}{1 \text{ (part)}} = \frac{1500 \text{ (mL)}}{y \text{ (mL)}}$$

y = 500 mL of liquid with specific gravity of 0.875, *answers.*

### Practice Problems

1. If 250 mL of a 1:800 (v/v) solution are diluted to 1000 mL, what will be the ratio strength (v/v)?

2. Aluminum acetate solution contains 5% (w/v) of aluminum acetate. When 100 mL are diluted to a liter, what will be the ratio strength (w/v)?

3. If 400 mL of a 20% (w/v) solution are diluted to 2 liters, what will be the percentage strength (w/v)?

4. If a 0.067% (w/v) methylbenzethonium chloride lotion is diluted with an equal volume of water, what will be the ratio strength (w/v) of the dilution?

5. In preparing a solution for a wet dressing, two 0.3-g tablets of potassium permanganate are dissolved in 1 gallon of distilled water. What will be the percentage strength (w/v) of the solution?

6. If 150 mL of a 17% (w/v) concentrate of benzalkonium chloride are diluted to 5 gallons, what will be the ratio strength (w/v) of the dilution?

7. What is the strength of a sodium chloride solution obtained by evaporating 800 g of a 10% (w/w) solution to 250 g?

8. How many grams of 10% (w/w) phosphoric acid can be made from 1 kg of 85% (w/w) acid?

9. How many milliliters of 0.45% (w/v) sodium hypochlorite solution can be prepared from 800 mL of an 11.25% (w/v) solution?

10. If 100 g of belladonna leaf, assaying 0.35% (w/w) alkaloids, are required to make 1000 mL of belladonna tincture, how many milliliters of the tincture can be made from 5 lb (avoir.) of belladonna leaf containing 0.4% (w/w) of alkaloids?

11. How many milliliters of 0.9% (w/v) sodium chloride solution can be prepared from 250 mL of 25% (w/v) solution?

12. How many milliliters of a 1:50 (w/v) stock solution of a chemical should be used to prepare 1 liter of a 1:4000 (w/v) solution?

13. A certain product contains benzalkonium chloride in a concentration of 1:5000 (w/v). How many milliliters of a 17% solution of benzalkonium chloride should be used in preparing 4 liters of the product?

14. How many milliliters of a 10% stock solution of a chemical are needed to prepare 120 mL of a solution containing 10 mg of the chemical per mL?

15. How many milliliters of water should be added to 1 gallon of 70% isopropyl alcohol to prepare a 30% solution for soaking sponges?

16. How many milliliters of sterile distilled water must be added to 10 liters of a 50% (w/v) sterile dextrose solution to reduce the concentration to 30% (w/v)?

17. The formula for a buffer solution contains 1.24% (w/v) of boric acid. How many milliliters of a 5% (w/v) boric acid solution should be used to obtain the boric acid needed in preparing 1 liter of the buffer solution?

18. Menthol 0.1%
Hexachlorophene 0.1%
Glycerin 10.0%
Alcohol 70%, to make 500 mL
Label: Menthol and Hexachlorophene Lotion.

How many milliliters of a 5% (w/v) solution of menthol in alcohol should be used to obtain the amount of menthol needed in preparing the lotion?

19. ℞ Certified Red Color 1:10000
Amphogel ad 180 mL
Sig. Tsp. in water.

How many milliliters of a 1% solution of a certified red color should be used in compounding the prescription?

20. ℞ Gentian Violet Solution 500 mL
1:100,000
Sig. Mouth wash.

How many milliliters of ½% solution of gentian violet should be used in compounding the prescription?

21. How many milliliters of Burow's Solution (containing 5% w/v of aluminum acetate) should be used in preparing 2 liters of a 1:800 (w/v) solution to be used as a wet dressing?

22. How many milliliters of solution containing 0.275 mg of histamine phosphate per mL should be used in preparing 15 mL of a 1:10000 histamine phosphate solution?

23. ℞ Calamine Lotion
Boric Acid Solution (3%)
White Lotion aa ad 240.0
Sig. Apply.

How many milliliters of 5% boric acid solution and how much water should be used in compounding the prescription?

24. A physician writes for an ophthalmic suspension to contain 100 mg of cortisone acetate in 8 mL of normal saline solution. The pharmacist has on hand a 2.5% suspension of cortisone acetate in normal saline solution. How many milliliters of this and how many milliliters of normal saline solution should be used in preparing the prescribed suspension?

25. ℞ Burow's Solution
(1:8 aqueous dilution)
Isopropyl Alcohol aa ad 120.0
Sig. Apply locally as directed.

How many milliliters of Burow's Solution should be used in compounding the prescription?

26. The formula for a mouth wash calls for 0.05% by volume of methyl salicylate. How many milliliters of a 10% (v/v) stock solution of methyl salicylate in alcohol will be needed to prepare 1 gallon of the mouth wash?

27. ℞ Benzalkonium Chloride Solution 240 mL
Make a solution such that 10 mL diluted to a liter equals a 1:5000 solution.
Sig. 10 mL diluted to a liter for external use.

How many milliliters of a 17% solution of benzalkonium chloride should be used in compounding the prescription?

28. Calculate the quantity of chemicals required to make 16 fluidounces of an aqueous solution so that 1 fluidounce added to 3 fluidounces of water will represent 1:500 of ephedrine sulfate and 1:3000 of chlorobutanol.

29. How many milliliters of water should be added to 100 mL of a 1:125 (w/v) solution to make a solution such that 25 mL diluted to 100 mL will yield a 1:4000 dilution?

30. How many milliliters of a 0.1% (w/v) thimerosal solution should be used to prepare 500 mL of a 1:5000 solution for irrigation?

31. How much water should be added to a liter of 1:3000 (w/v) solution to make a 1:8000 (w/v) solution?

32. How many milliliters of water should be added to 30 mL of a 17% (w/v) benzalkonium chloride solution to produce a 1:500 (w/v) solution?

33. How much water should be added to 2500 mL of 83% (v/v) alcohol to prepare 50% (v/v) alcohol?

34. How many milliliters of water should be mixed with 1200 g of 65% (w/w) alcohol to make 45% (w/w) alcohol?

35. ℞ Methyl Salicylate 60.0 mL
Chloroform Liniment 60.0 mL
Alcohol 80% ad 240.0 mL
Sig. Apply to parts.

How many milliliters of 95% (v/v) alcohol and how much water should be used in compounding the prescription?

36. ℞ Castor Oil 5.0 mL
Euresol 15.0 mL
Alcohol 85% ad 240.0 mL
Sig. For the scalp.

How many milliliters of 95% (v/v) alcohol and how much water should be used in compounding the prescription?

37. How many milliliters of 95% (w/w) sulfuric acid having a specific gravity of 1.820 should be used in preparing 2 liters of 10% (w/v) acid?

38. How many milliliters of 37% (w/w) hydrochloric acid having a specific gravity of 1.18 should be used in preparing 1000 mL of 10% (w/v) acid?

39. How many milliliters of 28% (w/w) ammonia water having a specific gravity of 0.89 should be used in preparing 2000 mL of 10% (w/w) ammonia water with a specific gravity of 0.96?

40. How many milliliters of a 70% (w/w) sorbitol solution, specific gravity 1.30, should be used in preparing 1 gallon of a 10% (w/v) solution?

41. In using isoproterenol hydrochloride solution (1:5000 w/v), 1 mL of the solution is diluted to 10 mL with sodium chloride injection prior to intravenous administration. What is the percentage concentration of the diluted solution?

42. For bladder and urethral irrigation, it is recommended that a 1:750

(w/v) solution of benzalkonium chloride be diluted with distilled water in a ratio of 3 parts of the benzalkonium solution and 77 parts of distilled water. What is the ratio strength of benzalkonium chloride in the final dilution?

43. In filling a medication order for 500 mL of diluted phosphoric acid, a pharmacist used 50 mL of 85% phosphoric acid with a specific gravity of 1.71. What was the percentage strength (w/v) of the finished product?

44. A sample of opium contains 28% of moisture and 10% of morphine. How many grams of morphine could be obtained from 350 g of the dry opium?

45. How many grams of lactose should be added to 75 g of belladonna extract assaying 1.50% (w/w) of alkaloids to reduce its strength to 1.40% (w/w)?

46. ℞ Benzocaine Ointment ℥ii
2.5%
Sig. Apply.

How many grains of 20% benzocaine ointment and how many grains of white petrolatum should be used in compounding the prescription?

47. ℞ Hydrocortisone Acetate Ointment 10 g
0.25%
Sig. Apply to the eye.

How many grams of 2.5% ophthalmic hydrocortisone acetate ointment and how many grams of ophthalmic base (diluent) should be used in compounding the prescription?

48. How many grams of zinc oxide should be added to 3400 g of a 10% zinc oxide ointment to prepare a product containing 15% of zinc oxide?

49. How many grams of petrolatum should be added to 250 g of a 25% ichthammol ointment to make a 5% ointment?

50. ℞ Zinc Oxide 1.5
Hydrophilic Petrolatum 2.5
Distilled Water 5.0
Hydrophilic Ointment ad 30.0
Sig. Apply to affected areas.

How much zinc oxide should be added to the product in order to make an ointment containing 10% of zinc oxide?

51. ℞ Coal Tar 5%
Lassar's Paste ad 50.0
Sig. Apply as directed.

In compounding, a pharmacist added 2.5 g of coal tar to 50 g of Lassar's Paste. Calculate the concentration of coal tar in the finished product.

52. A vaginal douche powder concentrate contains 2% (w/w) of active ingredient. What would be the percentage concentration (w/v) of the resultant solution after one 5-gram packet of powder is dissolved in enough water to make a quart of solution?

53. If one tablespoonful of a 0.2% (w/v) solution of phenylmercuric acetate is diluted to a quart with water, what would be the resultant percentage concentration (w/v) of the solution?

54. Liquefied phenol contains 90% of phenol and 10% of water. How many fluidounces of water should be added to 5 lb of phenol crystals to prepare liquefied phenol?

55. How many grams of coal tar should be added to 925 g of Zinc Oxide Paste to prepare an ointment containing 6% of coal tar?

56. How many grams of lactose and how many milligrams of atropine sulfate should be used to make 4 g of a 1:10 trituration of atropine sulfate?

57. A prescription calls for 0.005 g of atropine sulfate. How much of a 1:10 trituration should be used to obtain the atropine sulfate?

58. ℞ Atropine Sulfate 0.130 mg
Acetylsalicylic Acid 0.3 g
Ft. pulv. tal. no. 20
Sig. One b.i.d.

How many milligrams of a 1:10 trituration of atropine sulfate should be used in compounding the prescription?

59. Four equal amounts of belladonna extract, containing 1.15%, 1.30%, 1.35%, and 1.20% of alkaloids, respectively, were mixed. What was the percentage strength of the mixture?

60. What is the percentage of alcohol in a lotion containing 1500 mL of witch hazel (14% alcohol), 2000 mL of glycerin, and 5000 mL of 50% alcohol?

61. A pharmacist mixes 200 g of 10% ichthammol ointment, 450 g of

5% ichthammol ointment, and 1000 g of petrolatum (diluent). What is the percentage of ichthammol in the finished product?

62. Coal Tar Solution 80 mL (85% alcohol)
Glycerin 160 mL
Alcohol 500 mL (95% alcohol)
Boric Acid Solution ad 1000 mL
Label: Medicated lotion.

Calculate the percentage of alcohol in the lotion.

63. ℞ Phenobarbital Elixir 30 mL (15% alcohol)
Belladonna Tincture 50 mL (65% alcohol)
Aromatic Elixir 120 mL (22% alcohol)
Distilled Water ad 250 mL
Sig. Teaspoonful t.i.d.

Calculate the percentage of alcohol in the prescription.

64. What is the percentage of zinc oxide in an ointment prepared by mixing 2 lb (avoir.) of a 20% zinc oxide ointment, 3 lb (avoir.) of white petrolatum, and 1000 g of zinc oxide paste (25% of zinc oxide)?

65. ℞ Chloroform Spirit 50.0 mL (88% alcohol)
Aromatic Elixir 150.0 mL (22% alcohol)
Terpin Hydrate Elixir 300.0 mL (40% alcohol)
Sig. 5 mL for cough.

Calculate the percentage of alcohol in the prescription.

66. Calculate the percentage of alcohol in a lotion containing 2 liters of witch hazel (14% of alcohol), 1 liter of alcohol (95%), and enough boric acid solution to make 5 liters.

67. What is the percentage of alcohol in a liniment containing 1 pint of aconite fluidextract (60% of alcohol), 1 pint of 95% alcohol, 1 pint of chloroform, and 5 pints of soft soap liniment (60% of alcohol)?

68. In what proportion should 95% alcohol be mixed with 30% alcohol to make 70% alcohol?

69. In what proportion should 10% and 2% coal tar ointments be mixed to prepare a 5% ointment?

70. In what proportion should a 20% zinc oxide ointment be mixed with white petrolatum to produce a 3% zinc oxide ointment?

71. In what proportion should 30% and 1.5% hydrogen peroxide solutions be mixed to prepare a 3% hydrogen peroxide solution?

72. The solvent for the extraction of a vegetable drug is 70% alcohol.

In what proportion may 95%, 60%, and 50% alcohol be mixed in order to prepare a solvent of the desired concentration?

73. How many milliliters of 50% (w/v) solution should be mixed with 2175 mL of 10% (w/v) solution to make a 20% (w/v) solution?

74. What is the percentage of iodine in a mixture of 3 liters of 7% (w/v) iodine solution, 10 pints of 2% (w/v) solution, and 2270 mL of 3.5% (w/v) solution?

75. A manufacturing pharmacist has four lots of ichthammol ointment, containing 50%, 25%, 10%, and 5% of ichthammol. How many grams of each may he use to prepare 4800 g of a 20% ichthammol ointment?

76. How many milliliters of a 2.5% (w/v) thiamylal sodium solution and how many milliliters of 0.9% (w/v) normal saline should be used to prepare 500 mL of a 0.3% (w/v) thiamylal sodium solution?

77. How many milliliters of a 2% (w/v) solution of lidocaine hydrochloride should be used in preparing 500 mL of a solution containing 4 mg of lidocaine hydrochloride per mL of solution?

78. Dopamine hydrochloride solution is available in 5-mL ampuls containing 40 mg of dopamine hydrochloride per mL. The solution must be diluted prior to administration. If a physician wishes to use sodium chloride injection as the diluent and wants a dilution containing 0.04% (w/v) of dopamine hydrochloride, how many milliliters of sodium chloride injection should be added to 5 mL of the solution?

79. A solution of benzalkonium chloride is available in a concentration of 1:750 (w/v). How many milliliters of distilled water should be added to 30 mL of the solution to prepare a 1:5000 benzalkonium chloride solution for use as a wet dressing to the skin?

80. If an antibiotic injection contains 5% (w/v) of the drug, how many milliliters of diluent should be added to 5 mL of the injection to prepare a concentration of 5 mg of the antibiotic per mL?

81. A vial of kanamycin sulfate injection contains 500 mg per 2 mL. If 1.6 mL of the injection are diluted to 200 mL with normal saline solution, how many milliliters of the dilution should be administered daily to a child weighing 22 lb if the daily dose is 15 mg/kg of body weight?

82. How many grams of coal tar should be added to a mixture of 1000 g of zinc oxide paste and 500 g of wool fat to make an ointment containing 10% of coal tar?

83. How many milliliters of phenytoin sodium suspensions contain-

ing 30 mg per 5 mL and 125 mg per 5 mL should be used in preparing 480 mL of a suspension containing 10 mg of phenytoin sodium per mL?

84. If wool fat absorbs twice its weight of water, how much additional water will be absorbed by 4000 g of hydrous wool fat containing 25% of water?

85. You have on hand 500 mL of a 12% and 1 liter of a 6% solution of sodium hypochlorite. How many milliliters of water should be added to a mixture of the two solutions to prepare a solution containing 0.5% of sodium hypochlorite?

86. ℞ Zinc Oxide 20.0
Wool Fat 60.0
Water ad 120.0
Sig. Apply.

No wool fat is available. How many grams of hydrous wool fat containing 25% of water and how many milliliters of water should be used in compounding the prescription?

87. You have on hand 800 g of a 5% coal tar ointment and 1200 g of a 10% coal tar ointment. (a) If the two ointments are mixed, what is the concentration of coal tar in the finished product? (b) How many grams of coal tar should be added to the product to obtain an ointment containing 15% of coal tar?

88. What is the specific gravity of a mixture containing 1000 mL of water, 500 mL of glycerin having a specific gravity of 1.25, and 1500 mL of alcohol having a specific gravity of 0.81? (Assume that there is no contraction when the liquids are mixed.)

89. How many milliliters of a liquid with a specific gravity of 1.48 and of a liquid with a specific gravity of 0.71 should be mixed to prepare 100 mL of a mixture with a specific gravity of 1.05?

90. How many milliliters of each of two liquids with specific gravities respectively of 1.32 and 1.12 should be mixed to make 1000 mL of a mixture with a specific gravity of 1.20?

91. How many milliliters of a syrup having a specific gravity of 1.350 should be mixed with 3000 mL of a syrup having a specific gravity of 1.250 to obtain a product having a specific gravity of 1.310?

92. How many grams of sorbitol solution having a specific gravity of 1.285 and how many grams (milliliters) of water should be used in preparing 500 g of a sorbitol solution having a specific gravity of 1.225?

# 12

# Isotonic Solutions

When a solvent passes through a semipermeable membrane from a dilute solution into a more concentrated one with the result that the concentrations tend to become equalized, the phenomenon is known as *osmosis*. The pressure responsible for this phenomenon is called *osmotic pressure,* and it proves to be caused by and to vary with the solute.

If the solute is a non-electrolyte, its solution will contain only molecules, and the osmotic pressure of the solution will vary only with the concentration of the solute. If, on the other hand, the solute is an electrolyte, its solution will contain ions, and the osmotic pressure of the solution will vary not only with the concentration, but also with the degree of dissociation of the solute. Obviously then, substances that dissociate have a relatively greater number of particles in solution and should exert a greater osmotic pressure than could undissociated molecules.

Like osmotic pressure, the other colligative properties of solutions, namely, vapor pressure, boiling point, and freezing point, depend upon the number of particles in solution. These properties, therefore, are related, and a change in any one of them will be attended by corresponding changes in the others.

Two solutions that have the same osmotic pressure are termed *isosmotic*. It is generally agreed that many solutions designed to be mixed with body fluids should have the same osmotic pressure for greater comfort, efficacy, and safety. A solution having the same osmotic pressure as a body fluid is said to be *isotonic,* meaning of equal tone.

Solutions of lower osmotic pressure than that of a body fluid are *hypotonic,* whereas those having a higher osmotic pressure are *hypertonic*. Blood and the fluids of the eye and nose have so far been principally concerned, and of these the pharmacist is most likely to be asked to make ophthalmic solutions, or *collyria,* isotonic with lachrymal fluid.

The calculations involved in preparing isotonic solutions may be made in terms of data relating to the colligative properties of solutions. Theoretically, any one of these properties may be used as a basis for determining tonicity. Practically and most conveniently, a comparison of freezing points may be used for this purpose. At one time, $-0.56°C$ and $-0.80°C$ were generally accepted as the freezing points of blood serum and lachrymal fluid, respectively. However, most investigators now agree that the freezing point of blood serum is $-0.52°C$ and not $-0.56°C$ as previously measured, and that the freezing point of lachrymal fluid is the same as that of blood serum.

When one gram molecular weight of any non-electrolyte—that is, a substance with negligible dissociation, such as boric acid—is dissolved in 1000 g of water, the freezing point of the solution is about 1.86°C below the freezing point of pure water. By simple proportion, therefore, we may calculate the weight of any non-electrolyte that should be dissolved in each 1000 g of water if the solution is to be isotonic with the body fluids.

Boric acid, for example, has a molecular weight of 61.8, and hence (in theory) 61.8 g in 1000 g of water should produce a freezing point of $-1.86°$ C. Therefore:

$$\frac{1.86\ (°C)}{0.52\ (°C)} = \frac{61.8\ (g)}{x\ (g)}$$

$$x = 17.3\ g$$

In short, 17.3 g of boric acid in 1000 g of water, having a weight-in-volume strength of approximately 1.73%, should make a solution isotonic with lachrymal fluid.

With electrolytes, the problem is not quite so simple. Since osmotic pressure depends rather upon the number than upon the kind of particles, substances that dissociate have a tonic effect that increases with the degree of dissociation, and the greater the dissociation, the smaller the quantity required to produce any given osmotic pressure. If we assume that sodium chloride in weak solutions is about 80% dissociated, then each 100 molecules yield 180 particles, or 1.8 times as many particles as are yielded by 100 molecules of a non-electrolyte. This dissociation factor, commonly symbolized by the letter $i$, must be included in the proportion when we seek to determine the strength of an isotonic solution of sodium chloride (molecular weight, 58.5):

$$\frac{1.86\ (°C) \times 1.8}{0.52\ (°C)} = \frac{58.5\ (g)}{x\ (g)}$$

$$x = 9.09\ g$$

Hence, 9.09 g of sodium chloride in 1000 g of water should make a solution isotonic with blood or lachrymal fluid. Actually, a 0.90% (w/v) sodium chloride solution is taken to be isotonic with the body fluids.

Simple isotonic solutions, then, may be calculated by this general formula:

$$\frac{0.52 \times \text{molecular weight}}{1.86 \times \text{dissociation } (i)} = \text{g of solute per 1000 g of water}$$

The value of $i$ for many a medicinal salt has not been experimentally determined. Some salts (such as zinc sulfate, with only some 40% dissociation and an $i$ value therefore of 1.4) are exceptional; but most medicinal salts approximate the dissociation of sodium chloride in weak solutions, and if the number of ions is known we may use the following values, lacking better information:

| | |
|---|---|
| Non-electrolytes and substances of slight dissociation | : 1.0 |
| Substances that dissociate into 2 ions | : 1.8 |
| Substances that dissociate into 3 ions | : 2.6 |
| Substances that dissociate into 4 ions | : 3.4 |
| Substances that dissociate into 5 ions | : 4.2 |

A special problem arises when a prescription directs us to make a solution isotonic by adding the proper amount of some substance other than the active ingredient or ingredients. Given a 0.5% (w/v) solution of sodium chloride, we may easily calculate that 0.9 g − 0.5 g = 0.4 g of additional sodium chloride should be contained in each 100 mL if the solution is to be made isotonic with a body fluid. But how much sodium chloride should be used in preparing 100 mL of a 1% (w/v) solution of atropine sulfate, which is to be made isotonic with lachrymal fluid? The answer depends upon *how much sodium chloride is in effect represented by the atropine sulfate.*

The relative tonic effect of two substances—that is, the quantity of one that is the equivalent in tonic effects to a given quantity of the other—may be calculated if the quantity of one having a certain effect in a specified quantity of solvent be divided by the quantity of the other having the same effect in the same quantity of solvent. For example, we have calculated above that 17.3 g of boric acid per 1000 g of water and that 9.09 g of sodium chloride per 1000 g of water are both instrumental in making an aqueous solution isotonic with lachrymal fluid. But if 17.3 g of boric acid are equivalent in tonicity to 9.09 g of sodium chloride, then 1 g of boric acid must be the equivalent of 9.09 g ÷ 17.3 g or 0.52 g of sodium chloride. And similarly, 1 g of sodium chloride must be the tonicic equivalent of 17.3 g ÷ 9.09 g or 1.90 g of boric acid.

We have seen that there is one quantity of any substance that should in theory have a constant tonic effect if dissolved in 1000 g of water: this is one gram molecular weight of the substance divided by its $i$ or dissociation value. Hence, the relative quantity of sodium chloride that is the tonicic equivalent of a quantity of boric acid may be calculated by these ratios:

$$\frac{58.5 \div 1.8}{61.8 \div 1.0} \text{ or } \frac{58.5 \times 1.0}{61.8 \times 1.8}$$

and we may formulate a convenient rule: *quantities of two substances that are tonicic equivalents are proportional to the molecular weights of each multiplied by the* i *value of the other.*

To return to the problem involving 1 g of atropine sulfate in 100 mL of solution:

Molecular weight of sodium chloride = 58.5; $i$ = 1.8
Molecular weight of atropine sulfate = 695; $i$ = 2.6

$$\frac{695 \times 1.8}{58.5 \times 2.6} = \frac{1\ (g)}{x\ (g)}$$

x = 0.12 g of sodium chloride represented by 1 g of atropine sulfate

Since a solution isotonic with lachrymal fluid should contain the equivalent of 0.90 g of sodium chloride in each 100 mL of solution, the difference to be added must be 0.90 g − 0.12 g = 0.78 g of sodium chloride.

The Table on pages 197–198 gives the sodium chloride equivalents of each of the substances listed. These values were calculated according to the rule stated above. If the number of grams (or grains) of a substance included in a prescription is multiplied by its sodium chloride equivalent, the amount of sodium chloride represented by that substance is determined.

The procedure for the *calculation of isotonic solutions with sodium chloride equivalents* may be outlined as follows:

*Step 1.* Calculate the amount (in g or gr) of sodium chloride represented by the ingredients in the prescription. This may be done by multiplying the amount (in g or gr) of each substance by its sodium chloride equivalent.

*Step 2.* Calculate the amount (in g or gr) of sodium chloride, alone, that would be contained in an isotonic solution of the volume specified in the prescription—namely, *the amount of sodium chloride in a 0.9% solution of the specified volume.* (Such a solution would contain 0.009 g per mL, or 4.1 gr per f℥.)

*Step 3.* Subtract the amount of sodium chloride represented by the ingredients in the prescription (Step 1) from the amount of sodium chloride, alone, that would be represented in the specific volume of an isotonic solution (Step 2). The answer represents the amount (in g or gr) of sodium chloride to be added to make the solution isotonic.

*Step 4.* If an agent other than sodium chloride, such as boric acid, dextrose, sodium or potassium nitrate, is to be used to make a solution isotonic, divide the amount of sodium chloride (Step 3) by the sodium chloride equivalent of the other substance.

**To calculate the dissociation (i) factor of an electrolyte:**

*Examples:*

*Zinc sulfate is a 2-ion electrolyte, dissociating 40% in a certain concentration. Calculate its dissociation* (i) *factor.*

On the basis of 40% dissociation, 100 particles of zinc sulfate will yield:

40 zinc ions
40 sulfate ions
60 undissociated particles
or 140 particles

Since 140 particles represent 1.4 times as many particles as there were before dissociation, the dissociation *(i)* factor is 1.4, *answer.*

*Zinc chloride is a 3-ion electrolyte, dissociating 80% in a certain concentration. Calculate its dissociation* (i) *factor.*

On the basis of 80% dissociation, 100 particles of zinc chloride will yield:

80 zinc ions
80 chloride ions
80 chloride ions
20 undissociated particles
or 260 particles

Since 260 particles represent 2.6 times as many particles as there were before dissociation, the dissociation *(i)* factor is 2.6, *answer.*

**To calculate the sodium equivalent of a substance:**

Remember that the sodium chloride equivalent of a substance may be calculated as follows:

$$\frac{\text{molecular weight of sodium chloride}}{i\text{ factor of sodium chloride}} \times \frac{i\text{ factor of the substance}}{\text{molecular weight of the substance}} = \text{sodium chloride equivalent}$$

*Example:*

*Papaverine hydrochloride* (molecular weight 376) *is a 2-ion electrolyte, dissociating 80% in a given concentration. Calculate its sodium chloride equivalent.*

Since papaverine hydrochloride is a 2-ion electrolyte, dissociating 80%, its $i$ factor is 1.8.

$$\frac{58.5}{1.8} \times \frac{1.8}{376} = 0.156, \text{ or } 0.16, \textit{ answer.}$$

**To calculate the amount of tonicic agent required:**

*Examples:*

*How much sodium chloride should be used in compounding the following prescription?*

| ℞ Pilocarpine Nitrate | | 0.3 g |
|---|---|---|
| Sodium Chloride | | q.s. |
| Distilled Water | ad | 30.0 mL |
| Make isoton. sol. | | |
| Sig. For the eye. | | |

*Step 1.* 0.22 × 0.3 g = 0.066 g of sodium chloride represented by the pilocarpine nitrate

*Step 2.* 30 × 0.009 = 0.270 g of sodium chloride in 30 mL of an isotonic sodium chloride solution

*Step 3.* 0.270 g (from Step 2)
− 0.066 g (from Step 1)
0.204 g of sodium chloride to be used, *answer.*

*How many grains of sodium chloride should be used in compounding the following prescription?*

| ℞ Atropine Sulfate | | gr v |
|---|---|---|
| Sodium Chloride | | q.s. |
| Distilled Water | ad | ℥i |
| Make isoton. sol. | | |
| Sig. One drop in right eye. | | |

*Step 1.* 0.12 × 5 gr = 0.6 gr of sodium chloride represented by the atropine sulfate

*Step 2.* 1 × 455 × 0.009 = 4.1 gr of sodium chloride in ℥i of an isotonic sodium chloride solution

*Step 3.* 4.1 gr (from Step 2)
− 0.6 gr (from Step 1)
3.5 gr of sodium chloride to be used, *answer.*

*How much boric acid should be used in compounding the following prescription?*

| ℞ | | | |
|---|---|---|---|
| | Holocaine Hydrochloride | | 1% |
| | Chlorobutanol | | ½% |
| | Boric Acid | | q.s. |
| | Distilled Water | ad | 60.0 |
| | Make isoton. sol. | | |
| | Sig. One drop in each eye. | | |

The prescription calls for 0.6 g of holocaine hydrochloride and 0.3 g of chlorobutanol.

*Step 1.* 0.17 × 0.6 g = 0.102 g of sodium chloride represented by holocaine hydrochloride
0.18 × 0.3 g = 0.054 g of sodium chloride represented by chlorobutanol
Total: 0.156 g of sodium chloride represented by both ingredients

*Step 2.* 60 × 0.009 = 0.540 g of sodium chloride in 60 mL of an isotonic sodium chloride solution

*Step 3.* 0.540 g (from Step 2)
−0.156 g (from Step 1)
0.384 g of sodium chloride required to make the solution isotonic

But since the prescription calls for boric acid:

*Step 4.* 0.384 g ÷ 0.52 (sodium chloride equivalent of boric acid) = 0.738 g of boric acid to be used, *answer.*

*How much sodium nitrate could be used to make the following prescription isotonic?*

| ℞ | | |
|---|---|---|
| | Sol. Silver Nitrate 1:500 w/v | 60.0 |
| | Make isoton. sol. | |
| | Sig. For eye use. | |

The prescription contains 0.120 g of silver nitrate.

*Step 1.* 0.34 × 0.120 g = 0.041 g of sodium chloride represented by silver nitrate

*Step 2.* $60 \times 0.009 = 0.540$ g of sodium chloride in 60 mL of an isotonic sodium chloride solution

*Step 3.* 0.540 g (from Step 2)
−0.041 g (from Step 1)

0.499 g of sodium chloride required to make solution isotonic

Since, in this solution, sodium chloride is incompatible with silver nitrate, the tonic agent of choice is sodium nitrate. Therefore,

*Step 4.* 0.499 g ÷ 0.69 (sodium chloride equivalent of sodium nitrate) = 0.720 g of sodium nitrate to be used, *answer.*

*How much sodium chloride should be used in compounding the following prescription?*

| ℞ | | |
|---|---|---|
| Ingredient X | | 0.5 |
| Sodium Chloride | | q.s. |
| Distilled Water | ad | 50.0 |
| Make isoton. sol. | | |
| Sig. Eye drops. | | |

Let us assume that Ingredient X is a new substance for which no sodium chloride equivalent is to be found in the Table, and that its molecular weight is 295 and its *i* factor is 2.4.

The sodium chloride equivalent of Ingredient X may be calculated as follows:

$$\frac{58.5}{1.8} \times \frac{2.4}{295} = 0.26, \text{ the sodium chloride equivalent for Ingredient X}$$

Then,

*Step 1.* $0.26 \times 0.5$ g $= 0.130$ g of sodium chloride represented by Ingredient X

*Step 2.* $50 \times 0.009 = 0.450$ g of sodium chloride in 50 mL of an isotonic sodium chloride solution

*Step 3.* 0.450 g (from Step 2)
−0.130 g (from Step 1)

0.320 g of sodium chloride to be used, *answer.*

## TABLE OF SODIUM CHLORIDE EQUIVALENTS

| *Substance* | *Molecular weight* | *Ions* | *i* | *Sodium chloride equivalent* |
|---|---|---|---|---|
| Achromycin (See Tetracycline hydrochloride) | | | | |
| Antazoline phosphate | 363 | 2 | 1.8 | 0.16 |
| Antipyrine | 188 | 1 | 1.0 | 0.17 |
| Antistine (See Antazoline phosphate) | | | | |
| Atropine sulfate. $H_2O$ | 695 | 3 | 2.6 | 0.12 |
| Aureomycin (See Chlortetracycline hydrochloride) | | | | |
| Benzalkonium chloride | 360 | 2 | 1.8 | 0.16 |
| Benzyl alcohol | 108 | 1 | 1.0 | 0.30 |
| Borax (See Sodium borate) | | | | |
| Boric acid | 61.8 | 1 | 1.0 | 0.52 |
| Carbachol | 183 | 2 | 1.8 | 0.33 |
| Carbamylcholine chloride (See Carbachol) | | | | |
| Chloramphenicol | 323 | 1 | 1.0 | 0.10 |
| Chlorobutanol | 177 | 1 | 1.0 | 0.18 |
| Chloromycetin (See Chloramphenicol) | | | | |
| Chlortetracycline hydrochloride | 515 | 2 | 1.8 | 0.11 |
| Cocaine hydrochloride | 340 | 2 | 1.8 | 0.17 |
| Cyclogyl (See Cyclopentolate hydrochloride) | | | | |
| Cyclopentolate hydrochloride | 328 | 2 | 1.8 | 0.18 |
| Dextrose (anhydrous) | 180 | 1 | 1.0 | 0.18 |
| Dextrose. $H_2O$ | 198 | 1 | 1.0 | 0.16 |
| Dionin (See Ethylmorphine hydrochloride) | | | | |
| Ephedrine hydrochloride | 202 | 2 | 1.8 | 0.29 |
| Ephedrine sulfate | 429 | 3 | 2.6 | 0.20 |
| Epinephrine hydrochloride | 220 | 2 | 1.8 | 0.27 |
| Epinephrine bitartrate | 333 | 2 | 1.8 | 0.18 |
| Eserine salicylate (See Physostigmine salicylate) | | | | |
| Eserine sulfate (See Physostigmine sulfate) | | | | |
| Ethylmorphine hydrochloride. $2H_2O$ | 386 | 2 | 1.8 | 0.15 |
| Eucatropine hydrochloride | 328 | 2 | 1.8 | 0.22 |
| Fluorescein sodium | 376 | 3 | 2.6 | 0.22 |
| Glycerin | 92.1 | 1 | 1.0 | 0.36 |
| Holocaine hydrochloride (See Phenacaine hydrochloride) | | | | |
| Homatropine hydrobromide | 356 | 2 | 1.8 | 0.16 |
| Hydroxyamphetamine hydrobromide | 232 | 2 | 1.8 | 0.25 |
| Hyoscine hydrobromide (See Scopolamine hydrobromide) | | | | |
| Hyoscine hydrochloride (See Scopolamine hydrochloride) | | | | |
| Lidocaine hydrochloride | 289 | 2 | 1.8 | 0.22 |
| Metycaine hydrochloride | 298 | 2 | 1.8 | 0.20 |
| Morphine hydrochloride. $3H_2O$ | 376 | 2 | 1.8 | 0.16 |
| Morphine sulfate. $5H_2O$ | 759 | 3 | 2.6 | 0.11 |
| Naphazoline hydrochloride | 247 | 2 | 1.8 | 0.27 |
| Neo-synephrine hydrochloride (See Phenylephrine hydrochloride) | | | | |

TABLE OF SODIUM CHLORIDE EQUIVALENTS *Continued*

| *Substance* | *Molecular weight* | *Ions* | *i* | *Sodium chloride equivalent* |
|---|---|---|---|---|
| Nupercaine hydrochloride | 380 | 2 | 1.8 | 0.15 |
| Ophthaine (See Proparacaine hydrochloride) | | | | |
| Oxytetracycline hydrochloride | 497 | 2 | 1.8 | 0.12 |
| Paredrine (See Hydroxyamphetamine hydrobromide) | | | | |
| Phenacaine hydrochloride | 353 | 2 | 1.8 | 0.17 |
| Phenylephrine hydrochloride | 204 | 2 | 1.8 | 0.29 |
| Physostigmine salicylate | 413 | 2 | 1.8 | 0.14 |
| Physostigmine sulfate | 649 | 3 | 2.6 | 0.13 |
| Pilocarpine hydrochloride | 245 | 2 | 1.8 | 0.24 |
| Pilocarpine nitrate | 271 | 2 | 1.8 | 0.22 |
| Pontocaine hydrochloride (See Tetracaine hydrochloride) | | | | |
| Potassium biphosphate | 136 | 2 | 1.8 | 0.43 |
| Potassium chloride | 74.6 | 2 | 1.8 | 0.78 |
| Potassium iodide | 166 | 2 | 1.8 | 0.35 |
| Potassium nitrate | 101 | 2 | 1.8 | 0.58 |
| Potassium penicillin G | 372 | 2 | 1.8 | 0.16 |
| Privine hydrochloride (See Naphazoline hydrochloride) | | | | |
| Procaine hydrochloride | 273 | 2 | 1.8 | 0.21 |
| Proparacaine hydrochloride | 331 | 2 | 1.8 | 0.18 |
| Scopolamine hydrobromide.$3H_2O$ | 438 | 2 | 1.8 | 0.13 |
| Scopolamine hydrochloride.$2H_2O$ | 376 | 2 | 1.8 | 0.16 |
| Silver nitrate | 170 | 2 | 1.8 | 0.34 |
| Sodium bicarbonate | 84 | 2 | 1.8 | 0.70 |
| Sodium bisulfite | 104 | 3 | 2.6 | 0.81 |
| Sodium borate.$10H_2O$ | 381 | 5 | 4.2 | 0.36 |
| Sodium carbonate | 106 | 3 | 2.6 | 0.80 |
| Sodium carbonate.$H_2O$ | 124 | 3 | 2.6 | 0.68 |
| Sodium chloride | 58 | 2 | 1.8 | 1.00 |
| Sodium citrate.$2H_2O$ | 294 | 4 | 3.4 | 0.38 |
| Sodium iodide | 150 | 2 | 1.8 | 0.39 |
| Sodium lactate | 112 | 2 | 1.8 | 0.52 |
| Sodium nitrate | 85 | 2 | 1.8 | 0.69 |
| Sodium phosphate, dibasic, anhydrous | 142 | 3 | 2.6 | 0.53 |
| Sodium phosphate, dibasic.$7H_2O$ | 268 | 3 | 2.6 | 0.31 |
| Sodium phosphate, monobasic, anhydrous | 120 | 2 | 1.8 | 0.49 |
| Sodium phosphate, monobasic.$H_2O$ | 138 | 2 | 1.8 | 0.42 |
| Sodium sulfite | 126 | 3 | 2.6 | 0.64 |
| Terramycin (See Oxytetracycline hydrochloride) | | | | |
| Tetracaine hydrochloride | 301 | 2 | 1.8 | 0.19 |
| Tetracycline hydrochloride | 481 | 2 | 1.8 | 0.12 |
| Tetrahydrozoline hydrochloride | 237 | 2 | 1.8 | 0.25 |
| Tyzine (See Tetrahydrozoline hydrochloride) | | | | |
| Urea | 60.1 | 1 | 1.0 | 0.54 |
| Xylocaine hydrochloride (See Lidocaine hydrochloride) | | | | |
| Zephiran (See Benzalkonium chloride) | | | | |
| Zinc chloride | 136 | 3 | 2.6 | 0.62 |
| Zinc sulfate.$7H_2O$ | 288 | 2 | 1.4 | 0.16 |

## Practice Problems

1. Isotonic Sodium Chloride Solution contains 0.9% of sodium chloride. If the sodium chloride equivalent of boric acid is 0.52, what is the percentage strength of an isotonic solution of boric acid?

2. Sodium chloride is a 2-ion electrolyte, dissociating 90% in a certain concentration. Calculate (a) its dissociation factor and (b) the freezing point of a molal solution.

3. A solution of anhydrous dextrose (mol. wt. 180) contains 25 g in 500 mL of water. Calculate the freezing point of the solution.

4. Procaine hydrochloride (mol. wt. 273) is a 2-ion electrolyte, dissociating 80% in a certain concentration. (a) Calculate its dissociation factor. (b) Calculate its sodium chloride equivalent. (c) Calculate the freezing point of a molal solution of procaine hydrochloride.

5. The freezing point of a molal solution of a non-electrolyte is −1.86°C. What is the freezing point of an 0.1% solution of zinc chloride (mol. wt. 136), dissociating 80%?[1]

6. The freezing point of a 5% solution of boric acid is −1.55°C. How much boric acid should be used in preparing 1000 mL of an isotonic solution?

7. ℞ Ephedrine Sulfate gr iv
Sodium Chloride q.s.
Distilled Water ad ℥i
Make isoton. sol.
Sig. Use as directed.

How many grains of sodium chloride should be used in compounding the prescription?

8. ℞ Dionin ½%
Scopolamine Hydrobromide ⅓%
Sodium Chloride q.s.
Distilled Water ad 30.0
Make isoton. sol.
Sig. Use in the eye.

[1]For lack of more definite information, the student must assume that the volume of the molal solution is approximately 1 liter.

How much sodium chloride should be used in compounding the prescription?

9. ℞ Zinc Sulfate 0.06
Boric Acid q.s.
Distilled Water ad 30.0
Make isoton. sol.
Sig. Drop in eyes.

How much boric acid should be used in compounding the prescription?

10. ℞ Atropine Sulfate 1%
Boric Acid q.s.
Distilled Water ad 30.0
Make isoton. sol.
Sig. One drop in each eye.

How much boric acid should be used in compounding the prescription?

11. Dextrose, anhydrous 2.5%
Sodium Chloride q.s.
Sterile Water for Injection ad 1000 mL
Label: Isotonic Dextrose and Saline Solution.

How many grams of sodium chloride should be used in preparing the solution?

12. ℞ Sol. Silver Nitrate 15.0
0.5%
Make isoton. sol.
Sig. For the eyes.

How much sodium nitrate could be used to make the prescription isotonic?

13. ℞ Cocaine Hydrochloride 0.150
Sodium Chloride q.s.
Distilled Water ad 15.0
Make isoton. sol.
Sig. One drop in left eye.

How much sodium chloride should be used in compounding the prescription?

14. ℞

| | | |
|---|---|---|
| Cocaine Hydrochloride | | 0.6 |
| Eucatropine Hydrochloride | | 0.6 |
| Chlorobutanol | | 0.1 |
| Sodium Chloride | | q.s. |
| Distilled Water | ad | 30.0 |

Make isoton. sol.
Sig. For the eye.

How much sodium chloride should be used in compounding the prescription?

15. ℞

| | | |
|---|---|---|
| Tetracaine Hydrochloride | | 0.1 |
| Zinc Sulfate | | 0.05 |
| Boric Acid | | q.s. |
| Distilled Water | ad | 30.0 |

Make isoton. sol.
Sig. Drop in eye.

How much boric acid should be used in compounding the prescription?

16. ℞

| | |
|---|---|
| Sol. Homatropine Hydrobromide 1% | 15.0 |

Make isoton. sol. with boric acid.
Sig. For the eye.

How much boric acid should be used in compounding the prescription?

17. ℞

| | | |
|---|---|---|
| Procaine Hydrochloride | | 1% |
| Sodium Chloride | | q.s. |
| Sterile Distilled Water | ad | 100.0 |

Make isoton. sol.
Sig. For injection.

How much sodium chloride should be used in compounding the prescription?

18. ℞

| | | |
|---|---|---|
| Phenylephrine Hydrochloride | | 1.0 |
| Chlorobutanol | | 0.5 |
| Sodium Bisulfite | | 0.2 |
| Sodium Chloride | | q.s. |
| Distilled Water | ad | 100.0 |

Make isoton. sol.
Sig. Use as directed.

How many milliliters of an 0.9% solution of sodium chloride should be used in compounding the prescription?

19. ℞ Holocaine Hydrochloride ½%
Hyoscine Hydrobromide ⅓%
Boric Acid Solution q.s.
Distilled Water ad 60.0
Make isoton. sol.
Sig. For the eyes.

How many milliliters of a 5% solution of boric acid should be used in compounding the prescription?

20. ℞ Ephedrine Hydrochloride 0.5
Chlorobutanol 0.25
Dextrose q.s.
Rose Water ad 50.0
Make isoton. sol.
Sig. Nose drops.

How much dextrose should be used in compounding the prescription?

21. ℞ Dionin 5%
Sodium Chloride q.s.
Distilled Water ad ℥i
Make isoton. sol.
Sig. Use as directed in the eye.

How many grains of sodium chloride should be used in compounding the prescription?

22. ℞ Oxytetracycline Hydrochloride 0.050
Chlorobutanol 0.1
Sodium Chloride q.s.
Distilled Water ad 30.0
Make isoton. sol.
Sig. Eye drops.

How many milligrams of sodium chloride should be used in compounding the prescription?

23. ℞ Tetracaine Hydrochloride 0.5%
Sol. Epinephrine Hydrochloride 1:1000 10.0
Boric Acid q.s.
Distilled Water ad 30.0
Make isoton. sol.
Sig. Eye drops.

The solution of epinephrine hydrochloride (1:1000) is already isotonic. How much boric acid should be used in compounding the prescription?

24. Monobasic Sodium Phosphate, anhydrous 5.6 g
    Dibasic Sodium Phosphate, anhydrous 2.84 g
    Sodium Chloride q.s.
    Sterile Distilled Water ad 1000 mL
    Label: Isotonic Buffer Solution, pH 6.5.

How many grams of sodium chloride should be used in preparing the solution?

25. How many grams of anhydrous dextrose should be used in preparing 1 liter of a ½% isotonic ephedrine sulfate nasal spray?

26. ℞ Ephedrine Sulfate 1%
    Chlorobutanol ½%
    Distilled Water ad 100.0
    Make isoton. sol. and buffer to pH 6.5
    Sig. Nose drops.

You have on hand an isotonic buffered solution, pH 6.5. How many milliliters of distilled water and how many milliliters of the buffered solution should be used in compounding the prescription?

27. ℞ Oxytetracycline Hydrochloride 0.5%
    Tetracaine Hydrochloride Sol. 2% 15.0 mL
    Sodium Chloride q.s.
    Distilled Water ad 30.0 mL
    Make isoton. sol.
    Sig. For the eye.

The 2% solution of tetracaine hydrochloride is already isotonic. How many milliliters of an 0.9% solution of sodium chloride should be used in compounding the prescription?

# 13

# Electrolyte Solutions

As noted in Chapter 12, the molecules of chemical compounds in solution may remain intact, or they may dissociate into particles known as *ions* which carry an electric charge. Substances that are not dissociated in solution are called *non-electrolytes,* and those with varying degrees of dissociation are called *electrolytes.* Urea and dextrose are examples of non-electrolytes in the body water; sodium chloride in body fluids is an example of an electrolyte.

Sodium chloride in solution provides $Na^+$ and $Cl^-$ ions which carry electric charges. If electrodes carrying a weak current are placed in the solution, the ions move in a direction opposite to their charges. $Na^+$ ions move to the negative electrode (*cathode*) and are called *cations.* $Cl^-$ ions move to the positive electrode (*anode*) and hence are called *anions.*

Electrolyte ions in the blood plasma include the cations $Na^+$, $K^+$, $Ca^{++}$, and $Mg^{++}$ and the anions $Cl^-$, $HCO_3^-$, $HPO_4^{--}$, $SO_4^{--}$, organic acids$^-$, and protein$^-$. Electrolytes in body fluids play an important role in maintaining the acid-base balance in the body. They play a part, too, in controlling body water volumes, and they also help to regulate body metabolism.

*Electrolyte solutions* are liquid preparations used for the treatment of disturbances in the electrolyte and fluid balance of the body. The concentration of these solutions, like the concentration of body electrolytes, used to be commonly expressed in terms of different units, such as g per 100 mL, volumes %, and mg%. The term "mg%" refers to the number of mg per 100 mL and represents the older concept of measuring electrolytes in units of weight or *physical units.* However, this concept does not take into consideration chemical equivalence and, consequently, does not indicate the measurement of the chemical combining power of the electrolyte in solution. More significantly, it does not give any direct information as to the number of ions or the charges that they carry. Since the chemical combining power depends not only on the number of particles in solution but also on the total number of ionic charges, the valence of the ions in solution must be taken into consideration in order to make the measurement a meaningful one.

A *chemical unit,* the *milliequivalent,* is now used almost exclusively by clinicians, physicians, and manufacturers to express the concentration of electrolytes in solution. This unit of measure is related to the total number of ionic charges in solution, and it takes note of the valence of the ions. In other words, it is a unit of measurement of the amount of *chemical activity* of an electrolyte.

Under normal conditions blood plasma contains 155 milliequivalents of cations and an equal number of anions. The total concentration of cations always equals the total concentration of anions. Any number of milliequivalents of $Na^+$, $K^+$, or any cation$^+$ always reacts with precisely the same number of milliequivalents of $Cl^-$, $HCO_3^-$, or any anion$^-$.

In preparing a solution of $K^+$ ions, a potassium salt is dissolved in water. In addition to the $K^+$ ions, the solution will also contain ions of opposite negative charge. These two components will be chemically equal in that the milliequivalents of one are equal to the milliequivalents of the other. The interesting point is that if we dissolve enough potassium chloride in water to give us 40 milliequivalents of $K^+$ per liter, we also have exactly 40 milliequivalents of $Cl^-$, but the solution will *not* contain the *same weight* of each ion.

A *milliequivalent*, abbreviated mEq, represents the amount, in mg, of a solute equal to $\frac{1}{1000}$ of its gram equivalent weight.

**To convert the concentration of electrolytes in solution expressed as milliequivalents per unit volume to weight per unit volume:**

*Examples:*

*What is the concentration, in mg per mL, of a solution containing 2 mEq of potassium chloride (KCl) per mL?*

Molecular weight of KCl = 74.5

Equivalent weight of KCl = 74.5

1 mEq of KCl = $\frac{1}{1000}$ × 74.5 g = 0.0745 g = 74.5 mg

2 mEq of KCl = 74.5 mg × 2 = 149 mg per mL, *answer.*

*What is the concentration, in g per mL, of a solution containing 4 mEq of calcium chloride ($CaCl_2.2H_2O$) per mL?*

It should be recalled that the equivalent weight of a binary compound may be found by dividing the formula weight by the *total valence* of the positive or negative radical.

Formula weight of $CaCl_2.2H_2O$ = 147

Equivalent weight of $CaCl_2.2H_2O$ = $\frac{147}{2}$ = 73.5

1 mEq of $CaCl_2.2H_2O$ = $\frac{1}{1000}$ × 73.5 g = 0.0735 g

4 mEq of $CaCl_2.2H_2O$ = 0.0735 g × 4 = 0.294 g per mL, *answer.*

*What is the percent (w/v) concentration of a solution containing 100 mEq of ammonium chloride per liter?*

Molecular weight of $NH_4Cl$ = 53.5

Equivalent weight of $NH_4Cl$ = 53.5

1 mEq of $NH_4Cl$ = $\frac{1}{1000} \times 53.5$ = 0.0535 g

100 mEq of $NH_4Cl$ = 0.0535 g × 100 = 5.35 g per liter
or 0.535 g per 100 mL, or 0.535%, *answer.*

**To convert the concentration of electrolytes in solution expressed as milligrams percent to milliequivalents per liter:**

*Examples:*

*A solution contains 10 mg% of $K^+$ ions. Express this concentration in terms of mEq per liter.*

Atomic weight of $K^+$ = 39

Equivalent weight of $K^+$ = 39

1 mEq of $K^+$ = $\frac{1}{1000} \times 39$ g = 0.039 g = 39 mg

10 mg% of $K^+$ = 10 mg of $K^+$ per 100 mL or
100 mg of $K^+$ per liter

100 mg ÷ 39 = 2.56 mEq per liter, *answer.*

*A solution contains 10 mg% of $Ca^{++}$ ions. Express this concentration in terms of mEq per liter.*

Atomic weight of $Ca^{++}$ = 40

Equivalent weight of $Ca^{++}$ = $\frac{40}{2}$ = 20

1 mEq of $Ca^{++}$ = $\frac{1}{1000} \times 20$ g = 0.020 g = 20 mg

10 mg% of $Ca^{++}$ = 10 mg of $Ca^{++}$ per 100 mL or
100 mg of $Ca^{++}$ per liter

100 mg ÷ 20 = 5 mEq per liter, *answer.*

**To convert the concentration of electrolytes in solution expressed as milliequivalents per liter to milligrams percent:**

*Example:*

*The normal magnesium ($Mg^{++}$) level in blood plasma is 2.5 mEq per liter. Express this concentration in terms of milligrams percent.*

Atomic weight of $Mg^{++} = 24$

Equivalent weight of $Mg^{++} = {}^{24}\!/_{2} = 12$

1 mEq of $Mg^{++} = {}^{1}\!/_{1000} \times 12\ g = 0.012\ g = 12\ mg$

2.5 mEq of $Mg^{++} = 30\ mg$

30 mg per liter or 3 mg per 100 mL = 3 mg%, *answer.*

**To convert the weight of an electrolyte to milliequivalents:**

*Examples:*

*How many milliequivalents of potassium chloride are represented in a 15-mL dose of a 10% (w/v) potassium chloride elixir?*

Molecular weight of KCl = 74.5

Equivalent weight of KCl = 74.5

1 mEq of KCl = ${}^{1}\!/_{1000} \times 74.5\ g = 0.0745\ g = 74.5\ mg$

15-mL dose of 10% (w/v) elixir = 1.5 g or 1500 mg of KCl

$$\frac{74.5\ (mg)}{1500\ (mg)} = \frac{1\ (mEq)}{x\ (mEq)}$$

x = 20.1 mEq, *answer.*

*How many milliequivalents of magnesium sulfate are represented in 1.0 g of anhydrous magnesium sulfate ($MgSO_4$)?*

Molecular weight of $MgSO_4 = 120$

Equivalent weight of $MgSO_4 = 60$

1 mEq of $MgSO_4 = {}^{1}\!/_{1000} \times 60\ g = 0.060\ g = 60\ mg$

1.0 g of $MgSO_4 = 1000\ mg$

$$\frac{60\ (mg)}{1000\ (mg)} = \frac{1\ (mEq)}{x\ (mEq)}$$

x = 16.7 mEq, *answer.*

**To calculate the amount of electrolyte or its solution in given concentration to provide a specified milliequivalent level:**

*Example:*

*A person is to receive 2 mEq of sodium chloride per kilogram of body weight. If the person weighs 132 lb, how many milliliters of an 0.9% sterile solution of sodium chloride should be administered?*

Molecular weight of NaCl = 58.5

Equivalent weight of NaCl = 58.5

1 mEq of NaCl = $\frac{1}{1000} \times 58.5$ g = 0.0585 g

2 mEq of NaCl = 0.0585 g × 2 = 0.117 g

1 kg = 2.2 lb   Weight of person in kg = $\frac{132 \text{ lb}}{2.2 \text{ lb}}$ = 60 kg

Since the person is to receive 2 mEq per kg,

then 2 mEq or 0.117 g × 60 = 7.02 g of NaCl needed

and since 0.9% sterile solution of sodium chloride contains 9.0 g of NaCl per liter,

then

$$\frac{9.0 \text{ (g)}}{7.02 \text{ (g)}} = \frac{1000 \text{ (mL)}}{x \text{ (mL)}}$$

x = 780 mL, *answer.*

## OSMOTIC ACTIVITY

Electrolytes play their part in controlling body water volumes by establishing osmotic pressure. This pressure is proportional to the *total number* of particles in solution. The unit that is used to measure *osmotic concentration* is the *milliosmole,* abbreviated mOsmol. For dextrose, a nonelectrolyte, 1 millimole (1 formula weight in mg) represents 1 milliosmole. However, this relationship is not the same with electrolytes, since the total number of particles in solution depends upon the degree of dissociation of the substance in question. Assuming complete dissociation, 1 millimole of NaCl represents 2 milliosmoles ($Na^+$ + $Cl^-$) of total particles, and 1 millimole of $CaCl_2$ represents 3 milliosmoles ($Ca^{++}$ + $2Cl^-$) of total particles.

The milliosmolar value of *separate* ions of an electrolyte may be obtained by dividing the concentration, in mg per liter, of the ion by its atomic weight; but the milliosmolar value of the *whole* electrolyte in solution is equal to the sum of the milliosmolar values of the separate ions.

**To calculate milliosmolar values:**

*Examples:*

*A solution contains 5% of anhydrous dextrose in water for injection. How many milliosmoles per liter are represented by this concentration?*

Formula weight of anhydrous dextrose = 180

1 millimole of anhydrous dextrose (180 mg) = 1 milliosmole

5% solution contains 50 g or 50000 mg per liter

50000 mg ÷ 180 = 278 mOsmol per liter, *answer.*

*A solution contains 156 mg of $K^+$ ions per 100 mL. How many milliosmoles are represented in a liter of the solution?*

Atomic weight of $K^+$ = 39

1 millimole of $K^+$ (39 mg) = 1 milliosmole

156 mg of $K^+$ per 100 mL = 1560 mg of $K^+$ per liter

1560 mg ÷ 39 = 40 mOsmol, *answer.*

*A solution contains 10 mg% of $Ca^{++}$ ions. How many milliosmoles are represented in 1 liter of the solution?*

Atomic weight of $Ca^{++}$ = 40

1 millimole of $Ca^{++}$ (40 mg) = 1 milliosmole

10 mg% of $Ca^{++}$ = 10 mg of $Ca^{++}$ per 100 mL or 100 mg of $Ca^{++}$ per liter.

100 mg ÷ 40 = 2.5 mOsmol, *answer.*

*How many milliosmoles are represented in a liter of an 0.9% sodium chloride solution?*

Osmotic concentration (in terms of milliosmoles) is a function of the total number of particles present.

Assuming complete dissociation, 1 millimole of sodium chloride (NaCl) represents 2 milliosmoles of total particles ($Na^+$ + $Cl^-$).

Formula weight of NaCl = 58.5

1 millimole of NaCl (58.5 mg) = 2 milliosmoles

$$1000 \times 0.009 = 9 \text{ g or } 9000 \text{ mg of NaCl per liter}$$

$$\frac{58.5 \text{ (mg)}}{9000 \text{ (mg)}} = \frac{2 \text{ (milliosmoles)}}{x \text{ (milliosmoles)}}$$

x = 307.7, or 308 mOsmol, *answer.*

**VALUES FOR SOME IMPORTANT IONS**

| *Ion* | *Formula* | *Valence* | *Atomic or Formula Weight* | *Milliequivalent Weight (mg)* |
|---|---|---|---|---|
| Sodium | $Na^+$ | 1 | 23 | 23 |
| Potassium | $K^+$ | 1 | 39 | 39 |
| Calcium | $Ca^{++}$ | 2 | 40 | 20 |
| Magnesium | $Mg^{++}$ | 2 | 24 | 12 |
| Ammonium | $NH_4^+$ | 1 | 18 | 18 |
| Lithium | $Li^+$ | 1 | 7 | 7 |
| Chloride | $Cl^-$ | 1 | 35.5 | 35.5 |
| Bicarbonate | $HCO_3^-$ | 1 | 61 | 61 |
| Sulfate | $SO_4^{--}$ | 2 | 96 | 48 |
| Carbonate | $CO_3^{--}$ | 2 | 60 | 30 |
| Phosphate | $H_2PO_4^-$ | 1 | 97 | 97 |
| | $HPO_4^{--}$ | 2 | 96 | 48 |
| Acetate | $C_2H_3O_2^-$ | 1 | 59 | 59 |
| Citrate | $C_6H_5O_7^{---}$ | 3 | 189 | 63 |
| Gluconate | $C_6H_{11}O_7^-$ | 1 | 195 | 195 |
| Lactate | $C_3H_5O_3^-$ | 1 | 89 | 89 |

## Practice Problems

1. What is the concentration, in mg per mL, of a solution containing 5 mEq of potassium chloride (KCl) per mL?

2. A solution contains 298 mg of potassium chloride (KCl) per mL. Express this concentration in terms of milliequivalents of potassium chloride.

3. A 10-mL ampul of potassium chloride contains 2.98 g of potassium chloride (KCl). What is the concentration of the solution in terms of mEq per mL?

4. A person is to receive 36 mg of ammonium chloride per kg of body weight. If the person weighs 154 lb, how many milliliters of a sterile solution of ammonium chloride ($NH_4Cl$—mol. wt. 53.5) containing 0.4 mEq per mL should be administered?

5. A sterile solution of potassium chloride (KCl) contains 2 mEq per mL. If a 20-mL ampul of the solution is diluted to a liter with sterile distilled water, what is the percentage strength of the resulting solution?

6. A certain electrolyte solution contains, as one of the ingredients, the equivalent of 4.6 mEq of calcium per liter. How many grams of calcium chloride ($CaCl_2.2H_2O$—mol. wt. 147) should be used in preparing 20 liters of the solution?

7. Sterile solutions of ammonium chloride containing 21.4 mg per mL are available commercially in 500- and 1000-mL intravenous infusion containers. Calculate the amount, in terms of milliequivalents, of ammonium chloride ($NH_4Cl$—mol. wt. 53.5) in the 500-mL container.

8. A solution contains, in each 5 mL, 0.5 g of potassium acetate ($C_2H_3KO_2$—mol. wt. 98), 0.5 g of potassium bicarbonate ($KHCO_3$—mol. wt. 100), and 0.5 g of potassium citrate ($C_6H_5K_3O_7.H_2O$—mol. wt. 324). How many mEq of potassium ($K^+$) are represented in each 5 mL of the solution?

9. How many grams of sodium chloride (NaCl) should be used in preparing 20 liters of a solution containing 154 mEq per liter?

10. Sterile solutions of potassium chloride (KCl) containing 5 mEq per mL are available in 20-mL containers. Calculate the amount, in grams, of potassium chloride in the container.

11. How many milliliters of a solution containing 2 mEq of potassium chloride (KCl) per mL should be used to obtain 2.98 g of potassium chloride?

12. A patient is to be given 1 g of sodium methicillin ($C_{17}H_{19}NaO_6S.H_2O$—mol. wt. 420) every six hours for 5 doses. How many mEq of sodium are represented in the prescribed amount of sodium methicillin?

13. A 40-mL vial of a sodium chloride solution was diluted to a liter with sterile distilled water. The concentration (w/v) of sodium chloride (NaCl) in the finished product was 0.585%. What was the concentration, in mEq per mL, of the original solution?

14. How many grams of sodium bicarbonate ($NaHCO_3$—mol. wt. 84) should be used in preparing a liter of a solution to contain 44.6 mEq per 50 mL?

15. A solution contains 20 mg% of $Ca^{++}$ ions. Express this concentration in terms of mEq per liter.

16. Sterile sodium lactate solution is available commercially as a ⅙-molar solution of sodium lactate in water for injection. How many mEq of sodium lactate ($C_3H_5NaO_3$—mol. wt. 112) would be provided by a liter of the solution?

17. A solution contains 322 mg of $Na^+$ ions per liter. How many milliosmoles are represented in the solution?

18. A certain electrolyte solution contains 0.9% of sodium chloride in 10% dextrose solution. (a) Express the concentration of sodium chloride (NaCl) in terms of mEq per liter. (b) How many milliosmoles of dextrose are represented in 1 liter of the solution?

19. ℞ Potassium Chloride 10%
Cherry Syrup q.s. ad 480 mL
Sig. Tablespoonful b.i.d.

How many milliequivalents of potassium chloride are represented in each prescribed dose?

20. How many milliequivalents of potassium are there in 5 million units of Penicillin V Potassium ($C_{16}H_{17}KN_2O_6S$—mol. wt. 388)? One mg of Penicillin V Potassium represents 1380 Penicillin V Units.

21. The normal potassium level in the blood plasma is 17 mg%. Express this concentration in terms of mEq per liter.

22. How many grams of potassium citrate ($C_6H_5K_3O_7$-$H_2O$—mol. wt. 324) should be used in preparing 500 mL of a potassium ion elixir so as to supply 15 mEq of $K^+$ in each 5-mL dose?

23. A potassium supplement tablet contains 2.5 g of potassium bicarbonate ($KHCO_3$—mol. wt. 100). How many milliequivalents of potassium ($K^+$) are supplied by the tablet?

24. Ringer's Injection contains 0.86% of sodium chloride, 0.03% of potassium chloride, and 0.033% of calcium chloride. How many milliequivalents of each chloride are contained in 1 liter of the injection?

25. Calculate the sodium ($Na^+$) content, in terms of milliequivalents, of 1 g of ampicillin sodium ($C_{16}H_{18}N_3NaO_4S$—mol. wt. 371).

26. A 20-mL vial of a concentrated ammonium chloride solution containing 5 mEq per mL is diluted to a liter with sterile distilled water. Calculate (a) the total mEq value of the ammonium ion in the dilution and (b) the percentage strength of the dilution.

27. Ringer's Solution contains 0.33 g of calcium chloride per liter. (a) Express the concentration in terms of mEq of calcium chloride per liter. (b) How many milliosmoles of calcium are represented in each liter of the solution?

28. How many milliosmoles of sodium chloride are represented in 1 liter of 3% hypertonic sodium chloride solution? Assume complete dissociation.

29. A solution of sodium chloride contains 77 mEq per liter. Calculate its osmolar strength in terms of milliosmoles per liter. Assume complete dissociation.

30. How many milliequivalents of potassium would be supplied daily by the usual dose (0.3 mL three times a day) of saturated potassium iodide solution? Saturated potassium iodide solution contains 100 g of potassium iodide per 100 mL.

31. Calculate the osmolar concentration, in terms of milliosmoles, represented by a liter of a 10% (w/v) solution of anhydrous dextrose (mol. wt. 180) in water.

32. A hyperalimentation formula calls for the addition of 25 mEq of sodium bicarbonate. How many milliliters of 8.4% (w/v) sodium bicarbonate injection should be added to the formula?

33. Calcium gluconate ($C_{12}H_{22}CaO_{14}$—mol. wt. 430) injection 10% is available in a 10-mL ampul. How many milliequivalents of $Ca^{++}$ does the ampul contain?

34. A flavored potassium chloride packet contains 1.5 g of potassium chloride. How many milliequivalents of potassium chloride are represented in each packet?

35. How many milliequivalents of $Li^{+}$ are provided by a daily dose of four 300-mg tablets of lithium carbonate ($Li_2CO_3$—mol. wt. 74)?

36. How many milliequivalents of ammonium ($NH_4^{+}$) ion are contained in a liter of 4.2% (w/v) solution of ammonium chloride?

37. A patient is to receive 10 mEq of potassium gluconate ($C_6H_{11}KO_7$—mol. wt. 234) four times a day for 3 days. If the dose is to be a teaspoonful in a cherry syrup vehicle, (a) how many grams of potassium gluconate should be used and (b) what volume, in milliliters, should be dispensed to provide the prescribed dosage regimen?

38. A physician wishes to administer 1,200,000 units of penicillin G potassium every 4 hours. If 1 unit of penicillin G potassium ($C_{16}H_{17}KN_2O_4S$—mol. wt. 372) equals 0.6 μg, how many milliequivalents of $K^{+}$ will the patient receive in a 24-hour period?

39. Five (5) mL of lithium citrate syrup contain the equivalent of 8 mEq of $Li^{+}$. Calculate the equivalent, in terms of milligrams, of lithium carbonate ($Li_2CO_3$—mol. wt. 74) in each 5-mL dose of the syrup.

40. How many milligrams of magnesium sulfate ($MgSO_4$—mol. wt. 120) should be added to an intravenous solution to provide 5 mEq of $Mg^{++}$ per liter?

41. A slow-release potassium chloride tablet is stated by its manufac-

turer to contain 600 mg of potassium chloride in a wax matrix. How many milliequivalents of potassium chloride are supplied by a dosage of one tablet three times a day?

42. An electrolyte solution contains 222 mg of sodium acetate ($C_2H_3NaO_2$—mol. wt. 82) and 15 mg of magnesium chloride ($MgCl_2$—mol. wt. 95) in each 100 mL. Express these concentrations in terms of milliequivalents of $Na^+$ and $Mg^{++}$ per liter.

43. Ammonium chloride ($NH_4Cl$—mol. wt. 53.5) is to be used as a urinary acidifier with a dose of 150 mEq. How many 500-mg tablets should be administered?

44. A patient has a sodium deficit of 168 mEq. How many milliliters of isotonic sodium chloride solution (0.9% w/v) should be administered to replace the deficit?

45. A normal 70 kg (154 lb) adult has 80 to 100 g of sodium. It is primarily distributed in the extracellular fluid. Body retention of 1 g additional of sodium results in excess body water accumulation of approximately 310 mL. If a person retains 100 mEq of extra sodium, how many milliliters of additional water could be expected to be retained?

46. A patient receives 3 liters of an electrolyte fluid containing 234 mg of sodium chloride ($NaCl$—58.5), 125 mg of potassium acetate ($C_2H_3KO_2$—mol. wt. 98), and 21 mg of magnesium acetate ($C_4H_6MgO_4$—mol. wt. 142) per 100 mL. How many milliequivalents each of $Na^+$, $K^+$, and $Mg^{++}$ does the patient receive?

47. How many milliliters of a 2% (w/v) solution of ammonium chloride ($NH_4Cl$—mol. wt. 53.5) should be administered intravenously to a patient to provide 75 mEq?

# 14

# Some Calculations Involving Parenteral Admixtures

The preparation of parenteral admixtures usually involves the addition of one or more drugs to large volume solutions such as intravenous and nutrient fluids. The administration or infusion of large amounts of fluids containing basic nutrients sufficient to achieve active tissue synthesis and growth is referred to as *parenteral hyperalimentation.* Nutrient fluids are often designated as *TPN* solutions because they are intended to provide *total parenteral nutrition.*

## ADDITIVES

Although a wide variety of drugs and drug combinations have been used in preparing dilute infusions for intravenous therapy and in formulating hyperalimentation solutions, some of the more commonly used additives include electrolytes, antibiotics, vitamins, trace minerals, heparin, and in some instances insulin.

In any properly administered parenteral admixture program, all basic fluids (large volume solutions), additives (already in solution or extemporaneously reconstituted), and *calculations* must be very carefully checked against the medication orders. The discussion which follows concerns itself *solely* with some calculations that may be encountered in the extemporaneous preparation of typical parenteral admixtures.

**To calculate the amount of additive(s) to be admixed with a large volume intravenous or nutrient fluid to produce an infusion containing a required quantity of a drug or combination of drugs:**

*Examples:*

*A medication order for a patient weighing 154 lb calls for 0.25 mg of amphotericin B per kg of body weight to be added to 500 mL of 5% dextrose injection. If the amphotericin B is to be obtained from a reconstituted injection that contains 50 mg per 10 mL, how many milliliters should be added to the dextrose injection?*

$$1 \text{ kg} = 2.2 \text{ lb}$$

$$\frac{154 \text{ (lb)}}{2.2 \text{ (lb)}} = 70 \text{ kg}$$

$$0.25 \text{ mg} \times 70 = 17.5 \text{ mg}$$

Reconstituted solution contains 50 mg per 10 mL

$$\frac{50 \text{ (mg)}}{17.5 \text{ (mg)}} = \frac{10 \text{ (mL)}}{\text{x (mL)}}$$

x = 3.5 mL, *answer.*

*An intravenous infusion is to contain 15 mEq of potassium ion and 20 mEq of sodium ion in 500 mL of 5% dextrose injection. Using an injection of potassium chloride containing 6 g per 30 mL and 0.9% injection of sodium chloride, how many milliliters of each should be used to supply the required ions?*

15 mEq of $K^+$ ion will be supplied by 15 mEq of KCl

and 20 mEq of $Na^+$ ion will be supplied by 20 mEq of NaCl

1 mEq of KCl = 74.5 mg

15 mEq of KCl = 1117.5 mg or 1.118 g

$$\frac{6 \text{ (g)}}{1.118 \text{ (g)}} = \frac{30 \text{ (mL)}}{\text{x (mL)}}$$

x = 5.59 or 5.6 mL, *and*

1 mEq of NaCl = 58.5 mg

20 mEq of NaCl = 1170 mg or 1.170 g

$$\frac{0.9 \text{ (g)}}{1.17 \text{ (g)}} = \frac{100 \text{ (mL)}}{\text{x (mL)}}$$

x = 130 mL, *answers.*

*A medication order for a child weighing 44 lb calls for polymyxin B sulfate to be administered by the intravenous drip method in a dosage of 7500 units per kg of body weight in 500 mL of 5% dextrose injection. Using a vial containing 500,000 units of polymyxin B sulfate and sodium chloride injection as the solvent, explain how you would obtain the polymyxin B sulfate needed in preparing the infusion.*

$$1 \text{ kg} = 2.2 \text{ lb}$$

$$\frac{44}{2.2} = 20 \text{ kg}$$

$$7500 \text{ units} \times 20 = 150{,}000 \text{ units}$$

*Step 1.* Dissolve contents of vial (500,000 units) in 10 mL of sodium chloride injection.

*Step 2.* Add 3 mL of reconstituted solution to 500 mL of 5% dextrose injection, *answer.*

## HYPERALIMENTATION SOLUTIONS

**To calculate the amount of component source(s) to be added to or admixed with a large volume intravenous or nutrient fluid to provide the required amount of additive(s) specified in a medication order:**

*Examples:*

*The following is a formula for a desired hyperalimentation solution. Using the source of each drug as indicated, calculate the amount of each component required in preparing the solution.*

| Hyperalimentation Solution Formula | Component Source |
|---|---|
| *(a)* Sodium Chloride 35 mEq | Vial, 5 mEq per 2 mL |
| *(b)* Potassium Acetate 35 mEq | Vial, 10 mEq per 5 mL |
| *(c)* Magnesium Sulfate 8 mEq | Vial, 4 mEq per mL |
| *(d)* Calcium Gluconate 9.6 mEq | Vial, 4.7 mEq per 10 mL |
| *(e)* Potassium Chloride 5 mEq | Vial, 40 mEq per 20 mL |
| *(f)* Folic Acid 1.7 mg | Ampul, 5 mg per mL |
| *(g)* Multiple Vitamin Infusion 10 mL | Ampul, 10 mL |
| To be added to: | |
| Amino Acids Infusion (8.5%) | 500 mL |
| Dextrose Injection (50%) | 500 mL |

(a) $$\frac{5 \text{ (mEq)}}{35 \text{ (mEq)}} = \frac{2 \text{ (mL)}}{x \text{ (mL)}}$$

x = 14 mL, *and*

(b) $$\frac{10 \text{ (mEq)}}{35 \text{ (mEq)}} = \frac{5 \text{ (mL)}}{x \text{ (mL)}}$$

x = 17.5 mL, *and*

(c) $$\frac{4 \text{ (mEq)}}{8 \text{ (mEq)}} = \frac{1 \text{ (mL)}}{x \text{ (mL)}}$$

x = 2 mL, *and*

(d) $$\frac{4.7 \text{ (mEq)}}{9.6 \text{ (mEq)}} = \frac{10 \text{ (mL)}}{x \text{ (mL)}}$$

x = 20.4 mL, *and*

(e) $$\frac{40 \text{ (mEq)}}{5 \text{ (mEq)}} = \frac{20 \text{ (mL)}}{x \text{ (mL)}}$$

x = 2.5 mL, *and*

(f) $$\frac{5 \text{ (mg)}}{1.7 \text{ (mg)}} = \frac{1 \text{ (mL)}}{x \text{ (mL)}}$$

x = 0.34 mL, *and*

(g) 10 mL, *answers.*

*The formula for a TPN solution calls for the addition of 2.7 mEq of $Ca^{++}$ and 20 mEq of $K^{+}$ per liter. How many milliliters of an injection containing 20 mg of calcium chloride per mL and how many milliliters of a 15% (w/v) potassium chloride injection should be used to provide the desired additives?*

1 mEq of $Ca^{++}$ = 20 mg

2.7 mEq of $Ca^{++}$ = 20 mg × 2.7 = 54 mg

54 mg of $Ca^{++}$ are furnished by 198.45 or 198 mg of calcium chloride

Since the injection contains 20 mg of calcium chloride per mL, then $198 \div 20 = 9.9$ mL, *and*

$$1 \text{ mEq of } K^+ = 39 \text{ mg}$$

$$20 \text{ mEq of } K^+ = 39 \text{ mg} \times 20 = 780 \text{ mg}$$

780 mg of $K^+$ are furnished by 1.49 g of potassium chloride

15% (w/v) solution contains 15 g of potassium chloride per 100 mL

then
$$\frac{15 \text{ (g)}}{1.49 \text{ (g)}} = \frac{100 \text{ (mL)}}{x \text{ (mL)}}$$

$x = 9.9$ mL, *answers.*

*A potassium phosphate injection contains a mixture of 224 mg of monobasic potassium phosphate ($KH_2PO_4$) and 236 mg of dibasic potassium phosphate ($K_2HPO_4$) per mL. If 10 mL of the injection are added to 500 mL of $D_5W$ (5% dextrose in water for injection), (a) how many milliequivalents of $K^+$ and (b) how many millimoles of total phosphate are represented in the prepared solution?*

Formula weight of $KH_2PO_4 = 136$

1 millimole (mmol) of $KH_2PO_4 = 136$ mg

10 mL of injection contain 2240 mg of $KH_2PO_4$

and thus provide $2240 \div 136 = 16.4$ or 16 mmol of $KH_2PO_4$

or 16 mmol of $K^+$ and 16 mmol of $H_2PO_4^{--}$

Formula weight of $K_2HPO_4 = 174$

1 millimole (mmol) of $K_2HPO_4 = 174$ mg

10 mL of injection contain 2360 mg of $K_2HPO_4$

and thus provide $2360 \div 174 = 13.6$ or 14 mmol of $K_2HPO_4$

or 14 (mmol) $\times$ 2 ($K^+$) = 28 mmol of $K^+$, and 14 mmol of $HPO_4^{--}$

thus 10 ml of injection provide a total of:

44 mmol of $K^+$ or (since the valence of $K^+$ is 1) 44 mEq of $K^+$,

*and*

30 mmol of total phosphate, *answers.*

## RATE OF FLOW OF INTRAVENOUS FLUIDS

It should be clearly understood that the physician specifies the rate of flow of intravenous fluids in mL per minute, drops per minute, or more frequently, as the approximate time of administration of the total volume of the infusion. In the latter instance, the pharmacist may be requested to make or to check the calculations involved in converting the desired total time interval into a flow rate of drops per minute.

**To calculate the rate of flow needed to administer a large volume intravenous fluid during a desired time interval:**

*Examples:*

*A medication order calls for 1000 mL of $D_5W$ to be administered over an 8-hour period. Using an IV administration set which delivers 10 drops per mL, how many drops per minute should be delivered to the patient?*

Volume of fluid = 1000 mL

8 hours = 480 minutes

$$\frac{1000\ (\text{mL})}{480\ (\text{min})} = 2.1 \text{ mL per minute}$$

2.1 mL/min × 10 (drops per mL) = 21 drops per minute, *answer.*

*Ten (10) mL of 10% calcium gluconate injection and 10 mL of multivitamin infusion are mixed with 500 mL of a 5% dextrose injection. The infusion is to be administered over a period of five hours. If the dropper in the venoclysis set calibrates 15 drops per mL, at what rate, in drops per minute, should the flow be adjusted in order to administer the infusion over the desired time interval?*

Total volume of infusion =

10 mL + 10 mL + 500 mL = 520 mL

Dropper calibrates 15 drops per mL

520 × 15 drops = 7800 drops

$$\frac{7800\ (\text{drops})}{300\ (\text{minutes})} = 26 \text{ drops per minute, } \textit{answer.}$$

*An intravenous infusion contains 10 mL of a 1:5000 solution of isoproterenol hydrochloride and 500 mL of a 5% dextrose injection. At what flow rate should the infusion be administered to provide 5 μg of isopro-*

*terenol hydrochloride per minute and what time interval will be necessary for the administration of the entire infusion?*

10 mL of a 1:5000 solution contain 2 mg

2 mg or 2000 μg are contained in a volume of 510 mL

$$\frac{2000\ (\mu g)}{5\ (\mu g)} = \frac{510\ (mL)}{x\ (mL)}$$

$$x = 1.275 \text{ or } 1.28 \text{ mL per minute, } \textit{and}$$

$$\frac{1.28\ (mL)}{510\ (mL)} = \frac{1\ (minute)}{x\ (minutes)}$$

$$x = 398 \text{ minutes or approx. } 6\tfrac{1}{2} \text{ hours, } \textit{answers.}$$

RATE OF FLOW vs. QUANTITY OF INFUSION SOLUTION vs. TIME
Taken from Scientific Tables, 7th ed. p. 529, Ciba-Geigy Limited, Basle

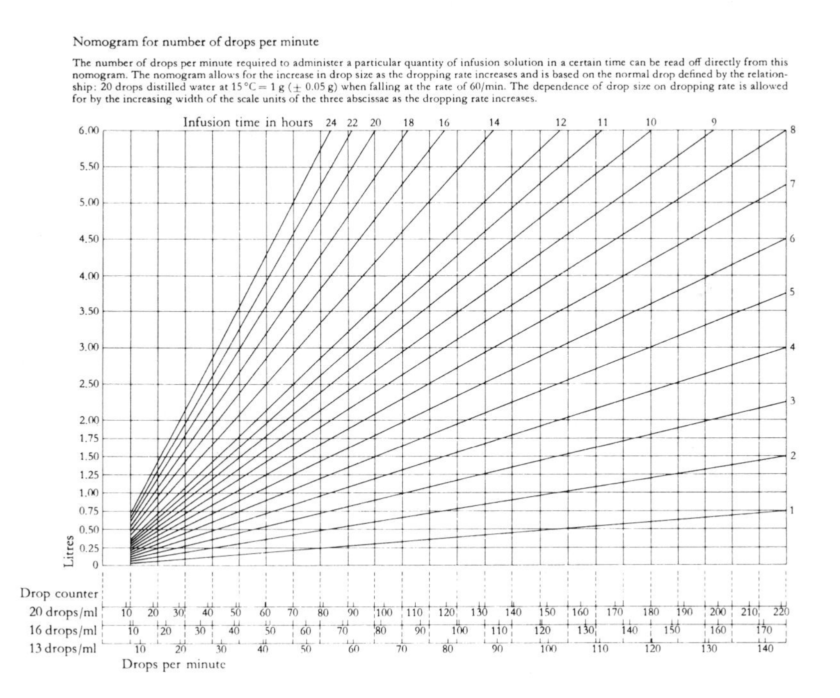


Reproduced from *Documenta Geigy* Scientific Tables. 8th Edition. With kind permission of Ciba-Geigy Limited, Basle (Switzerland).

## Practice Problems

1. A medication order for an intravenous infusion for a patient weighing 110 lb calls for 0.3 mEq of ammonium chloride per kg of body

weight to be added to 500 mL of 5% dextrose injection. How many milliliters of a sterile solution containing 100 mEq of ammonium chloride per 20 mL should be used in preparing the infusion?

2. An intravenous infusion for a child weighing 60 lb is to contain 20 mg of vancomycin hydrochloride per kg of body weight in 200 mL of sodium chloride injection. Using a 10-mL vial containing 500 mg of vancomycin hydrochloride (dry powder), explain how you would obtain the amount needed in preparing the infusion.

3. An intravenous infusion for a patient weighing 132 lb calls for 7.5 mg of kanamycin sulfate per kg of body weight to be added to 250 mL of 5% dextrose injection. How many milliliters of a kanamycin sulfate injection containing 500 mg per 2 mL should be used in preparing the infusion?

4. A medication order calls for a liter of hyperalimentation solution to contain 2.125% of amino acids and 20% of dextrose. How many milliliters each of 8.5% amino acids injection, 50% dextrose injection, and sterile water for injection should be used to prepare the solution?

5. A physician orders a 2-g vial of cephalothin sodium to be added to 500 mL of $D_5W$ (5% dextrose in water for injection). If the administration rate is 125 mL per hour, how many milligrams of cephalothin sodium will a patient receive per minute?

6. A certain hyperalimentation fluid measures 1 liter. If the solution is to be administered over a period of 6 hours and if the administration set is calibrated at 25 drops per mL, at what rate should the set be adjusted to administer the solution during the designated time interval?

7. A physician orders 35 mg of amphotericin B and 25 units of heparin to be administered intravenously in 1000 mL of $D_5W$ over an 8-hour period to a hospitalized patient. In filling the medication order, the available sources of the additives are a vial containing 50 mg of amphotericin B in 10 mL and a syringe containing 10 units of heparin per mL. *(a)* How many milliliters of each additive should be used in filling the medication order? *(b)* How many milliliters of the intravenous fluid per minute should the patient receive in order that the fluid be administered over the designated time interval?

8. A reconstituted solution containing 500,000 units of polymyxin B sulfate in 10 mL of water for injection is added to 250 mL of 5% dextrose injection. The infusion is to be administered over a period of two hours. If the dropper in the venoclysis set calibrates 15 drops per mL, at what rate, in drops per minute, should the flow be adjusted in order to administer the infusion over the designated time interval?

9. Five hundred (500) mL of a 2% sterile solution of ammonium

chloride are to be administered by intravenous infusion over a period of four hours. If the dropper in the venoclysis set calibrates 20 drops per mL, at what rate, in drops per minute, should the flow be adjusted in order to administer the infusion over the desired time interval?

10. A liter of a 0.3% intravenous infusion of potassium chloride is to be administered over a period of four hours. (a) How many milliequivalents of potassium are represented in the infusion? (b) If the dropper in the venoclysis set calibrates 20 drops per mL, calculate the rate of flow, in drops per minute, needed to administer the infusion over the desired time interval.

11. Five hundred (500) mL of an intravenous solution contain 0.2% of succinylcholine chloride in sodium chloride injection. At what flow rate should the infusion be administered to provide 2.5 mg of succinylcholine chloride per minute?

12. A physician orders 2 g of an antibiotic to be placed in 1000 mL of $D_5W$. Using a reconstituted injection which contains 300 mg of the antibiotic per 2 mL, how many milliliters should be added to the dextrose solution in filling the medication order?

13. A physician orders 750 mg of chloramphenicol to be added to 100 mL of sterile sodium chloride solution and infused into a patient over a period of 6 hours. Using a reconstituted injection which contains the equivalent of 1 g of chloramphenicol per 10 mL, how many milliliters should be added to the sterile sodium chloride solution?

14. A medication order for a TPN solution calls for additives as indicated in the following formula. Using the sources designated below, calculate the amount of each component required in filling the medication order.

| TPN Solution Formula | Component Source |
|---|---|
| Sodium Chloride 40 mEq | 10-mL vial of 30% solution |
| Potassium Acetate 15 mEq | 20-mL vial containing 40 mEq |
| Vitamin $B_{12}$ 10 μg | vial containing 1 mg in 10 mL |
| Insulin 8 units | vial of Insulin U-100 |

To be added to:

500 mL of 50% dextrose injection
500 mL of 7% protein hydrolysate injection

15. In preparing an intravenous infusion containing sodium bicarbonate, 50 mL of a 7.5% sodium bicarbonate injection were added to 500 mL of 5% dextrose injection. How many milliequivalents of sodium were represented in the total volume of the infusion?

16. A potassium phosphate solution contains 0.9 g of potassium dihy-

drogen phosphate and 4.7 g of potassium monohydrogen phosphate in 30 mL. If 15 mL of this solution are added to a liter of $D_5W$, how many milliequivalents of potassium phosphate will be represented in the infusion?

17. How many milliliters of a reconstituted injection containing 1 g of drug in 4 mL should be used in filling a medication order requiring 275 mg of the drug to be added to 500 mL of $D_5W$ solution? If the solution is administered at the rate of 1.6 mL per minute, how many milligrams of the drug will the patient receive in 1 hour?

18. A physician orders 20 mg of ampicillin per kg of body weight to be administered intravenously in 500 mL of sodium chloride injection. How many milliliters of a reconstituted solution containing the equivalent of 250 mg of ampicillin per mL should be used in filling the medication order for a 110-lb patient?

19. A solution of potassium phosphate contains a mixture of 164 mg of monobasic potassium phosphate and 158 mg of dibasic potassium phosphate per mL. *(a)* If a hyperalimentation fluid calls for the addition of 45 mEq of $K^+$, how many milliliters of the solution should be used to provide this level of potassium? *(b)* How many millimoles of total phosphate will be represented in the calculated volume of potassium phosphate solution?

20. Using the component sources as indicated, calculate the amount of each component required in preparing 1000 mL of the following hyperalimentation fluid:

| Hyperalimentation Fluid Formula | Component Source |
|---|---|
| *(a)* Amino Acids 2.125% | 500 mL of 8.5% amino acids injection |
| *(b)* Dextrose 20% | 500 mL of 50% dextrose injection |
| *(c)* Sodium Chloride 30 mEq | 20-mL vial of 15% solution |
| *(d)* Calcium Gluconate 2.5 mEq | 10-mL vial containing 4.6 mEq |
| *(e)* Insulin 15 units | vial of U-100 insulin |
| *(f)* Heparin 2500 units | 5-mL vial containing 1000 units per ml |
| *(g)* Sterile Water for Injection to make 1000 mL | 500 mL of sterile water for injection |

21. An intravenous fluid of 1000 mL of Lactated Ringer's Injection was started in a patient at 8 a.m. and was scheduled to run for 12 hours. At 3 p.m. it was found that 800 mL of the fluid remained in the bottle. At what rate of flow should the remaining fluid be regulated using an

IV set that delivers 15 drops per mL in order to complete the administration of the fluid in the scheduled time?

22. If a physician orders 5 units of insulin to be added to a 1-liter intravenous solution of $D_5W$ to be administered over an 8-hour period, (a) how many drops per minute should be administered using an IV set that delivers 15 drops per mL, and (b) how many units of insulin would be administered in each 30-minute period?

# 15

# Some Calculations Involving Hydrogen-ion Concentration and pH

When the hydrogen-ion concentration of solutions is expressed quantitatively, it varies from a value of nearly 1 for a normal solution of a strong acid to about $1 \times 10^{-14}$ for a normal solution of a strong alkali. Consequently, there is a variation of about 100,000,000,000,000 in the numerical values within these two limits. The use of ordinary notation for handling numbers of such magnitude in computations that involve hydrogen-ion concentration is impractical.

In order to simplify the statement of hydrogen-ion concentration, it is convenient to use logarithmic notation, with the mantissa usually rounded off to one or two places of decimals. It has become customary, therefore, to speak of the hydrogen-ion concentration of a given solution in terms of its pH value which is defined as the *logarithm of the reciprocal of the hydrogen-ion concentration.* Mathematically, this statement may be expressed as

$$\mathrm{pH} = \log \frac{1}{[\mathrm{H}^+]}$$

and since the logarithm of a reciprocal equals the negative logarithm of a number, this equation may also be written

$$\mathrm{pH} = -\log\, [\mathrm{H}^+]$$

Therefore pH value may also be defined as the *negative logarithm of the hydrogen-ion concentration.*

Now, the reciprocal, or negative, of a logarithm always contains a *negative mantissa. Log* $(7 \times 10^{-8})$, for example, equals $\bar{8}.8451$ or approximately $\bar{8}.8$, which is interpreted as $-8 + 0.8$. Its reciprocal is $-(-8 + 0.8)$, or $8 - 0.8$. In expressing pH value we eliminate the negative by borrowing *1* from the characteristic and adding it to the mantissa:

$$8 - 0.8 = (8 - 1) + (1 - 0.8) = 7 + 0.2, \text{ or } 7.2$$

If you say this is merely an elaborate way of subtracting *0.8* from *8.0*, you are quite right; but the importance of doing it this way becomes clear when you reverse the process.

Given *pH* = *7.2*, to convert it to $-\log [H^+]$ as the first step in ascertaining the hydrogen-ion concentration, you must add *1* to the characteristic and subtract it from the mantissa:

$$7.2 \text{ or } 7 + 0.2 = (7 + 1) + (0.2 - 1) = 0.8$$

Now you can proceed: if $8 - 0.8 = -\log [H^+]$, then $\log [H^+] = -(8 - 0.8) = -8 + 0.8$ or $\bar{8}.8$.

**To calculate the pH value of a solution, given its hydrogen-ion concentration:**

*Examples:*

*The hydrogen-ion concentration of a certain solution is* $5 \times 10^{-6}$. *Calculate the pH value of the solution.*

$$\text{pH} = -\log [H^+] = -\log (5 \times 10^{-6})$$
$$\log (5 \times 10^{-6}) = \bar{6}.6990 \text{ or } \bar{6}.7, \text{ or } -6 + 0.7$$
$$-\log (5 \times 10^{-6}) = -(-6 + 0.7) = 6 - 0.7$$
$$\text{pH} = (6 - 1) + (1 - 0.7) = 5.3, \textit{ answer.}$$

*The hydrogen-ion concentration of a certain solution is 0.00012 gram-ion per liter. Calculate the pH value of the solution.*

$$0.00012 = 1.2 \times 10^{-4}$$
$$\text{pH} = -\log [H^+], = -\log (1.2 \times 10^{-4})$$
$$\log (1.2 \times 10^{-4}) = \bar{4}.08, \text{ or } -4 + 0.08$$
$$-\log (1.2 \times 10^{-4}) = -(4 + 0.08) = 4 - 0.08$$
$$\text{pH} = (4 - 1) + (1 - 0.08) = 3.92, \textit{ answer.}$$

**To calculate the hydrogen-ion concentration of a solution, given its pH value:**

*Examples:*

*The pH value of a certain solution is 11.1. Calculate the hydrogen-ion concentration of the solution.*

$$\text{pH} = 11.1 = -\log [H^+]$$
$$-\log [H^+] = (11 + 1) + (0.1 - 1) = 12 - 0.9$$
$$\log [H^+] = -(12 - 0.9) = -12 + 0.9, \text{ or } \overline{12}.9$$
$$\text{hydrogen-ion concentration} = \text{antilog } \overline{12}.9 = 7.94 \times 10^{-12}, \textit{ answer.}$$

*The pH value of a certain solution is 5.7. Express the hydrogen-ion concentration of the solution as gram-ion per liter.*

$$\text{pH} = 5.7 = -\log [H^+]$$
$$-\log [H^+] = (5 + 1) + (0.7 - 1) = 6 - 0.3$$
$$\log [H^+] = -(6 - 0.3) = -6 + 0.3 = \bar{6}.3$$
$$\text{hydrogen-ion concentration} = \text{antilog } \bar{6}.3 = 2.0 \times 10^{-6}, \text{ or}$$

0.000002 gram-ion per liter, *answer.*

### Practice Problems

1. The hydrogen-ion concentration of a certain solution is $2.5 \times 10^{-11}$. Calculate the pH value of the solution.

2. The hydrogen-ion concentration of a certain buffer solution is $2.85 \times 10^{-10}$. Calculate the pH value of the solution.

3. The hydrogen-ion concentration of a certain buffer solution is 0.000000603 gram-ion per liter. Calculate the pH of the solution.

4. The hydrogen-ion concentration of a certain solution is 0.0000036 gram-ion per liter. Calculate the pH of the solution.

5. The hydrogen-ion concentration of a buffer solution is $4.4 \times 10^{-8}$. Calculate the pH value of the solution.

6. Calculate the pH of a buffer solution which has a hydrogen-ion concentration of $6.5 \times 10^{-7}$.

7. The hydrogen-ion concentration of a 0.1 molar acetic acid solution was found to be $1.32 \times 10^{-3}$. Calculate the pH of the solution.

8. The pH value of a certain solution is 6.5. Calculate the hydrogen-ion concentration of the solution.

9. The pH value of an 0.1 molar boric acid solution is 5.1. Express the hydrogen-ion concentration of the solution as gram-ion per liter.

10. A prescription for a collyrium calls for a buffer solution having a pH value of 7.2. Calculate the hydrogen-ion concentration of the buffer solution.

11. A 1:200 solution of quinidine sulfate has a pH value of 6.4. Calculate the hydrogen-ion concentration of the solution.

12. The average normal pH of blood plasma is 7.4. Calculate the hydrogen-ion concentration of blood plasma.

13. An intravenous fluid has a pH of 6.2. Express the hydrogen-ion concentration of the fluid as gram-ion per liter.

# 16

# Some Calculations Involving Buffer Solutions

## BUFFERS AND BUFFER SOLUTIONS

When a minute trace of hydrochloric acid is added to pure water, a very significant increase in *hydrogen-ion* concentration occurs immediately. In a similar manner, when a minute trace of sodium hydroxide is added to pure water, it will cause a correspondingly large increase in the *hydroxyl-ion* concentration. These changes take place because water alone cannot neutralize even traces of acid or base. In other words, it has no ability to resist changes in hydrogen-ion concentration or pH. A solution of a neutral salt, such as sodium chloride, also lacks this ability, and therefore it is said to be *unbuffered.*

The presence of certain substances or combinations of substances in aqueous solution imparts to the system the ability to maintain a desired pH at a relatively constant level even upon the addition of materials which may be expected to change the hydrogen-ion concentration. These substances or combinations of substances are called *buffers;* their ability to resist changes in pH is referred to as *buffer action;* their efficiency is measured by the function known as *buffer capacity;* and solutions of them are called *buffer solutions.* By definition, then, a *buffer solution* is a system, usually an aqueous solution, which possesses the property of resisting changes in pH upon the addition of small amounts of a strong acid or base.

Buffers are used to establish and maintain an ion activity within rather narrow limits. In pharmaceutical practice, the most common buffer systems are used (1) in the preparation of dosage forms that approach isotonicity and (2) in the manufacture of formulations in which the pH must be maintained at a relatively constant level in order to insure maximum stability.

Buffer solutions are usually composed of a *weak acid and a salt of the acid,* as for example, acetic acid and sodium acetate, or a *weak base and a salt of the base,* such as ammonium hydroxide and ammonium chloride. Typical buffer systems which may be used in pharmaceutical formulations include the following pairs: acetic acid and sodium acetate, boric acid and sodium borate, and disodium phosphate and sodium acid phosphate. Formulas for several other buffer systems, including those which are suggested for use in ophthalmic solutions, are given in the *United States Pharmacopeia.*

In the selection of a buffer system, due consideration must be given to the dissociation constant of the weak acid or base so as to insure maximum buffer capacity. This dissociation constant, in the case of an acid, is a measure of the strength of the acid; the more readily the acid dissociates the higher its dissociation constant and the stronger the acid. Selected dissociation constants or $K_a$ values are given in the accompanying table.

**Table of Dissociation Constants of Some Weak Acids at 25° C**

| *Acid* | $K_a$ |
|---|---|
| Acetic | $1.75 \times 10^{-5}$ |
| Barbituric | $1.05 \times 10^{-4}$ |
| Benzoic | $6.30 \times 10^{-5}$ |
| Boric | $6.4 \times 10^{-10}$ |
| Formic | $1.76 \times 10^{-4}$ |
| Lactic | $1.38 \times 10^{-4}$ |
| Mandelic | $4.29 \times 10^{-4}$ |
| Salicylic | $1.06 \times 10^{-3}$ |

The dissociation constant or $K_a$ value of a weak acid is given by the equation:

$$K_a = \frac{(H^+)(A^-)}{(HA)} \qquad \text{where } A^- = \text{salt}, \quad HA = \text{acid}$$

Since the numerical values of most dissociation constants are small numbers and may vary over many powers of 10, it is more convenient to express them as negative logarithms, i.e.,

$$pK_a = -\log K_a$$

When equation $K_a = \frac{(H^+)(A^-)}{(HA)}$ is expressed in logarithmic form, it is written:

$$pK_a = -\log (H^+) - \log \frac{\text{salt}}{\text{acid}}$$

and since $pH = -\log (H^+)$

then $pK_a = pH - \log \frac{\text{salt}}{\text{acid}}$

and $pH = pK_a + \log \frac{\text{salt}}{\text{acid}}$

## BUFFER EQUATION

The equation just derived is the Henderson-Hasselbalch equation for weak acids, commonly known as the *buffer equation*.

Similarly, the dissociation constant or $K_b$ value of a weak base is given by the equation:

$$K_b = \frac{(B^+)\,(OH^-)}{(BOH)} \qquad \text{where } B^+ = \text{salt}$$

$$\text{and BOH} = \text{base}$$

and the buffer equation for weak bases which is derived from this relationship may be expressed as:

$$pH = pK_w - pK_b + \log \frac{\text{base}}{\text{salt}}$$

The buffer equation is useful (1) for calculating the pH of a buffer system if its composition is known and (2) for calculating the molar ratio of the components of a buffer system required to give a solution of a desired pH. The equation may also be used to calculate the change in pH of a buffered solution upon the addition of a given amount of acid or base.

**To calculate the $pK_a$ value of a weak acid, given its dissociation constant, $K_a$:**

*Example:*

*The dissociation constant of acetic acid is $1.75 \times 10^{-5}$ at 25°C. Calculate its $pK_a$ value.*

$$K_a = 1.75 \times 10^{-5}$$

and

$$\log K_a = \log 1.75 + \log 10^{-5}$$

$$= 0.2430 - 5 = -4.757 \text{ or } -4.76$$

Since

$$pK_a = -\log K_a$$

$$pK_a = -(-4.76) = 4.76, \textit{ answer.}$$

**To calculate the pH value of a salt/acid buffer system:**

*Example:*

*What is the pH of a buffer solution prepared with 0.05 M sodium borate and 0.005 M boric acid? The $pK_a$ value of boric acid is 9.24 at 25°C.*

It should be noted that the ratio of the components of the buffer solution is given in molar concentrations.

Using the buffer equation for weak acids,

$$pH = pK_a + \log \frac{\text{salt}}{\text{acid}}$$

$$= 9.24 + \log \frac{0.05}{0.005}$$

$$= 9.24 + \log 10$$

$$= 9.24 + 1$$

$$= 10.24, \textit{ answer.}$$

**To calculate the pH value of a base/salt buffer system:**

*Example:*

*What is the pH of a buffer solution prepared with 0.05 M ammonia and 0.05 M ammonium chloride? The $K_b$ value of ammonia is $1.80 \times 10^{-5}$ at 25°C.*

Using the buffer equation for weak bases,

$$pH = pK_w - pK_b + \log \frac{\text{base}}{\text{salt}}$$

Since the $K_w$ value for water is $10^{-14}$ at 25°C, $pK_w = 14$.

$$K_b = 1.80 \times 10^{-5}$$

and

$$\log K_b = \log 1.8 + \log 10^{-5}$$

$$= 0.2553 - 5 = -4.7447 \text{ or } -4.74$$

$$pK_b = -\log K_b$$

$$= -(-4.74) = 4.74$$

and

$$pH = 14 - 4.74 + \log \frac{0.05}{0.05}$$

$$= 9.26 + \log 1$$

$$= 9.26, \textit{ answer.}$$

**To calculate the molar ratio of salt/acid required to prepare a buffer system having a desired pH value:**

*Example:*

*What molar ratio of salt/acid is required to prepare a sodium acetate-acetic acid buffer solution having a pH of 5.76? The $pK_a$ value of acetic acid is 4.76 at 25°C.*

Using the buffer equation,

$$pH = pK_a + \log \frac{\text{salt}}{\text{acid}}$$

$$\log \frac{\text{salt}}{\text{acid}} = pH - pK_a$$

$$= 5.76 - 4.76 = 1$$

$$\text{antilog of } 1 = 10$$

$$\text{ratio} = 10/1 \text{ or } 10:1, \textit{ answer.}$$

**To calculate the amounts of the components of a buffer solution required to prepare a desired volume, given the molar ratio of the components and the total buffer concentration:**

*Example:*

*The molar ratio of sodium acetate to acetic acid in a buffer solution having a pH of 5.76 is 10:1. Assuming that the total buffer concentration is $2.2 \times 10^{-2}$ mole/liter, how many grams of sodium acetate (mol. wt. – 82) and how many grams of acetic acid (mol. wt. – 60) should be used in preparing a liter of the solution?*

Since the molar ratio of sodium acetate to acetic acid is 10:1,

$$\text{the mole fraction of sodium acetate} = \frac{10}{1 + 10} \text{ or } \frac{10}{11}$$

$$\text{and the mole fraction of acetic acid} = \frac{1}{1 + 10} \text{ or } \frac{1}{11}$$

$$\text{If the total buffer concentration} = 2.2 \times 10^{-2} \text{ mole/liter,}$$

$$\text{the concentration of sodium acetate} = \frac{10}{11} \times (2.2 \times 10^{-2})$$

$$= 2.0 \times 10^{-2} \text{ mole/liter}$$

$$\text{and the concentration of acetic acid} = \frac{1}{11} \times (2.2 \times 10^{-2})$$

$$= 0.2 \times 10^{-2} \text{ mole/liter}$$

then $2.0 \times 10^{-2}$ or $0.02 \times 82 = 1.64$ g of sodium acetate per liter of solution, *and*

$0.2 \times 10^{-2}$ or $0.002 \times 60 = 0.120$ g of acetic acid per liter of solution, *answers.*

The efficiency of buffer solutions, that is their specific ability to resist changes in pH, is measured in terms of *buffer capacity;* and the *smaller* the pH change upon the addition of a given amount of acid or base, the *greater* the buffer capacity of the system. Among other factors, the buffer capacity of a system depends upon (1) the relative concentration of the buffer components and (2) the ratio of the components. For example, a 0.5 M acetate buffer at a pH of 4.76 would have a higher buffer capacity than a 0.05 M buffer.

Now, if a strong base such as sodium hydroxide is added to a buffer system consisting of equimolar concentrations of sodium acetate and acetic acid, the base is neutralized by the acetic acid forming more sodium acetate, and the resulting *increase* in pH is slight. Actually, the addition of the base increases the concentration of sodium acetate and decreases *by an equal amount* the concentration of acetic acid.

In a similar manner, the addition of a strong acid to a buffer system consisting of a weak base and its salt would produce only a small *decrease* in pH.

**To calculate the change in pH of a buffer solution upon the addition of a given amount of acid or base:**

*Example:*

*Calculate the change in pH upon adding 0.04 mole of sodium hydroxide to a liter of a buffer solution containing 0.2 M concentrations of sodium acetate and acetic acid. The $pK_a$ value of acetic acid is 4.76 at 25°C.*

The pH of the buffer solution is calculated by using the buffer equation as follows:

$$pH = pK_a + \log \frac{\text{salt}}{\text{acid}}$$

$$= 4.76 + \log \frac{0.2}{0.2}$$

$$= 4.76 + \log 1$$

$$= 4.76$$

The addition of 0.04 mole of sodium hydroxide converts 0.04 mole of acetic acid to 0.04 mole of sodium acetate. Consequently, the concentration of acetic acid is *decreased* and the concentration of sodium acetate is *increased* by equal amounts according to the following equation:

$$pH = pK_a + \log \frac{\text{salt} + \text{base}}{\text{acid} - \text{base}}$$

and

$$pH = pK_a + \log \frac{0.2 + 0.04}{0.2 - 0.04}$$

$$= pK_a + \log \frac{0.24}{0.16}$$

$$= 4.76 + 0.1761 = 4.9361 \text{ or } 4.94$$

Since the pH before the addition of the sodium hydroxide was 4.76, the change in pH = 4.94 − 4.76 = 0.18 unit, *answer.*

**Practice Problems**

1. The dissociation constant of lactic acid is $1.38 \times 10^{-4}$ at 25°C. Calculate its $pK_a$ value.

2. Calculate the $pK_a$ value of an acid having a dissociation constant of $1.75 \times 10^{-10}$ at 25°C.

3. The dissociation constant of ethanolamine is $2.77 \times 10^{-5}$ at 25°C. Calculate its $pK_b$ value.

4. Calculate the $pK_b$ value of urea which has a dissociation constant of $1.5 \times 10^{-14}$ at 25°C.

5. What is the pH of a buffer solution prepared with 0.055 M sodium acetate and 0.01 M acetic acid? The $pK_a$ value of acetic acid is 4.76 at 25°C.

6. Calculate the pH of a buffer solution containing 0.1 mole of acetic acid and 0.2 mole of sodium acetate per liter. The $pK_a$ value of acetic acid is 4.76 at 25°C.

7. What is the pH of a buffer solution prepared with 0.5 M disodium phosphate and 1 M sodium acid phosphate? The $pK_a$ value of sodium acid phosphate is 7.21 at 25°C.

8. What is the pH of a buffer solution prepared by using 0.001 molar sodium benzoate and 0.01 molar benzoic acid? The $pK_a$ value of benzoic acid is 4.20 at 25°C.

9. What molar ratio of salt to acid would be required to prepare a buffer solution having a pH of 4.5? The $pK_a$ value of the acid is 4.05 at 25°C.

10. What molar ratio of base to salt would be required to prepare a buffer solution having a pH of 6.8? The dissociation constant of the base is $4.47 \times 10^{-5}$ at 25°C.

11. What is the change in pH upon adding 0.02 mole of sodium hydroxide to a liter of a buffer solution containing 0.5 M of sodium acetate and 0.5 M acetic acid? The $pK_a$ value of acetic acid is 4.76 at 25°C.

12. What molar ratio of salt/acid is required to prepare a sodium borate-boric acid buffer solution having a pH of 9.44? The $pK_a$ value of boric acid is 9.24 at 25°C.

13. The molar ratio of salt to acid needed to prepare a sodium acetate-acetic acid buffer solution is 1:1. Assuming that the total buffer concentration is 0.1 mole/liter, how many grams of sodium acetate (mol. wt. $-82$) and how many grams of acetic acid (mol. wt. $-60$) should be used in preparing 2 liters of the solution?

14. What is the change in pH upon the addition of 0.01 hydrochloric acid to a liter of a buffer solution containing 0.05 M of ammonia and 0.05 M of ammonium chloride? The $K_b$ value of ammonia is $1.80 \times 10^{-5}$ at 25°C.

# 17

# Some Calculations Involving Radioactive Pharmaceuticals

## RADIOISOTOPES

The atoms of a given element are not necessarily alike. In fact, certain elements actually consist of several different components, called *isotopes,* which are chemically identical but which physically may differ slightly in mass. Isotopes, then, may be defined as atoms having the same nuclear charge, and hence the same atomic number, but having masses differing from each other. The mass number physically characterizes a particular isotope.

Isotopes may be classified as stable and unstable. Those that are stable never change unless affected by some outside force; but those that are unstable are distinguishable by radioactive transformations and hence are said to be radioactive. The radioactive isotopes of the elements are called *radioisotopes* or *radionuclides.* They may be divided into two different types: the naturally occurring and the artificially produced radionuclides.

The use of naturally occurring radioisotopes in medicine dates back some 65 years when radium was first introduced in radiologic practice. However, it was not until after 1946 that artificially produced radioisotopes became readily available to hospitals and to the medical profession. Since that time radionuclides have become important tools in medical research, and selected radioisotopes have been recognized as extremely valuable diagnostic and therapeutic agents. Monographs on thirty-eight radioactive pharmaceuticals are now official in the *United States Pharmacopeia.* Examples of some of these are listed in the following table:

**EXAMPLES OF OFFICIAL RADIOACTIVE PHARMACEUTICALS**

Chromic Phosphate P 32 Suspension
Cyanocobalamin Co 57 Capsules
Cyanocobalamin Co 57 Solution
Cyanocobalamin Co 60 Capsules
Cyanocobalamin Co 60 Solution
Ferrous Citrate Fe 59 Injection
Gallium Citrate Ga 57 Injection

**EXAMPLES OF OFFICIAL RADIOACTIVE PHARMACEUTICALS** ***Continued***

Indium In 111 Pentetate Injection
Iodinated I 125 Albumin Injection
Iodinated I 131 Albumin Injection
Iodinated I 131 Albumin Aggregated Injection
Iodohippurate Sodium I 131 Injection
Rose Bengal Sodium I 131 Injection
Selenomethionine Se 75 Injection
Sodium Chromate Cr 51 Injection
Sodium Iodide I 123 Capsules
Sodium Iodide I 123 Solution
Sodium Iodide I 125 Capsules
Sodium Iodide I 125 Solution
Sodium Iodide I 131 Capsules
Sodium Iodide I 131 Solution
Sodium Pertechnetate Tc 99m Injection
Sodium Phosphate P 32 Solution
Technetium Tc 99m Injection
Technetium Tc 99m Albumin Aggregated Injection
Technetium Tc 99m Etidronate Injection
Technetium Tc 99m Ferpentetate Injection
Technetium Tc 99m Gluceptate Injection
Technetium Tc 99m Medronate Injection
Technetium Tc 99m Oxidronate Injection
Technetium Tc 99m Succimer Injection
Technetium Tc 99m Pentetate Injection
Technetium Tc 99m Pyrophosphate Injection
Technetium Tc 99m Sulfur Colloid Injection
Thallous Chloride Tl 201 Injection
Xenon Xe 133 Injection
Ytterbium Yb 169 Pentetate Injection

These and many other radioactive pharmaceutical products are commercially available to properly trained and licensed personnel. Pharmacists, especially those engaged in hospital practice, who have a knowledgeable background in nuclear pharmacy may be required to make certain modifications and dilutions of the products which are usually available from pharmaceutical manufacturers. They may also be required to make certain corrections for radioactive decay in making dosage calculations.

## RADIOACTIVITY

The breakdown of an unstable isotope is characterized by radioactivity. In the process of radioactivity an unstable isotope undergoes changes until a stable state is reached and in the transformation emits energy in the form of radiation. This radiation may consist of *alpha particles, beta particles,* and *gamma rays.* The stable state is reached as a result of *radioactive decay* which is characteristic of all types of radioactivity. Individual radioisotopes differ in the rate of radioactive decay, but in each case a definite time is required for half of the original atoms to decay. This time is called the *half-life* of the radioisotope. Each radioisotope, then, has a distinct half-life. The half-lives of some commonly used radioisotopes are given in the accompanying table:

**TABLE OF HALF-LIVES OF SOME RADIOISOTOPES**

| *Radioisotope* | *Half-life* |
|---|---|
| $^{198}Au$ | 2.70 days |
| $^{14}C$ | 5,700 years |
| $^{45}Ca$ | 180 days |
| $^{57}Co$ | 270 days |
| $^{60}Co$ | 5.27 years |
| $^{51}Cr$ | 27.8 days |
| $^{59}Fe$ | 45.1 days |
| $^{67}Ga$ | 78.3 hours |
| $^{203}Hg$ | 46.6 days |
| $^{123}I$ | 13.2 hours |
| $^{125}I$ | 60 days |
| $^{131}I$ | 8.08 days |
| $^{111}In$ | 2.83 days |
| $^{42}K$ | 12.4 hours |
| $^{81m}Kr$ | 13.1 seconds |
| $^{99}Mo$ | 2.6 years |
| $^{22}Na$ | 2.6 years |
| $^{24}Na$ | 15.0 hours |
| $^{32}P$ | 14.3 days |
| $^{35}S$ | 87.2 days |
| $^{75}Se$ | 120 days |
| $^{85}Sr$ | 64 days |
| $^{99m}Tc$ | 6.0 hours |
| $^{201}Tl$ | 73.1 hours |
| $^{133}Xe$ | 5.24 days |
| $^{169}Yb$ | 32.0 days |

The rate of decay is always a constant fraction of the total number of undecomposed atoms present. Mathematically, the rate of disintegration may be expressed as follows:

$$-\frac{dN}{dt} = \lambda N \qquad (1)$$

where N is the number of undecomposed atoms at time t, and $\lambda$ is the decay constant or the fraction disintegrating per unit of time.

The constant may be expressed in any unit of time, *i.e.*, reciprocal seconds, minutes, hours, etc. The numerical value of the decay constant will be 24 times as great when expressed in days, for example, as when expressed in hours. This equation may be integrated to give the expression of the *exponential decay law* which may be written,

$$N = N_0 e^{-\lambda t} \qquad (2)$$

where N is the number of atoms remaining at elapsed time t, $N_0$ is the number of atoms originally present (when t = 0), λ is the decay constant for the unit of time in terms of which the interval t is expressed, and e is the base of the natural logarithm 2.71828.[1]

Since the rate of decay may also be characterized by the half-life ($T_{1/2}$), the value of N in equation (2) at the end of a half period is $\frac{1}{2}N_0$. The equation then becomes,

$$\tfrac{1}{2}N_0 = N_0 e^{-\lambda T_{1/2}} \qquad (3)$$

Solving equation (3) by natural logarithms results in the following expression:

$$\ln \tfrac{1}{2} = -\lambda T_{1/2}$$

$$\text{or} \quad \lambda T_{1/2} = \ln 2$$

$$\text{then} \quad \lambda T_{1/2} = 2.303 \log 2$$

$$\text{and} \quad T_{1/2} = \frac{0.693}{\lambda} \qquad (4)$$

The half-life ($T_{1/2}$), then, is related to the disintegration constant (λ) by equation (4). Hence, if one value is known, the other can be readily calculated.

## UNITS OF RADIOACTIVITY

The quantity of activity of a radioisotope is expressed in absolute units (total number of atoms disintegrating per unit time). The basic unit is the *curie* (Ci) which is defined as that quantity of a radioisotope in which $3.7 \times 10^{10}$ (37 billion) atoms disintegrate per second. The *millicurie* (mCi) is one-thousandth of a curie and the *microcurie* (μCi) is one-millionth of a curie. The *nanocurie* (nCi), also known as the *millimicrocurie,* is one-billionth of a curie ($10^{-9}$ Ci). The doses of the official radioactive pharmaceuticals are expressed in terms of millicuries and microcuries.

Other units which may be encountered in practice—but which will not be used in the calculations that follow—include the roentgen and the rad. The *roentgen* is the international unit of X rays or gamma ra-

[1]See p. 302.

diation. It is the quantity of X rays or gamma radiation that will produce under standard conditions of temperature and pressure ions carrying 1 electrostatic unit of electrical charge of either sign. The *rad* (acronym for radiation absorbed dose) is a unit of measurement of the absorbed dose of ionizing radiation. It corresponds to an energy transfer of 100 ergs per gram of any absorbing material (including tissues).

**To calculate the half-life of a radioisotope when its disintegration constant is given:**

*Example:*

*The disintegration constant of a radioisotope is 0.02496 day$^{-1}$. Calculate the half-life of the radioisotope.*

$$T_{1/2} = \frac{0.693}{\lambda}$$

$$\text{Substituting, } T_{1/2} = \frac{0.693}{0.02496 \text{ day}^{-1}}$$

$$T_{1/2} = 27.76 \text{ or } 27.8 \text{ days, } \textit{answer.}$$

**To calculate the disintegration constant of a radioisotope when its half-life is given:**

*Example:*

*The half-life of $^{198}Au$ is 2.70 days. Calculate its disintegration constant.*

$$T_{1/2} = \frac{0.693}{\lambda}$$

$$\text{Substituting, } 2.70 \text{ days} = \frac{0.693}{\lambda}$$

$$\lambda = \frac{0.693}{2.70 \text{ days}} = 0.2567 \text{ day}^{-1}, \textit{ answer.}$$

**To calculate the disintegration constant and the half-life of a radioisotope when its initial activity and its activity at time *t* are given:**

*Example:*

*The original quantity of a radioisotope is given as 500 microcuries per mL. If the quantity remaining after 16 days is 125 microcuries per mL, calculate (a) the disintegration constant and (b) the half-life of the radioisotope.*

(a) Equation (2), written in logarithmic form, becomes

$$1n \frac{N}{N_0} = -\lambda t$$

or

$$\lambda = \frac{2.303}{t} \log \frac{N_0}{N}$$

Substituting,

$$\lambda = \frac{2.303}{16} \log \frac{500}{125}$$

$$\lambda = \frac{2.303}{16} \left(0.6021\right)$$

$$\lambda = 0.08666 \text{ day}^{-1}, \textit{ answer.}$$

(b) Equation (4) may now be used to calculate the half-life.

$$T_{1/2} = \frac{0.693}{\lambda}$$

Substituting,

$$T_{1/2} = \frac{0.693}{0.08666 \text{ day}^{-1}} = 8.0 \text{ days}, \textit{ answer.}$$

**To calculate the activity of a radioisotope remaining at any time *t* after the original assay:**

*Examples:*

*A sample of* $^{131}I$ *has an initial activity of 30 microcuries. Its half-life is 8.08 days. Calculate its activity, in microcuries, at the end of exactly 20 days.*

By substituting $\lambda = \frac{0.693}{T_{1/2}}$ and $e^{-0.693} = 2$

in equation (2), the activity of a radioactive sample decreases with time according to the following expression:

$$N = N_0 \left(2^{-t/T_{1/2}}\right) = N_0 \left(\frac{1}{2^{t/T_{1/2}}}\right)$$

Since

$$t/T\tfrac{1}{2} = \frac{20}{8.08} = 2.475$$

then

$$N = 30\left(\frac{1}{2^{2.475}}\right)$$

Solving by logarithms $\log N = \log 30 - \log 2\ (2.475)$

$$= 1.4771 - 0.7450$$

$$\log N = 0.7321$$

$$N = 5.39 \text{ or } 5.4 \text{ microcuries, } \textit{answer.}$$

*A vial of Sodium Phosphate P 32 Solution has a labeled activity of 500 microcuries per mL. How many milliliters of this solution should be administered exactly 10 days after the original assay to provide an activity of 250 microcuries? The half-life of $^{32}P$ is 14.3 days.*

The activity exactly 10 days after the original assay is given by

$$N = N_0 \left(\frac{1}{2^{t/T_{1/2}}}\right)$$

Since $$t/T_{1/2} = \frac{10}{14.3} = 0.6993$$

then $$N = 500 \left(\frac{1}{2^{0.6993}}\right)$$

$$\log N = \log 500 - \log 2\ (0.6993)$$

$$= 2.6990 - 0.2105$$

$$\log N = 2.4885$$

$$N = 308 \text{ microcuries per mL, activity after radioactive decay}$$

$$\frac{308\ (\mu Ci)}{250\ (\mu Ci)} = \frac{1\ (mL)}{x\ (mL)}$$

$$x = 0.81 \text{ mL, } \textit{answer.}$$

**Practice Problems**

1. Calculate the half-life of a radioisotope that has a disintegration constant of 0.00456 $day^{-1}$.

2. Calculate the half-life of $^{203}Hg$ which has a disintegration constant of 0.0149 $day^{-1}$.

3. Calculate the disintegration constant of $^{64}Cu$ which has a half-life of 12.8 hours.

4. Calculate the disintegration constant of $^{35}S$ which has a half-life of 87.2 days.

5. The original quantity of a radioisotope is given as 100 millicuries. If the quantity remaining after 6 days is 75 millicuries, calculate the disintegration constant and the half-life of the radioisotope.

6. A series of measurements on a sample of a radioisotope gave the following data:

| *Days* | *Counts per minute* |
|---|---|
| 0 | 5600 |
| 4 | 2000 |

Calculate the disintegration constant and the half-life of the radioisotope.

7. The original activity of a radioisotope is given as 10 millicuries per 10 mL. If the quantity remaining after exactly 15 days is 850 microcuries per mL, calculate the disintegration constant and the half-life of the radioisotope.

8. If the half-life of a radioisotope is 12 hours, what will be the activity after 4 days of a sample that has an original activity of 1 curie? Express the activity in terms of microcuries.

9. Sodium iodide I 131 capsules have a labeled potency of 100 microcuries. What will be their activity exactly 3 days after the stated assay date? The half-life of $^{131}I$ is 8.08 days.

10. A sodium chromate Cr 51 injection has a labeled activity of 50 millicuries at 5:00 p.m. on April 19. Calculate its activity at 5:00 p.m. on May 1. The half-life of $^{51}Cr$ is 27.8 days.

11. Iodinated I 125 Albumin Injection contains 0.5 millicurie of radioactivity per mL. How many milliliters of the solution should be administered exactly 30 days after the original assay to provide an activity of 60 microcuries? The half-life of $^{125}I$ is 60 days.

12. An Ytterbium Yb 169 Pentetate Injection has a labeled radioactivity of 5 millicuries per mL. How many milliliters of the injection should be administered 10 days after the original assay to provide an activity of 100 microcuries per kilogram of body weight for a person weighing 110 lb? The half-life of $^{169}Yb$ is 32.0 days.

13. A sodium pertechnetate Tc 99m injection has a labeled activity of 15 millicuries per mL. If the injection is administered 10 hours after the time of calibration, *(a)* what will be its activity and *(b)* how many milliliters of the injection will be required to provide a dose of 15 millicuries? The half-life of $^{99m}Tc$ is 6.0 hours.

14. A sodium phosphate P 32 solution contains 1 millicurie per mL at the time of calibration. How many milliliters of the solution will provide an activity of 500 microcuries one week after the original assay? The half-life of $^{32}P$ is 14.3 days.

# 18

# Basic Statistical Concepts

Statistics may be defined as the science of the collection, classification, and interpretation of facts on the basis of relative number or occurrence as a ground for induction. Accordingly, all statistical studies begin with the gathering of reliable data. This information, or "raw data," whether it deals with measurements in business or science, is subsequently tabulated and analyzed for significance and validity by means of a number of mathematical and graphical procedures.

In this brief presentation some of the elementary concepts that form the basis for these procedures will be discussed in order to acquaint the student with the fundamentals of the "statistical approach."

## THE ARRAY

When numerical facts are collected, they are initially recorded in haphazard fashion. But before the data can be effectively analyzed, a logical arrangement of it must be made. In other words, the "raw data" must be tabulated. One such simple arrangement is called the *array.* It consists of listing the items in a set of values in order of their magnitude from smallest to largest or from the largest to smallest. Thus, the array rearranges the values but does not summarize them. The data are organized but not reduced.

*Example:*

*Prepare an array of the following set of body temperatures (°F) of 20 individuals.*

| | | | | |
|---|---|---|---|---|
| 98.3 | 98.6 | 98.6 | 98.8 | 98.5 |
| 98.6 | 98.7 | 98.4 | 98.5 | 98.6 |
| 98.7 | 98.4 | 98.6 | 98.7 | 98.6 |
| 98.5 | 99.0 | 98.9 | 98.6 | 98.9 |

The array is made by listing the body temperatures (°F) from the lowest to the highest.

Temperature (°F)

| | | | | |
|---|---|---|---|---|
| 98.3 | 98.5 | 98.6 | 98.6 | 98.8 |
| 98.4 | 98.5 | 98.6 | 98.7 | 98.8 |
| 98.4 | 98.6 | 98.6 | 98.7 | 98.9 |
| 98.5 | 98.6 | 98.6 | 98.7 | 99.0 |

*answer.*

## THE FREQUENCY DISTRIBUTION

A more precise tabulation consists of arranging the given data in classes and listing their frequencies. Such an arrangement is called the *frequency distribution.* In this arrangement the data are both organized and reduced.

*Example:*

*Prepare a frequency distribution of the body temperatures given in the preceding example.*

The frequency distribution of the body temperatures is made by separating the values into classes and listing the number of times a value appears in each class. If 5 classes of 0.2 beginning with 98.15 are chosen, the tabulation is made in the following manner.

| *Class* | *Tally* | *Frequency* |
|---|---|---|
| 98.15–98.35 | \| | 1 |
| 98.35–98.55 | 𝍸 | 5 |
| 98.55–98.75 | 𝍸 𝍸 | 10 |
| 98.75–98.95 | \|\|\| | 3 |
| 98.95–99.15 | \| | 1 |
| | Total: | 20 |

This tabulation shows that there is a concentration of values in the 98.55–98.75 class.

In general, frequency distributions should have not less than 5 classes and not more than 15. Unequal class intervals should be avoided for ease of understanding.

## AVERAGES

### Mean, Median, and Mode

One of the commonly used summary measures, or measures of central tendency, is the *arithmetic mean* or *average.* This is computed by adding the values of all the items in a set of data and dividing by the number of items. The formula for the arithmetic mean or average is:

$$\overline{X} = \frac{\text{Sum of values (X)}}{\text{Number of values}} = \frac{\Sigma X}{n}$$

The notation $\overline{X}$ (read X-bar) is the symbol for the average. The symbol $\Sigma$ (the Greek capital letter sigma) means the summation of all the items of the variable X, and n refers to the number of values in the given set of data.

*Example:*

*Referring to the array of the set of body temperatures, find the arithmetic mean of the recorded values.*

$$\overline{X} = \frac{\Sigma X}{n}$$

$$\frac{1(98.3) + 2(98.4) + 3(98.5) + 7(98.6) + 3(98.7) + 2(98.8) + 1(98.9) + 1(99.0)}{20}$$

$$= \frac{1972.4}{20} = 98.6, \textit{ answer.}$$

Another type of average is called the *median*, sometimes referred to as the *middle* item in a series. It *is* the middle item if there is an odd number of items in the tabulation. However, in a tabulation with an even number of items, the median may be considered as the average of the two middle items or, if greater precision is desired, it is the *weighted average* of the two middle items.

*Example:*

*Referring to the array of the set of body temperatures, find the median of the recorded values.*

Average of the two middle temperatures =

$$\frac{98.6 + 98.7}{2} = \frac{197.3}{2} = 98.65, \text{ or } 98.7, \textit{ answer.}$$

or,

Weighted average of the two middle temperatures =

$$\frac{7\,(98.6) + 3(98.7)}{10} = \frac{986.3}{10} = 98.63, \text{ or } 98.6, \textit{ answer.}$$

A third type of summary measure is the *mode*. It is the item that appears most *frequently* in a set of values. The mode in the array of the set of body temperatures is 98.6 because that temperature appears the greatest number of times in the tabulation. The mode and the median are considered as "positional averages" since they are determined by location. The arithmetic mean is a "computed average."

## MEASURES OF VARIATION

### Range, Average Deviation, and Standard Deviation

The measures of central tendency that have been discussed offer one characteristic of a distribution. Another characteristic is the measure of variation within the distribution. The simplest measure of variation is the *range* or the difference between the largest and smallest item in a distribution. The range is symbolized by the capital letter *R*. For the body temperature distribution previously cited, $R = 0.7$.

The amount by which a given single item in a set of values differs from the mean of those values is the *deviation*. A deviation is considered positive if the item is larger than the mean, and negative if it is smaller. One of the measures used to describe how much, on an average, an item deviates from the mean is called the *average deviation*. It is obtained by summing all the deviations from the mean without regard to algebraic sign and dividing by the number of deviations. The formula for average deviations, abbreviated *A.D.*, is:

$$\text{A.D.} = \frac{\text{Sum of absolute deviations}}{\text{Number of deviations}} = \frac{\Sigma\,|X - \overline{X}|}{n} = \frac{\Sigma d}{n}$$

*Example:*

*Using a micrometer caliper, the diameter of a sample of a nylon suture material at different points on the strand was found to be: 0.230 mm, 0.265 mm, 0.225 mm, 0.240 mm, 0.250 mm, 0.240 mm, 0.260 mm,*

*0.235 mm, 0.225 mm, and 0.270 mm. Calculate the mean and the average deviation.*

| *Diameter* | *Absolute Deviation* |
|---|---|
| *mm* | *mm* |
| 0.230 | 0.014 |
| 0.265 | 0.021 |
| 0.225 | 0.019 |
| 0.240 | 0.004 |
| 0.250 | 0.006 |
| 0.240 | 0.004 |
| 0.260 | 0.016 |
| 0.235 | 0.009 |
| 0.225 | 0.019 |
| 0.270 | 0.026 |
| 2.440 | 0.138 |

$$\text{Mean} = \frac{2.440}{10} = 0.244 \text{ mm, } \textit{and}$$

$$\text{A.D.} = \frac{0.138}{10} = 0.0138 \text{ or } 0.014 \text{ mm, } \textit{answers.}$$

The more commonly used measure of variation is the *standard deviation* of the items in a given set of values. It is a measure of the precision of the mean and is obtained by (1) squaring the deviations, (2) summing the squared deviations and dividing by the number of deviations *minus one,* and (3) finding the square root of the quotient of the division. The formula for standard deviation, abbreviated S.D., is:

$$\text{S.D.} = \sqrt{\frac{\text{Sum of (deviations)}^2}{\text{Number of deviations minus one}}} = \sqrt{\frac{\Sigma d^2}{n - 1}}$$

(The minus one in this formula is referred to as a "degree of freedom.")

*Example:*

*In checking the weights of a set of divided powders, the following values were obtained: 304 mg, 295 mg, 310 mg, 305 mg, 290 mg, 306 mg,*

*298 mg, 293 mg, 302 mg, and 297 mg. Calculate the mean and the standard deviation.*

| *Weight* | *Deviation* | *(Deviation)²* |
|---|---|---|
| *mg* | *mg* | |
| 304 | + 4 | 16 |
| 295 | − 5 | 25 |
| 310 | +10 | 100 |
| 305 | + 5 | 25 |
| 290 | −10 | 100 |
| 306 | + 6 | 36 |
| 298 | − 2 | 4 |
| 293 | − 7 | 49 |
| 302 | + 2 | 4 |
| 297 | − 3 | 9 |
| 3000 | | 368 |

$$\text{Mean} = \frac{3000}{10} = 300 \text{ mg, } \textit{and}$$

$$\text{S.D.} = \sqrt{\frac{\Sigma d^2}{n - 1}} = \sqrt{\frac{368}{9}} = \sqrt{40.9} = 6.4 \text{ mg, } \textit{answers.}$$

In general, the following approximate relationships may be used to compare the accuracy of measures of variation:

(1) The average deviation is approximately ⅘ of the standard deviation.

(2) The range is never less than the standard deviation nor more than 7 times the standard deviation.

## SOME ASPECTS OF PROBABILITY

When you speak of "probability" you should make sure that both you and your listener know the sense in which you are using the word.

In our everyday speech, "probability" often expresses merely a hunch about some likelihood or possibility, and we may indicate the strength of our hunch in phrases ranging from "extremely probable" to "very unlikely." Sometimes the hunch can be supported—like the predictions of a competent weather prophet—by very good evidence. But sometimes we have no other evidence except a vague "feeling"—and this lacks the degree of reliability sought in the world of mathematics and science.

To the mathematician, "probability"—in a usage that has nicely been termed "classical"—is a kind of *certainty.* Not certainty that an event *E* will take place. Certainty, rather, about the *chance* that $E$ will take place in competition with a number $N$ of alternate events that might happen to take place instead. The mathematician envisions an ideal or abstract world in which the chances of every competing event are *absolutely equal.* This basic premise is called the *Principle of Indifference.* It can claim 100% accuracy in some formulas only when referring imaginatively to an infinite number of cases.

As soon as "classical" probability formulas were devised they were predictably seized by gamblers and financial speculators, and the literature abounds with references to coin tossing, dice rolling, and card dealing, as well as to expectations of births, deaths, and shipwrecks. But, warn the mathematicians, the rules apply only if we respect the Principle of Indifference: our coins must not be bent, nor our dice loaded, nor our cards marked or stacked.

The statistician, whose research now carries him into every field of human interest and activity, has been forced to recognize and overcome a two-fold handicap. For one thing, actual events rarely and perhaps never are patterned by the Principle of Indifference. For another thing, equally significant, the statistician deals with a total number of cases (which he likes to called his "population") that lies a long way this side of infinity.

True, when the "population" is enormous—such as the number of molecules of gas in a chamber, or even the far lesser number of fine particles in a trituration—you can regard the great postulate of science that *like causes always produce like effects* as if it were a certainty. As a chemist, for example, you may feel certain that your gas laws will not be broken by random molecules all at once heading toward one end of the chamber; and as a pharmacist you may feel certain that with proper trituration a small amount of a potent substance like atropine sulfate will be uniformly distributed throughout a larger amount of a diluent such as powdered lactose.

Even when dealing with much smaller "populations" the statistician has found a very satisfactory substitute for "classical" probability. His "applied" probability, as indicated in the definition of statistics in the opening paragraph of this chapter, is revealed by the *relative frequency* of an event shown by an *actual survey* of cases.

An extended treatment of the subject is beyond the scope of this book. The odds are that you will find delight and profit if you explore this increasingly important area of study. Meantime, you may be interested in the following elementary observations. You may find ways to apply them in your own practice.

(1) When an event $E$ is one of a total $N$ of equally likely alter-

natives, the chance, or probability $p$, of its occurrence is one in that total number:

$$p = \frac{1}{N} \text{ or 1 chance in N}$$

The fraction $\frac{1}{N}$ may be expressed as a percentage.

The so-called "odds" are 1 to $N - 1$.

*Example:*

*If a question on a multiple-choice examination directs you to underscore one of five alternative answers, what is your chance of guessing the correct answer?*

$$\frac{1}{N} = \frac{1}{5} \text{ or 1 chance in 5, or 20\%, } \textit{answer.}$$

*What are the odds in favor of a correct guess?*

1 to $N - 1 = 1$ to 4, *answer.*

(2) The probability $q$ of the non-occurrence of $E$ in the preceding example is

$$q = \frac{N - 1}{N} = N - 1 \text{ in } N = 4 \text{ in } 5, \text{ or } 80\%$$

The *odds* in favor of $q$ are $N - 1$ to $1 = 4$ to 1.

(3) If $E$ has several (or $n$) chances of occurring among a given total $N$ of alternatives, its chances are

$$p = \frac{n}{N} \text{ or n chances in N}$$

A "classic" example is the drawing of a playing card from a pack. The chance of drawing the Queen of Spades is 1 in 52, but the chances of drawing any *one* of the *four* queens are

$$\frac{n}{N} = \frac{4}{52} = \frac{1}{13} \text{ or 1 chance in 13}$$

*Example:*

*If you are asked to underscore the two correct answers among six alternatives in a multiple-choice examination, what are your chances of guessing one correct answer?*

$$\frac{n}{N} = \frac{2}{6} = \frac{1}{3} \text{ or 1 chance in 3, } \textit{answer.}$$

(4) A succession of events may or may not one by one exhaust the total of possible alternatives. If you draw a queen from a pack and then restore it before a second drawing, you have restored the $^4/_{52}$ or $^1/_{13}$ ratio. But if you withdraw a queen and then draw again, hoping for another queen, you have a new ratio: three remaining queens among 51 remaining cards gives 3 in 51 or 1 in 17. A third drawing after two queens have been removed faces a ratio of two queens in 50 cards, or 1 in 25, and if this succeeds, a fourth attempt will face 1 in 49. You combine odds by multiplying, and your chances of drawing four queens in succession are only 1 in 270,725. Perhaps you can figure out why your chances of drawing them in the order of spades, hearts, diamonds, clubs are only 1 in 6,497,400.

You must be alert to such shifting odds if you are to avoid one of the most treacherous pitfalls in the game of probability.

*Example:*

*Referring to the multiple-choice question cited in (3) above, what are your chances of guessing both correct answers among the six alternatives?*

By analysis of the chances you face in each step of your two-part answer, you may reckon chances of 2 in 6 or 1 in 3 for a correct first step; but then you face a chance of 1 in 5 for a correct second step. Combining the two ratios, you have the following chance of being twice correct:

$$\frac{1}{3} \times \frac{1}{5} = \frac{1}{15} \text{ or 1 chance in 15, } \textit{answer.}$$

A clear proof of this analytical calculation may be charted. Presented with six alternatives—a, b, c, d, e, f—you may pair them in fifteen possible ways, and only one pair will contain the two correct answers:

| | | | | |
|---|---|---|---|---|
| a | a | a | a | a |
| b | c | d | e | f |
| b | b | b | b | c |
| c | d | e | f | d |
| c | c | d | d | e |
| e | f | e | f | f |

Therefore you have only a 1 in 15 chance of guessing the correct pair.

(5) Often the probability of the occurrence of an event or the percentage of occurrences in a total number of cases cannot be calculated in advance of research. Recall that the *relative frequency* of the event is the number of times it actually occurs in a total number of *observations. Statistical probability* (in contrast to "classical" probability) may be defined as *the limit of the relative frequency as the number of observations increases.* To illustrate, you may be curious about the extent of your vocabulary. The mean average percentage of words you know on a few representative pages of your dictionary will enable you to calculate very roughly—perhaps within a limit of five percentage points more or less—how many words you know in the entire dictionary. Test yourself on several dozen more pages, and your score will approach a limit of one percentage point.

(6) When a limited number of samplings is supposed to represent an unattainable whole "population" the selection of samples should be as *random* as possible, so that every member of the whole (in theory at least) has an equal chance of being selected. A survey of public opinion should not be limited to the dwellers on one or two streets in a city, or to people whose names begin with *A*, or to members of a particular club.

*Example:*

*Criticize the procedure of a tablet maker who selected for assay every fiftieth tablet during the first part of a run.*

Since a machine might conceivably have regular cycles of varying dependability, the selection of samples should be at random intervals scattered throughout the entire run, *answer.*

(7) In any survey-by-sampling, the greater the number of measurements, the greater the probability that their mean average will approach the true one being sought. Therefore, in appraising the

value of a statistical report of apparent general reliability, be ready to question any "break-downs" into components that may be individually unreliable. For example, a survey of the hair-grooming habits of 5000 American males may appear to be representative of American males in general; but if it is "broken down" into special groups (460 lawyers, 57 clergymen, 275 teachers, 13 convicts, etc.) can we fairly generalize about American lawyers, clergymen, teachers, convicts, etc.?

For comparing two surveys of a similar kind it has been found that *the probability of a truer mean average varies as the square root of the number of measurements.*

*Example:*

*Two groups of researchers made a series of freezing point determinations on an 0.9% solution of sodium chloride which, theoretically, freezes at −0.52°C. Group A made 36 measurements, Group B 16. Assuming equal skill, which group probably found a truer average?*

$$\frac{A}{B} = \frac{\sqrt{36}}{\sqrt{16}} = \frac{6}{4} = \frac{3}{2}$$ or a 3 to 2 probability in favor of Group A, *answer.*

(8) Another means of comparing the reliability of two sets of measurements involves the average deviations from the mean averages. *The reliability varies inversely as the deviations.*

*Example:*

*In the preceding example, if given the average deviation of report A as 0.006°C and of report B as 0.012°C, you could compare their reliability as follows:*

$$\frac{A}{B} = \frac{\frac{1}{0.006}}{\frac{1}{0.012}} = \frac{0.012}{0.006} = \frac{2}{1}$$ or a 2 to 1 probability in favor of Group A, *answer.*

(9) If the results of two investigations differ both in number of measurements and in average deviation from the mean average, you can use both factors together in comparing relative trustworthiness, keeping in mind that this varies *directly with the square root of the number of measurements and inversely as the average deviation from the mean average.*

*Example:*

*Combine the data in the two preceding examples.*

$$\frac{A}{B} = \frac{\sqrt{36}}{\sqrt{16}} \times \frac{\frac{1}{0.006}}{\frac{1}{0.012}} = \frac{0.072}{0.024} = \frac{3}{1} \text{ or 3 to 1 in favor of A, } \textit{answer}.$$

Or, combining the separate answers in (7) and (8):

$$\frac{A}{B} = \frac{3}{2} \times \frac{2}{1} = \frac{6}{2} = \frac{3}{1} \text{ or 3 to 1 in favor of A, } \textit{answer}.$$

(10) In many a survey, particularly if of a social nature, the reliability of some of the measurements may be open to question, or a reported measurement may be irrelevant to the purpose of the survey. Any measurement that is widely out of line with others of its kind may be rejected, since its inclusion would have a disproportionate and misleading influence on the mean average and other calculations.

For example, a pharmacist in a small isolated town that had lost its only resident physician headed a committee to investigate the possibility of arranging a subsidy to attract some young general practitioner. The inhabitants consisted of several score householders, most of whom worked in a mill that was the only local industry. There were also an eccentric, uncooperative recluse, rumored to be rich, and the mill owner, a man of known considerable means. The committee decided that its survey to ascertain the average family income need not include the recluse and should not include the mill owner. The latter's income would have raised the mean average significantly.

## Practice Problems

1. The blood pressures of a group of 15 individuals were recorded as follows:

| | | | | |
|---|---|---|---|---|
| 125 | 130 | 127 | 136 | 132 |
| 126 | 134 | 125 | 120 | 125 |
| 138 | 119 | 130 | 126 | 124 |

Prepare an array of the data, calculate the mean, and find the median and the mode from the array.

2. A sample of catgut was measured for diameter by use of a micrometer caliper. The values obtained at 10 different points on the strand were:

| | | | |
|---|---|---|---|
| 0.230 mm | 0.225 mm | 0.240 mm | 0.250 mm |
| 0.225 mm | 0.260 mm | 0.270 mm | 0.265 mm |
| 0.235 mm | 0.255 mm | | |

Calculate the mean, the range, and the average deviation.

3. In checking the weights of a set of 15 tablets, the following values were obtained:

| | | | | |
|---|---|---|---|---|
| 95 mg | 100 mg | 98 mg | 103 mg | 100 mg |
| 102 mg | 105 mg | 104 mg | 97 mg | 99 mg |
| 104 mg | 101 mg | 105 mg | 96 mg | 101 mg |

Calculate the mean, the average deviation, and the standard deviation for the set of values.

4. In determining the viscosity of a liquid in terms of centipoises, 10 observations were made and the following values were recorded:

| | | | |
|---|---|---|---|
| 10.5 cps | 9.6 cps | 10.0 cps | 9.5 cps |
| 10.0 cps | 10.3 cps | 9.9 cps | 11.0 cps |
| 9.8 cps | 10.0 cps | | |

Calculate the mean, the average deviation, and the standard deviation for the recorded values.

5. A series of 15 samples of a solution were assayed. The results, in terms of percent of active ingredient, were as follows:

| | | | | |
|---|---|---|---|---|
| 5.05% | 4.92% | 4.85% | 5.23% | 5.05% |
| 4.89% | 5.05% | 5.20% | 5.15% | 4.96% |
| 4.95% | 5.00% | 5.02% | 5.10% | 4.87% |

Calculate the mean, and find the median and the mode for the recorded data.

6. During a year-long community centennial celebration, the local pharmacist collaborated by keeping 300 tags identifying his regular customers in a drum. Each week for 50 weeks a tag was drawn from the drum, a souvenir prize awarded, and the tag returned to the drum.

(a) In any drawing, what was any customer's chance of winning the prize?

(b) During the series of drawings, what was a customer's chance of winning two prizes?

(c) What was a customer's chance of winning two prizes in a row?

(d) If the tags, once drawn, had not been returned to the drum, what would have been a previously unawarded customer's chance of winning in the last drawing?

7. In choosing a sample of 25 subjects for a certain experiment, a researcher has a group of 50 individuals available to him from which he is to select the sample. He assigns a number to each of the 50 subjects corresponding to an identical number on each of 50 buttons. He shakes the buttons in a container, draws one button, shakes the remaining buttons, then draws another button, shakes the buttons again, draws a third one, and so on until he has 25 buttons. The subjects whose numbers correspond to the numbers on the buttons that were drawn are chosen for the experiment. Is this a random selection? Justify your answer.

8. Report A on a reduction in absenteeism in an industrial institution attributed to vaccination during an outbreak of influenza: among the 1,952 employees there were 183 cases (9.4%) of clinical influenza; in the vaccinated group of 847, only 15 cases (1.77%) appeared.

Report B on a similar study: in a total of 3,497 employees, of which 1,148 received vaccination, the influenza attack rate was 10.8% as compared with 15.02% in the controls.

Comparing only the total "population" in these reports, calculate the odds that Report B may have produced more reliable percentages.

9. An old-time check of the body temperature of 25 people "in normal health" found an average of 98.4°F with an average deviation of 0.18°F. A later check of 100 people found an average temperature of 98.6°F with an average deviation of 0.12°F. By comparing both "population" and average deviation, calculate the ratio of the reliability of the two checks.

10. An aptitude test being devised for undergraduate applicants to graduate school was experimentally tested on fifteen subjects. With a possible score of 200, the results were as follows:

| | | |
|---|---|---|
| 141 | 115 | 153 |
| 119 | 109 | 132 |
| 108 | 127 | 138 |
| 69 | 126 | 114 |
| 157 | 132 | 120 |

Compare the mean averages and average deviations calculated with and without the inclusion of the low 69. Which figures would probably be more reliable?

11. In checking the weight variation of a batch of uncoated tablets formulated to contain 250 mg of a drug substance, twenty (20) tablets were weighed individually and the following values were obtained:

| | | | | |
|---|---|---|---|---|
| 250 mg | 260 mg | 242 mg | 235 mg | 239 mg |
| 245 mg | 225 mg | 267 mg | 250 mg | 258 mg |
| 230 mg | 232 mg | 275 mg | 248 mg | 263 mg |
| 248 mg | 256 mg | 250 mg | 232 mg | 250 mg |

(a) Calculate the mean or average weight of the tablets sampled.

(b) If the designated weight tolerance, based on average weight, is 7.5%, do all the tablets sampled fall within this limit?

12. A series of belladonna tincture assays yielded the following values in terms of mg of total alkaloids per 100 mL:

| | | |
|---|---|---|
| 40 mg | 35 mg | 28 mg |
| 33 mg | 29 mg | 32 mg |
| 27 mg | 31 mg | 27 mg |
| 30 mg | 25 mg | 30 mg |

Calculate the mean, and find the median and the mode for the recorded values.

APPENDIX

# A

# Thermometry

A *thermometer* is an instrument for measuring temperature, or intensity of heat. For practical purposes, a liquid such as alcohol or mercury undergoes a constant and measurable expansion or contraction with a rising or lowering of temperature. If contained in a small rigid bulb attached to a hermetically sealed extension tube, the liquid forces a column upward in the tube upon expanding and draws the column down again upon contracting. If the tube has a uniform bore and we mark it with evenly spaced lines, we have a thermometer.

Obviously, any number of degrees of temperature may be marked off between any two fixed points on the tube, and similar degrees can then be uniformly extended above and below them. Late seventeeth-century physicists suggested the constant temperatures of melting ice and of pure water boiling under normal atmospheric pressure as offering the most convenient fixed points.

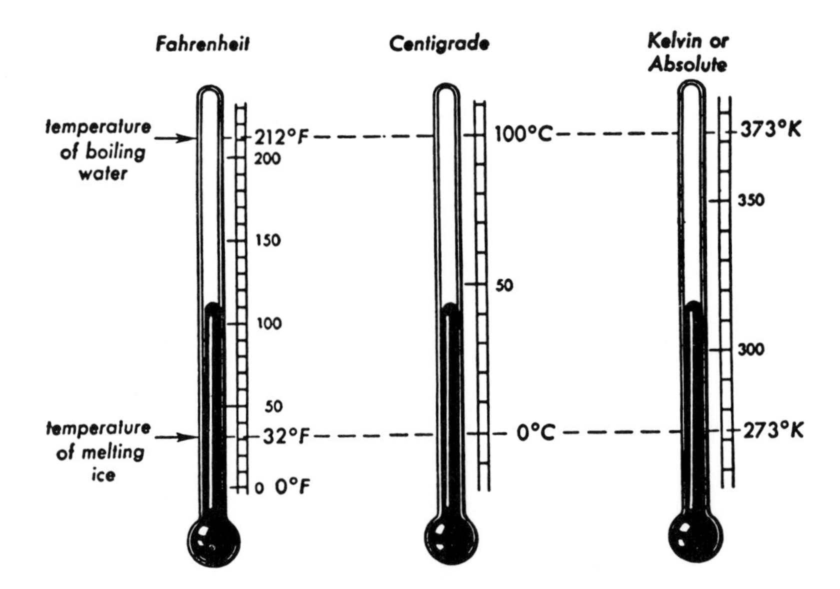


Mercury thermometers showing the Fahrenheit, Centigrade, and Kelvin scales (White's *Modern College Physics,* Copyright 1962, D. Van Nostrand Company, Inc., Princeton, N.J.).

In 1709, the German scientist Gabriel Fahrenheit (who improved the construction of thermometers and was the first to use mercury instead of alcohol) took for 0° the temperature of a mixture of snow and sal ammoniac (equal parts by weight). He discovered that by the scale he had marked on his thermometer ice melted at 32° and water boiled at 212°, with a difference of 180 degrees between these two points. The *Fahrenheit thermometer* is still commonly used in the United States.

In 1742, Anders Celsius, a Swedish astronomer, suggested the convenience of a thermometer with a scale having a difference of 100° between two fixed points, and the *centigrade thermometer* was devised, with 0° for the freezing and 100° for the boiling points of water.

On each thermometer, negative numbers are used to designate degrees "below" the arbitrarily selected zero.

Since 100 centigrade degrees (100° − 0°) measure the same difference in temperature that is measured by 180 Fahrenheit degrees (212° − 32°), each centigrade degree is the equivalent of 1.8 or $\frac{9}{5}$ the size of each Fahrenheit degree, and therefore, any given rise or fall in temperature is measured by $\frac{9}{5}$ as many Fahrenheit degrees as centigrade degrees. So, we may construct a general formula for converting from one system to the other:

$$\frac{\text{Number of centigrade degrees above or below any degree centigrade}}{\text{Number of Fahrenheit degrees above or below an equivalent degree Fahrenheit}} = \frac{5}{9}$$

In other words, every 5° change in temperature as measured by the centigrade thermometer is a 9° change as measured by the Fahrenheit.

To derive a specific working proportion, it remains for us only to select points on the two thermometers that are known to be equivalent, are easy to remember, and are convenient to use in calculations.

Here are some equivalent readings above and below the melting point of ice:

| | | | | | |
|---|---|---|---|---|---|
| 0°C | = | 32°F | 0°C | = | 32°F |
| 5°C | = | 41°F | −5°C | = | 23°F |
| 10°C | = | 50°F | −10°C | = | 14°F |
| 15°C | = | 59°F | −15°C | = | 5°F |
| 20°C | = | 68°F | −20°C | = | −4°F |
| 30°C | = | 86°F | −30°C | = | −22°F |
| 40°C | = | 104°F | −40°C | = | −40°F |
| 50°C | = | 122°F | −50°C | = | −58°F |
| 75°C | = | 167°F | −75°C | = | −103°F |
| 100°C | = | 212°F | −100°C | = | −148°F |
| and so on. | | | and so on. | | |

**First or fundamental method:**

Modern physicists not only have verified the hypothesis that "cold" is lower "heat" activity, but have found the point at which no such activity would be present, called *absolute zero.* Temperatures which are measured from this point are called *absolute temperatures* or temperatures on the *Kelvin scale.* Absolute zero has been computed as approximately −273° centigrade or −459.4° Fahrenheit. Consequently, this temperature may be considered the basic point of equivalence in the two systems:

$$-273°C = -459.4°F$$

By subtracting −273 from any given number of degrees centigrade we get the number of centigrade degrees above absolute zero. But subtracting a negative number is the same as adding its positive counterpart, so we may express this operation as C + 273. Similarly, any number of Fahrenheit degrees above absolute zero may be expressed as F + 459.4.

Our general proportion can now be specifically revised:

$$\frac{C + 273}{F + 459.4} = \frac{5}{9}$$

Using this proportion, if given the value of C we could compute the corresponding value of F, and *vice versa.*

But this can scarcely be called a working formula, since the numbers involved would not permit swift calculation. There are at least two other points of equivalence that are both easy to remember and easy to use: (1) the temperature at which both thermometers happen to register the same number of degrees and (2) the temperature of melting ice.

**Second method:**

The temperature registered as −40° centigrade happens also to be −40° Fahrenheit. The difference between any number of degrees centigrade and −40°C may be expressed as C + 40, and the difference between any number of degrees Fahrenheit and −40°F may be expressed as F + 40. By our general proportion, then,

$$\frac{C + 40}{F + 40} = \frac{5}{9}$$

Since this proportion is easy to remember, it is favored by many students, who usually sum up a working procedure as follows:

(1) To convert centigrade to Fahrenheit, *add 40 to the given number of centigrade degrees, multiply by* $9/5$*, and subtract 40.*

(2) To convert Fahrenheit to centigrade, *add 40 to the given number of Fahrenheit degrees, multiply by* $5/9$*, and subtract 40.*

These rules interpret the following derived equations:

$$(1) \quad F = \tfrac{9}{5}(C + 40) - 40$$

$$(2) \quad C = \tfrac{5}{9}(F + 40) - 40$$

**Third or standard method:**

The method of conversion most commonly employed, since its calculations are simplest, is based on the fact that 0° centigrade is equivalent to 32° Fahrenheit. Any number of centigrade degrees above or below 0°C may be expressed as C − 0, or simply C. Any number of Fahrenheit degrees above or below 32° Fahrenheit may be expressed as F − 32. Hence:

$$(1) \quad \frac{C}{F - 32} = \frac{5}{9}$$

$$(2) \quad C = \tfrac{5}{9}(F - 32)$$

$$(3) \quad F = 32 + \tfrac{9}{5} C$$

Perhaps a majority of scientists use equations (2) and (3), depending upon the direction of conversion, and resolve them by simple arithmetic.

**Fourth and easiest method:**

Here is a noteworthy fact: *no matter what specific proportion we select, if we multiply means and extremes and simplify the result we get the same working equation.*

$$(1) \quad \frac{C + 273}{F + 459.4} = \frac{5}{9}$$

$$9C + 2457 = 5F + 2297$$

$$9C = 5F - 160$$

$$(2) \quad \frac{C + 40}{F + 40} = \frac{5}{9}$$

$$9C + 360 = 5F + 200$$

$$9C = 5F - 160$$

$$(3) \quad \frac{C}{F - 32} = \frac{5}{9}$$

$$9C = F - 160$$

Once the principle is understood, therefore, it would seem advisable to use this equation (by the rules of elementary algebra) for conversion in either direction. It is easy to remember; it is convenient to use; it prevents the errors that frequently arise from careless interchange of $5/9$ and $9/5$ or confusion of the minus and plus signs in the other equations.

*Examples:*

*Convert 26°C to Fahrenheit.*

$$\begin{aligned} 9\,C &= 5\,F - 160 \\ 9 \times 26 &= 5\,F - 160 \\ 234 + 160 &= 5\,F \\ 5\,F &= 394 \\ F &= 78.8°, \textit{ answer.}[1] \end{aligned}$$

*Convert −12°C to Fahrenheit.*

$$\begin{aligned} 9\,C &= 5\,F - 160 \\ 9 \times -12 &= 5\,F - 160 \\ -108 + 160 &= 5\,F \\ 5F &= 52 \\ F &= 10.4°, \textit{ answer.} \end{aligned}$$

*Convert 162°F to centigrade.*

$$\begin{aligned} 9\,C &= 5F - 160 \\ 9\,C &= (5 \times 162) - 160 \\ 9\,C &= 650 \\ C &= 72\tfrac{2}{9}°, \textit{ answer.} \end{aligned}$$

*Convert −62°F to centigrade.*

$$\begin{aligned} 9\,C &= 5\,F - 160 \\ 9\,C &= (5 \times -62) - 160 \\ 9\,C &= -470 \\ C &= -52\tfrac{2}{9}°, \textit{ answer.} \end{aligned}$$

[1]When centigrade degrees are converted to Fahrenheit, fractions are fifths and are customarily expressed as decimals; but when Fahrenheit degrees are converted to centigrade, fractions are ninths.

Clinical thermometer showing the average normal oral body temperature (98.6°F).

## Practice Problems

1. Convert 10°C to Fahrenheit.

2. Convert −30°C to Fahrenheit.

3. Convert 4°C to Fahrenheit.

4. Convert −173°C to Fahrenheit.

5. Convert 77°F to centigrade.

6. Convert 240°F to centigrade.

7. The normal temperature of the human body is 98.6°F. Express this temperature on the centigrade scale.

8. A saturated solution of sodium chloride boils at 227.1°F. What is its boiling point on the centigrade scale?

9. The range of a centigrade thermometer is −5° to 300°. What is this range on the Fahrenheit scale?

10. Liquid petrolatum has a kinematic viscosity of 38.1 centistokes at 37.8°C. Express this temperature on the Fahrenheit scale.

11. The U.S.P. expression "excessive heat" refers to any temperature above 104°F. Express this temperature on the centigrade scale.

12. If a person shows a temperature of 102.5°F on a clinical thermometer, what temperature would this be on the centigrade scale?

13. If mercury freezes at −40°F, what is its freezing point on the centigrade scale?

14. The U.S.P. defines a *refrigerator* as a cold place in which the temperature is maintained thermostatically between 2° and 8°C. Express this temperature range on the Fahrenheit scale.

15. Theobroma oil melts between 30° and 35°C. What is the range of its melting point on the Fahrenheit scale?

16. If the maximum density of water is reached at 4°C, what would this point be on the Fahrenheit scale?

17. A specific gravity determination was made at 20°C. What was the temperature on the Fahrenheit scale?

18. Oxygen can be liquefied at −119°C. Express this temperature on *(a)* the Fahrenheit scale and *(b)* the absolute scale.

19. The U.S.P. defines a *freezer* as a cold place in which the temperature is maintained thermostatically between −20° and −10°C. Express this temperature range on the Fahrenheit scale.

20. A table of specifications states that a certain substance must congeal at −34.6°F. Express this temperature on the centigrade scale.

21. In preparing a vanishing cream, you are directed to heat the oil phase to 80°C and the aqueous phase to 82°C. Express these temperatures on the Fahrenheit scale.

22. The directions for the preparation of a certain formulation specified that the ingredients were to be heated for fifteen minutes at 70°F. This was a typographical error; it should have read 70°C. What is the difference in centigrade degrees between these two readings?

23. The critical temperature of a certain aerosol propellant is 388.4°F and its freezing point is −168°F. Express these temperatures on the centigrade scale.

24. Dry ice vaporizes at −112°F. What is the corresponding temperature on *(a)* the centigrade scale and *(b)* the Kelvin scale?

25. A pharmacist purchased a biological refrigerator which is equipped with a centigrade thermometer. At what temperature should the refrigerator be set for storing insulin which is directed to be kept at 40°F?

26. Rubber closures for containers for injections are sterilized preferably with moist heat in an autoclave at 121°C for 15 to 20 minutes. Express this temperature on the Fahrenheit scale.

APPENDIX

# B

# Proof Strength

It is customary to express the percentage strength of an aqueous solution of alcohol in volume-in-volume percentage, reckoned from the number of milliliters or minims or fluidounces of pure or *absolute* alcohol contained in 100 of the same unit. Consequently, if weight-in-weight percentage is specified, it should be clearly identified.

The legal and official temperature for the specific gravity of alcohol of all strengths is 60°F, or 15.56°C, at which temperature the specific gravity of absolute alcohol is 0.794.

*Proof spirit* is an aqueous solution containing 50% (v/v) of absolute alcohol. Alcohols of other percentage strengths are said to be *above proof* or *below proof*, depending upon whether they contain more or less than 50% (v/v) of absolute alcohol.

*Proof strength* of alcohol is expressed by taking 50% alcohol, or proof spirit, as *100 proof*. Then 100% or *absolute* alcohol is twice as strong, or 200 proof; 25% alcohol is half as strong, or 50 proof; and, inevitably, proof strength is always numerically twice as great as percentage strength (v/v). Hence, if percentage strength (v/v) is multiplied by 2, we have the corresponding proof strength—so 35% alcohol is 70 proof, 95% alcohol is 190 proof, and so on. Conversely, if proof strength is divided by 2, we have percentage strength (v/v)—so 160 proof alcohol is 80% (v/v) strength, 90 proof alcohol is of 45% (v/v) strength, and so on.

Alcohol and alcoholic beverages are generally measured in gallons, for purposes of taxation, whatever their percentage strengths; and for this and other reasons, a unit called the *proof gallon* is frequently used to measure, or evaluate, alcohols of given quantities and strengths. The tax on alcohol or alcoholic liquors is quoted at a definite figure per proof gallon. A *drawback* or refund of the tax paid on distilled spirits which are used in the manufacture of medicines and medicinal preparations is allowed by the government and may be obtained by eligible claimants. Like the tax on distilled spirits, the drawback is quoted at a definite rate per proof gallon.

A *proof gallon* is 1 wine gallon (a gallon by measure) of proof spirit. In other words, 1 proof gallon = 1 wine gallon of an alcohol solution containing ½ wine gallon of absolute alcohol and having therefore a strength of 100 proof or 50% (v/v). Any quantity of alcohol containing ½ wine gallon of absolute alcohol is said "to be the equivalent of" or "to contain" 1 proof gallon. So, 2 wine gallons of 50 proof or 25% (v/v) alcohol would contain ½ wine gallon of absolute alcohol, and would therefore be the equivalent of 1 proof gallon; but 3 wine gallons of such a solution would contain 1½ proof gallons.

**To calculate the number of proof gallons contained in a given quantity of alcohol of specified strength:**

Since a proof gallon has a percentage strength of 50% (v/v), the equivalent number of proof gallons may be calculated by the formula:

$$\text{Proof gallons} = \frac{\text{Wine gallons} \times \text{Percentage strength of solution}}{50\ (\%)}$$

And since proof strength is twice percentage strength, the formula may validly be revised as follows:

$$\text{Proof gallons} = \frac{\text{Wine gallons} \times \text{Proof strength of solution}}{100\ (\text{proof})}$$

*Example:*

*How many proof gallons are contained in 5 wine gallons of 75% (v/v) alcohol?*

First method:

1 proof gallon = 1 wine gallon of 50% (v/v) strength

$$\frac{5\ (\text{wine gallons}) \times 75\ (\%)}{50\ (\%)} = 7.5 \text{ proof gallons, } \textit{answer.}$$

Second method:

75% (v/v) = 150 proof

$$\frac{5\ (\text{wine gallons}) \times 150\ (\text{proof})}{100\ (\text{proof})} = 7.5 \text{ proof gallons, } \textit{answer.}$$

**To calculate the number of wine gallons of alcohol of specified strength equivalent to a given number of proof gallons:**

$$\text{Wine gallons} = \frac{\text{Proof gallons} \times 50\ (\%)}{\text{Percentage strength of solution}}$$

or,

$$\text{Wine gallons} = \frac{\text{Proof gallons} \times 100\ (\text{proof})}{\text{Proof strength of solution}}$$

*Example:*

*How many wine gallons of 20% (v/v) alcohol would be the equivalent of 20 proof gallons?*

First method:

1 proof gallon = 1 wine gallon of 50% (v/v) strength

$$\frac{20\ (\text{proof gallons}) \times 50\ (\%)}{20\ (\%)} = 50 \text{ wine gallons, } \textit{answer.}$$

Second method:

20% (v/v) = 40 proof

$$\frac{20\ (\text{proof gallons}) \times 100\ (\text{proof})}{40\ (\text{proof})} = 50 \text{ wine gallons, } \textit{answer.}$$

**To calculate the tax on a given quantity of alcohol of a specified strength:**

*Example:*

*If the tax on alcohol is quoted at $12.50 per proof gallon, how much tax would be collected upon 10 wine gallons of alcohol marked "190 proof"?*

$$\frac{10\ (\text{wine gallons}) \times 190\ (\text{proof})}{100\ (\text{proof})} = 19 \text{ proof gallons}$$

$$\$12.50 \times 19\ (\text{proof gallons}) = \$237.50, \textit{ answer.}$$

**Practice Problems**

1. How many proof gallons are represented by 54 wine gallons of 95% (v/v) alcohol?

2. How many gallons of proof spirit are there in 25 wine gallons of a sample that contains 70% (v/v) of pure alcohol?

3. How many proof gallons are contained in 500 wine gallons of Diluted Alcohol, N.F., that contain 49% (v/v) of pure alcohol?

4. During a certain month, a hospital pharmacist used 54 gallons of 95% alcohol and 5 gallons of absolute (100%) alcohol. How many proof gallons were used during the month?

5. A pharmaceutical manufacturer has 4,500 gallons of 95% (v/v) alcohol. How many proof gallons are represented by this quantity?

6. How many wine gallons of 95% (v/v) alcohol would contain 91.2 proof gallons?

7. Calculate the volume, in wine gallons, represented by 175 proof gallons of 70% (v/v) alcohol.

8. If a drum contains 54 wine gallons of 95% (v/v) alcohol, how much tax must be paid on it at the rate of $12.50 per proof gallon?

9. If the tax on alcohol is $12.50 per proof gallon, how much tax must be paid on 5 wine gallons of Alcohol, U.S.P., that contain 94.9% (v/v) of pure alcohol?

10. If alcohol is taxed at the rate of $12.50 per proof gallon, compute the tax on 6 wine gallons of 65% (v/v) alcohol.

11. The drawback on alcohol is $11.50 per proof gallon. If an eligible claimant used 18 gallons of 95% alcohol, how much drawback will be allowed?

12. A manufacturing pharmacist received a drawback of $1380 on the alcohol that was used during a certain period. If the drawback on alcohol is $11.50 per proof gallon, how many wine gallons of 95% alcohol were used during the period?

13. The formula for an elixir calls for 4 gallons of 95% alcohol. Alcohol (95%) costs $32.50 per gallon and the drawback is $11.50 per proof gallon. Calculate the net cost of the alcohol in the formula.

14. The drawback on a quantity of 95% alcohol used in the manufacture of a certain medicinal preparation was $218.50, and the net cost of the alcohol was $106.50. If the rate of drawback is $11.50 per proof gallon, what was the original purchase price per gallon of the alcohol?

15. On the first of the month, a hospital pharmacist had on hand a drum containing 54 gallons of 95% alcohol. During the month the following amounts were used:

(*a*) 10 gallons in the manufacture of bathing lotion.
(*b*) 20 gallons in the manufacture of medicated alcohol.
(*c*) 5 gallons in the manufacture of soap solution.

How many proof gallons of alcohol were on hand at the end of the month?

16. A hospital pharmacist had two drums (108 gallons) of 95% alcohol and 10 pints of absolute (100%) alcohol on hand on the first of the month. During the month 20 gallons of 70% (v/v) alcohol and 30 gallons of 50% (v/v) alcohol were prepared. Two pints of absolute alcohol were also dispensed. How many proof gallons did the alcohol inventory show at the end of the month?

APPENDIX

# C

# Solubility Ratios

The *solubility* of a substance is the ratio between the amount of it contained in a given amount of saturated solution (at a given temperature) and the amount of solvent therein. For instance, if 400 g of saturated solution contain 100 g of solute and 300 g of solvent, the solubility of the active ingredient (at that temperature) is 100:300 and may be expressed as 1:3. The relative amounts of solute and solvent may be calculated from various data, such as the ratio or percentage strength of the saturated solution.

The *Reference Tables* of the United States Pharmacopeia give approximate solubilities of U.S.P. and N.F. articles as 1 g of solute in so many mL of solvent (for example, *1 g of sodium chloride is soluble in 2.8 mL of water)*. Solubilities may also be expressed as so many grams of solute in 100 mL of a saturated solution.

**To calculate the solubility of a substance:**

This procedure will work for any kind of solution: (1) use the data to set up a proportion including the ratio *1:x*, *x* being the number of parts by weight containing *1* part by weight of active ingredient, and (2) if required, calculate the *volume* of *x* weight parts of solvent.

*Examples:*

*What is the solubility of an anhydrous chemical if 100 g of a saturated aqueous solution leave a residue of 25 g after evaporation?*

100 g − 25 g = 75 g of water

$$\frac{25\text{ (g)}}{75\text{ (g)}} = \frac{1\text{ (part)}}{\text{x (parts)}}$$

x = 3 parts of water, indicating a solubility of 1:3, or 1 g in 3 g or mL of water, *answer.*

*What is the solubility of an anhydrous chemical if 100 g of a saturated alcoholic solution leave a residue of 20 g after evaporation? (The sp. gr. of the alcohol is 0.80.)*

$100 \text{ g} - 20 \text{ g} = 80 \text{ g}$ of alcohol

$$\frac{20 \text{ (g)}}{80 \text{ (g)}} = \frac{1 \text{ (part)}}{x \text{ (parts)}}$$

x = 4 parts of alcohol, indicating a solubility of 1:4, or 1 g in 4 g of alcohol

4 g of water measure 4 mL

$\frac{4 \text{ mL}}{0.80} =$ 5 mL, indicating a solubility of 1 g in 5 mL of alcohol, *answer.*

*A saturated aqueous solution contains, in each 100 mL, 25 g of a substance. The specific gravity of the solution is 1.15. Calculate the solubility of the substance.*

100 mL of water weigh 100 g

$100 \text{ g} \times 1.15 = 115 \text{ g}$ (weight of 100 mL of saturated solution)

$115 \text{ g} - 25 \text{ g} = 90 \text{ g}$ of water

$$\frac{25 \text{ (g)}}{90 \text{ (g)}} = \frac{1 \text{ (part)}}{x \text{ (parts)}}$$

x = 3.6 parts of water, indicating a solubility of 1:3.6, or 1 g in 3.6 g or mL of water, *answer.*

*What is the solubility of the active ingredient if a saturated aqueous solution has a strength of 20% (w/w)?*

100 parts − 20 parts = 80 parts of solvent in every 100 parts of solution

$$\frac{20 \text{ (parts)}}{80 \text{ (parts)}} = \frac{1 \text{ (part)}}{x \text{ (parts)}}$$

x = 4 parts of solvent, indicating a solubility of 1:4, or 1 g in 4 g or mL of water, *answer.*

**To determine the percentage strength (w/w) of a saturated solution when the solubility is given:**

*Examples:*

*One gram of boric acid is soluble in 18 mL of water. What is the percentage strength (w/w) of a saturated aqueous solution?*

$1\text{ g} + 18\text{ g (18 mL of water)} = 19\text{ g}$

$$\frac{19\text{ (g)}}{1\text{ (g)}} = \frac{100\text{ (\%)}}{x\text{ (\%)}}$$

$x = 5.26\%$, *answer.*

*One gram of boric acid is soluble in 18 mL of alcohol. What is the percentage strength (w/w) of a saturated alcoholic solution? (The specific gravity of the alcohol is 0.80.)*

18 mL of water weigh 18 g

$18\text{ g} \times 0.80 = 14.4\text{ g}$, weight of 18 mL of alcohol

$1\text{ g} + 14.4\text{ g} = 15.4\text{ g}$ of solution

$$\frac{15.4\text{ (g)}}{1\text{ (g)}} = \frac{100\text{ (\%)}}{x\text{ (\%)}}$$

$x = 6.49\%$, *answer.*

## Practice Problems

1. What is the solubility of a substance in water if 125 g of a saturated aqueous solution yield a 20-g residue upon evaporation?

2. What is the solubility of a chemical if a saturated aqueous solution has a strength of 15% (w/w)?

3. A saturated aqueous solution contains 30 g of a substance in each 100 mL. The specific gravity of the solution is 1.10. Calculate the solubility of the substance.

4. One gram of calcium hydroxide is soluble in 630 mL of water at 25°C. Calculate the percentage strength (w/w) of a saturated solution.

5. The solubility of sodium borate is 1 g in 16 mL of water at 25°C. What is the percentage strength (w/w) of a saturated solution?

6. A saturated aqueous solution contains, in each 500 mL, 400 g of a substance. The specific gravity of the solution is 1.30. What is the solubility of the substance?

7. The solubility of a substance is 1 g in 3 mL of water. When 5 g of it are dissolved in 15 mL of water, the volume of the resulting solution is 16.8 mL. How many grams of the substance and how many milliliters of water should be used to make 200 mL of a saturated solution?

8. One gram of a substance is soluble in 0.55 mL of water. When 20 g of it are dissolved in 11 mL water, the volume of the resulting solution is 23.5 mL.

*(a)* How many grams of the substance and how many milliliters of water should be used in preparing 1000 mL of a saturated solution?

*(b)* Calculate the percentage strength (w/w) of the solution.

*(c)* Calculate the percentage strength (w/v) of the solution.

*(d)* What is the specific gravity of the saturated solution?

9. A saturated solution of potassium iodide contains, in each 100 mL, 100 g of potassium iodide. The specific gravity of the solution is 1.7. Calculate the solubility of potassium iodide.

10. The solubility of magnesium sulfate is 1 g in 0.8 mL of water at 25°C. How many grams of magnesium sulfate should be used in preparing a liter of a saturated solution? Assume a specific gravity of 1.30 for the saturated solution at 25°C.

11. If the percentage strength (w/v) of a saturated aqueous solution of sucrose is 85% and the specific gravity of the solution is 1.313, what is the solubility of sucrose in water?

APPENDIX

# D

# Emulsion Nucleus

In the preparation of emulsions by the *Continental Method* ("4-2-1 Method"), the proportions for the *nucleus* or *primary emulsion* are "fixed oil *4* parts by volume, water *2* parts by volume, and acacia *1* part by corresponding weight." The weight is measured in grams when volumes are measured in milliliters, and in apothecaries' ounces when volumes are measured in fluidounces. The mixture therefore contains one half as much water by volume as oil and one quarter as much acacia by "corresponding" weight.

When emulsions of volatile oils are prepared by this method, the proportions are "volatile oil *2* parts by volume, water *2* parts by volume, and acacia *1* part by corresponding weight."

**To calculate the quantities of ingredients required for a nucleus or primary emulsion:**

*Examples:*

*A castor oil emulsion contains 30% of castor oil. How much castor oil, water, and acacia are required to prepare the primary emulsion in the formulation of a liter of the emulsion?*

1 liter = 1000 mL

1000 mL × 30% = 300 mL of castor oil required

Since castor oil is a *fixed* oil, the ratio *4–2–1* is used.

| *4* — | *2* — | *1* |
|---|---|---|
| 300 mL | 150 mL | 75 g, *answers.* |
| oil | water | acacia |

In preparing the emulsion, the castor oil and acacia are mixed, the water is added, and the mixture is emulsified forming the primary emulsion which is then diluted to the required volume.

*A mineral oil emulsion contains 25% of mineral oil. How much mineral oil, water, and acacia are required to prepare the primary emulsion in the formulation of a pint of the emulsion?*

1 pint = 16 f℥

16 f℥ × 25% = 4 f℥ of mineral oil required

Since mineral oil is a *fixed* oil, the ratio *4–2–1* is used.

| *4* | — *2* | — *1* |
|---|---|---|
| 4 f℥ | 2 f℥ | 1 f℥ (480 grains), *answers.* |
| oil | water | acacia |

*A turpentine emulsion contains 15% of turpentine oil. How much turpentine oil, water, and acacia are required to prepare the primary emulsion in the formulation of 4 liters of the emulsion:*

4 liters = 4000 mL

4000 mL × 15% = 600 mL of turpentine oil required

Since turpentine oil is a *volatile* oil, the ratio *2–2–1* is used.

| *2* | — *2* | — *1* |
|---|---|---|
| 600 mL | 600 mL | 300 g, *answers.* |
| oil | water | acacia |

## Practice Problems

In each of the following formulas or prescriptions, calculate *(a)* the amount of acacia and *(b)* the amount of water to be used in preparing the nucleus or primary emulsion.

1. | | | |
|---|---|---|
| Mineral Oil | 500 mL | (A *fixed* oil.) |
| Acacia | q.s. | |
| Syrup | 100 mL | |
| Vanillin | 40 mg | |
| Alcohol | 60 mL | |
| Purified Water, to make | 1000 mL | |

   Label: Mineral Oil Emulsion.

2. Castor Oil (A *fixed* oil.)
   Chocolate Syrup aa 25%
   Acacia q.s.
   Purified Water, to make 2000 mL
   Label: Castor Oil Emulsion.

3. Cod Liver Oil 50% (A *fixed* oil.)
   Acacia q.s.
   Syrup 10%
   Peppermint Water, to make 5000 mL
   Label: Cod Liver Oil Emulsion.

4. Turpentine Oil 150 mL (A *volatile* oil.)
   Syrup 100 mL
   Acacia q.s.
   Purified Water, to make 1000 mL
   Label: Turpentine Oil Emulsion.

5. ℞ Aspidium Oleoresin 4.0 (Treat as a *volatile* oil.)
   Syrup 5.0
   Vanilla Tincture 2.0
   Acacia q.s.
   Water ad 60.0
   Sig. Take at one dose.

6. ℞ Castor Oil ℥iv (A *fixed* oil.)
   Chocolate Syrup ℥iv
   Acacia q.s.
   Water ad ℥xvi
   Sig. Emulsion of Castor Oil 25%.

7. ℞ Copaiba Balsam 20.0 (Treat as a *volatile* oil.)
   Olive Oil 30.0 (A *fixed* oil.)
   Glycyrrhiza Syrup 30.0
   Acacia q.s.
   Purified Water ad 240.0
   Sig. 5 mL t.i.d.

APPENDIX

# E

# HLB System: Problems Involving HLB Values

The systematic choice of emulsifying agents in the formulation of many emulsion systems depends upon their HLB (Hydrophile-Lipophile-Balance) values. These values form the basis of the so-called HLB System which was developed by Griffin.[1] The system presupposes a scale of HLB numbers and is based upon the facts (1) that every surfactant or emulsifier molecule is partly hydrophilic and partly lipophilic in character, and (2) that a certain balance between these two parts is necessary for various types of surfactant functions. In this scheme, each surfactant or emulsifying agent is assigned a number which varies from 1 to 20. The lower values are assigned to substances which are predominantly lipophilic (oil-loving) and which have a tendency to form water-in-oil (w/o) emulsions. The higher values are given to those materials which show hydrophilic (water-loving) characteristics and which favor the formation of oil-in-water (o/w) emulsions. Consequently, the HLB number of an emulsifying agent is an index of the type of emulsion which it has the greatest tendency to form. The HLB values of a few selected surfactants are given in the table which follows:

**TABLE OF HLB VALUES OF SOME SURFACTANTS**

| *Surfactant* | *HLB* |
|---|---|
| Sorbitan trioleate (Span 85)* | 1.8 |
| Sorbitan tristearate (Span 65)* | 2.1 |
| Sorbitan sesquioleate (Arlacel 83)* | 3.7 |
| Glyceryl monostearate, N.F. | 3.8 |
| Sorbitan monooleate, N.F., (Span 80)* | 4.3 |
| Sorbitan monostearate, N.F., (Span 60)* | 4.7 |
| Sorbitan monopalmitate, N.F., (Span 40)* | 6.7 |
| Sorbitan monolaurate, N.F., (Span 20)* | 8.6 |
| Polyoxyethylene sorbitan tristearate (Tween 65)* | 10.5 |
| Polyoxyethylene sorbitan trioleate (Tween 85)* | 11.0 |
| Polyethylene glycol 400 monostearate | 11.6 |
| Polysorbate 60, N.F., (Tween 60)* | 14.9 |

[1]Griffin, W.C., *J. Soc. Cos. Chem.*, *5*, 249 (1954).

**TABLE OF HLB VALUES OF SOME SURFACTANTS *(Continued)***

| *Surfactant* | *HLB* |
|---|---|
| Polyoxyethylene monostearate (Myrj 49)* | 15.0 |
| Polysorbate 80, N.F., (Tween 80)* | 15.0 |
| Polysorbate 40, N.F., (Tween 40)* | 15.6 |
| Polysorbate 20, N.F., (Tween 20)* | 16.7 |

*ICI Americas, Inc., Wilmington, Delaware.

Just as surfactants and emulsifiers are assigned HLB numbers, so, too, the ingredients to be emulsified have been given certain "required HLB" numbers. These have been determined experimentally and are necessary for the proper emulsification of the dispersed phase. The "required HLB" values for some of the more commonly used ingredients in emulsion formulation are given in the accompanying table:

**TABLE OF "REQUIRED HLB" VALUES OF SOME INGREDIENTS**

| *Ingredient* | *"Required HLB" for w/o emulsion* | *"Required HLB" for o/w emulsion* |
|---|---|---|
| Acid, Stearic | 6 | 15 |
| Alcohol, Cetyl | — | 15 |
| Alcohol, Stearyl | — | 14 |
| Lanolin, Anhydrous | 8 | 10 |
| Oil, Cottonseed | 5 | 10 |
| Oil, Mineral | 5 | 12 |
| Petrolatum | 5 | 12 |
| Wax, Beeswax | 4 | 12 |

### To calculate the HLB of a blend of emulsifying agents:

When two or more emulsifiers are combined, the HLB of the combination is determined arithmetically by adding the contribution that each makes to the HLB total of the mixture.

*Example:*

*What is the HLB of a mixture of 40% of Span 60 and 60% of Tween 60?*

HLB of Span 60 = 4.7
HLB of Tween 60 = 14.9

| | *HLB* | | *% of mixture* | |
|---|---|---|---|---|
| Span 60 | 4.7 | × | 40% | = 1.9 |
| Tween 60 | 14.9 | × | 60% | = 8.9 |

HLB of mixture = 10.8, *answer.*

**To calculate the "required HLB" of a combination of ingredients which are to be emulsified:**

The "required HLB" of each ingredient is multiplied by the percentage or the fraction of the oil phase that the ingredient represents; the products are then added to give the "required HLB" for emulsification of the oil phase.

*Example:*

*Calculate the "required HLB" for the oil phase of the following o/w emulsion.*

| | | |
|---|---|---|
| Cetyl Alcohol | | 15.0 g |
| White Wax | | 1.0 g |
| Lanolin, Anhydrous | | 2.0 g |
| Emulsifier | | q.s. |
| Glycerin | | 5.0 g |
| Distilled Water | ad | 100.0 g |

The oil phase represents *18 parts* of the entire formula.

Cetyl Alcohol = $\frac{15}{18}$ of the oil phase
White Wax = $\frac{1}{18}$ of the oil phase
Lanolin, Anhydrous = $\frac{2}{18}$ of the oil phase

| | *"Required HLB"* | | *Fraction of oil phase* | | |
|---|---|---|---|---|---|
| Cetyl Alcohol | 15 | × | $\frac{15}{18}$ | = | 12.5 |
| White Wax | 12 | × | $\frac{1}{18}$ | = | 0.7 |
| Lanolin, Anhydrous | 10 | × | $\frac{2}{18}$ | = | 1.1 |

"Required HLB" of the oil phase = 14.3, *answer.*

**To calculate the relative amounts of emulsifiers that should be used to obtain a "required HLB":**

Problems of this type are conveniently solved by alligation alternate (p. 172).

*Examples:*

*In what proportion should Tween 80 and Span 80 be blended to obtain a "required HLB" of 12.0?*

HLB of Tween 80 = 15.0
HLB of Span 80 = 4.3

By alligation,

| | | |
|---|---|---|
| 15.0 | | 7.7 parts of Tween 80 |
| | 12.0 | |
| 4.3 | | 3.0 parts of Span 80 |

Relative amounts: 7.7:3.0 or 72%:28%, *answer.*

*A formula for a cosmetic cream calls for 35 g of an emulsifier blend consisting of Tween 40 and Span 20. If the "required HLB" is 12.6, how many grams of each emulsifier should be used in preparing the cream?*

HLB of Tween 40 = 15.6
HLB of Span 20 = 8.6

By alligation,

| | | |
|---|---|---|
| 15.6 | | 4.0 parts of Tween 40 |
| | 12.6 | |
| 8.6 | | 3.0 parts of Span 20 |

Relative amounts 4:3 with a total of 7 parts

$$\frac{4 \text{ (parts)}}{7 \text{ (parts)}} = \frac{x \text{ (g)}}{35 \text{ (g)}}$$

x = 20 g of Tween 40, *and*

$$\frac{3 \text{ (parts)}}{7 \text{ (parts)}} = \frac{y \text{ (g)}}{35 \text{ (g)}}$$

y = 15 g of Span 20, *answers.*

## Practice Problems

1. What is the HLB of an emulsifier blend consisting of 25% of Span 20 and 75% of Tween 20?

2. Calculate the HLB of a mixture of 45 g of Span 80 and 55 g of Polysorbate 80.

3. What is the HLB of an emulsifier blend consisting of 20% of Span 60, 20% of Span 80, and 60% of Tween 60?

4. Calculate the "required HLB" for the oil phase of the following ointment.

| | | |
|---|---|---|
| Stearyl Alcohol | | 250 g |
| White Petrolatum | | 250 g |
| Propylene Glycol | | 120 g |
| Emulsifier | | q.s. |
| Preserved Water | ad | 1000 g |

5. Calculate the "required HLB" for the oil phase of the following oil-in-water type lotion.

| | | |
|---|---|---|
| Mineral Oil | | 30% |
| Lanolin, Anhydrous | | 2% |
| Cetyl Alcohol | | 3% |
| Emulsifier | | q.s. |
| Preserved Water | ad | 100% |

6. In what proportion should Tween 60 and Arlacel 83 be blended to obtain a "required HLB" of 11.5?

7. The "required HLB" of an oil phase is 13.2. What percentage of Tween 40 and of Span 40 should be used to give the "required HLB"?

8. The formula for a greaseless ointment calls for 100 g of an emulsifier blend consisting of Polysorbate 80 and Span 80. If the "required HLB" of the oil phase is 11.5, how many grams of each emulsifier should be used in preparing the ointment?

9. The formula for a cosmetic cream calls for 5% of an emulsifier blend consisting of Span 60 and Tween 20. If the "required HLB" of the oil phase is 14.0, how many grams of each emulsifier should be used in preparing 500 g of the cream?

10.

| | | |
|---|---|---|
| Stearic Acid | | 8.0% |
| Cetyl Alcohol | | 1.0% |
| Lanolin, Anhydrous | | 1.0% |
| Emulsifier | | 4.0% |
| Glycerin | | 10.0% |
| Preserved Water | ad | 100.0% |

(*a*) Calculate the "required HLB" of the oil phase.

(*b*) How many grams of Span 80 and how many grams of Tween 60 should be used in formulating 1000 g of the product?

APPENDIX

# F

# Some Calculations Involving the Use of Tablets and Capsules in Compounding Procedures

Pharmacists frequently find that proprietary tablets and capsules provide the only convenient source of medicinal agents needed to compound a prescription or medication order. Formerly, *dispensing tablets* and *tablet triturates* were used to provide pharmacists with convenient and measured quantities of potent drug substances for compounding purposes. Today, dispensing tablets are no longer in use and tablet triturates are only rarely used. Thus, in extemporaneous compounding the pharmacist may utilize commercially prepared tablets and capsules as the source of drug substance(s) required.

In addition to the use of tablets for compounding, some tablets are utilized as the measured source of a drug substance in the preparation of solutions. Official monographs describe *Tablets for Solution* (e.g., Halazone Tablets for Solution), *Tablets for Oral Solution* (e.g., Penicillin G Potassium Tablets for Oral Solution) and *Tablets for Topical Solution* (e.g., Cocaine Hydrochloride Tablets for Topical Solution) which are intended to be added to a given volume of water to produce a solution of a desired concentration.

**To obtain a desired quantity of a drug substance by the use of tablets:**

*Examples:*

*The only source of sodium chloride is in the form of tablets each containing 1 g. Explain how you would obtain the amount of sodium chloride needed for the following prescription.*

| ℞ | | |
|---|---|---|
| ℞ | Ephedrine Sulfate | 0.5 |
| | Isotonic Sodium Chloride Solution (0.9%) | 50.0 |
| | Sig. For the nose. | |

$50 \text{ (g)} \times 0.009 = 0.450 \text{ g}$ of sodium chloride needed

Since one tablet contains 1 g of sodium chloride or $^{20}/_{9}$ *times* the amount desired, $^{9}/_{20}$ of the tablet will contain the required quantity or 0.450 g. The required amount of sodium chloride may be obtained as follows:

*Step 1.* Dissolve *one* tablet in enough distilled water to make 20 mL of dilution.

*Step 2.* Take 9 mL of the dilution, *answer.*

*The only source of potassium permanganate is in the form of tablets for topical solution each containing 0.3 g. Explain how you would obtain the amount of potassium permanganate needed for the following prescription.*

℞ Potassium Pemanganate Solution 1:5000 250 mL
Sig. Use as directed.

$$1{:}5000 = 0.02\%$$

$$250 \text{ (g)} \times 0.0002 = 0.050 \text{ g or } 50 \text{ mg of potassium permanganate needed}$$

Since one tablet for topical solution contains 300 mg of potassium permanganate or 6 *times* the amount needed, $^{1}/_{6}$ of the tablet will contain the required amount or 50 mg. The required quantity of potassium permanganate may be obtained as follows:

*Step 1.* Dissolve *one* tablet for topical solution in enough distilled water to make 60 mL of dilution.

*Step 2.* Take 10 mL of the dilution, *answer.*

*Only capsules, each containing 25 mg of indomethacin, are available. How many capsules should be used to obtain the amount of indomethacin needed in preparing the following prescription?*

℞ Indomethacin 2 mg/mL
Cherry Syrup ad 150 mL
Sig. 5 mL b.i.d.

Since 2 mg/mL of indomethacin are prescribed, 300 mg are needed in filling the prescription.

And since each capsule contains 25 mg of indomethacin, then, 300 (mg) ÷ 25 (mg) = 12 capsules are needed, *answer.*

## Practice Problems

1. ℞ Potassium Permanganate Solution 1:10,000 500 mL
Sig. Use as directed.

Using tablets, each containing 0.3 g of potassium permanganate, explain how you would obtain the amount of potassium permanganate needed for the prescription.

2. A pediatric prescription calls for 250 mL of a solution, each teaspoonful to contain $\frac{1}{1000}$ gr of atropine sulfate. How many tablets, each containing $\frac{1}{150}$ gr of atropine sulfate, should be used in preparing the solution?

3. How many milliliters of a 0.9% solution of sodium chloride can be made from 10 tablets for solution each containing 2.25 g of sodium chloride?

4. ℞ Holocaine Hydrochloride Solution 1% 7.5 mL
Scopolamine Hydrobromide Solution 0.2% 7.5 mL
Sig. For the eye.

How many tablets, each containing 600 μg of scopolamine hydrobromide, should be used in compounding the prescription?

5. ℞ Hexachlorophene
Hydrocortisone aa 0.25%
Coal Tar Solution 30.0 mL
Hydrophilic Ointment ad 120.0 g
Sig. Apply.

How many tablets, each containing 20 mg of hydrocortisone, should be used in compounding the prescription?

6. ℞ Atropine Sulfate gr $\frac{1}{200}$ per teaspoonful
B Complex Elixir ad 240 mL
Sig. Teaspoonful in water.

Only $\frac{1}{150}$-gr tablets of atropine sulfate are available. How many tablets should be used to obtain the required amount of atropine sulfate?

7. ℞ Vitamin $B_{12}$ 0.6 mg
Lactated Pepsin Elixir
Phenobarbital Elixir aa 120 mL
Sig. 5 mL t.i.d.

How many tablets of vitamin $B_{12}$, each containing 25 μg, should be used in compounding the prescription?

8. How many tablets for solution, each containing 4 mg of halazone, should be added to 1 gallon of water to provide a concentration of 1:250,000 (w/v)?

9. How many tablets for topical solution, each containing 300 mg of potassium permanganate, should be added to 1 gallon of distilled water to provide a concentration of 0.012% (w/v)?

10. A prescription for 240 mL of a cough mixture calls for 2 mg of hydrocodone bitartrate per teaspoonful. How many tablets, each containing 5 mg of hydrocodone bitartrate, should be used in preparing the cough mixture?

11. ℞ Atropine Sulfate 0.3 mg
Aspirin 300 mg
Make 20 such capsules
Sig. One capsule as directed.

How many tablets, each containing 400 μg of atropine sulfate, should be used to obtain the atropine sulfate needed for the prescription?

12. ℞ Cocaine Hydrochloride 1 g
Isotonic Sodium Chloride Solution 100 mL
Sig. For the nose.

The only source of sodium chloride is in the form of tablets each containing 2.25 g. Explain how you would obtain the amount of sodium chloride needed for the prescription. Isotonic sodium chloride solution contains 0.9% of sodium chloride.

13. ℞ Colchicine gr $\frac{1}{150}$
Sodium Salicylate gr v
Make 20 such capsules
Sig. One for pain.

How many granules, each containing $\frac{1}{120}$ gr of colchicine, should be used to obtain the amount of colchicine required for the prescription?

14. The only source of sodium chloride is in the form of tablets, each containing 2.25 g. How many tablets should be used in preparing 1 liter of a stock solution of such strength that 20 mL diluted 100 mL with water will yield a 0.9% (w/v) solution?

15. ℞ Atropine Sulfate 300 μg
Phenobarbital 30 mg
Dextroamphetamine Sulfate 3 mg
Make 20 such capsules
Sig. One capsule as directed.

If the atropine sulfate is available only in the form of tablets, each containing $\frac{1}{150}$ gr, how many tablets should be used in compounding the prescription?

16. A physician prescribes thirty capsules, each containing 300 mg of ibuprofen, for a patient. The pharmacist has on hand 400 mg and 600 mg ibuprofen tablets. How many each of these tablets could be used to obtain the amount of ibuprofen needed in filling the prescription?

17. A pharmacist prepared a solution of atropine sulfate by dissolving 10 tablets, each containing $\frac{1}{150}$ gr, in enough distilled water to make 10 mL. How many milliliters of the solution would provide a patient with $\frac{1}{100}$ gr of atropine sulfate prior to surgery?

18. ℞ Minoxidil 0.3%
Vehicle/N ad 50 mL
Sig. Apply to affected areas of the scalp b.i.d.

Tablets, containing 2.5 mg and 10 mg of minoxidil, are available. Explain how you would obtain the amount of minoxidil needed in filling the prescription, using the available sources of the drug.

19. ℞ Nystatin 100,000 units/g
Chloramphenicol 250 mg
Unibase
Petrolatum aa ad 30 g
Sig. Apply to hands twice daily.

How many tablets, each containing 500,000 units of nystatin, could be used to obtain the nystatin needed in compounding the prescription?

20. ℞ Aminophylline 500 mg
Sodium Pentobarbital 75 mg
Carbowax Base ad 2 g
Ft. suppos. no. 12
Sig. Insert one at night.

How many capsules, each containing 100 mg of sodium pentobarbital, should be used to provide the sodium pentobarbital needed in compounding the prescription?

APPENDIX

# G

# Some Calculations Involving Units of Potency

The potency of many antibiotics and endocrine preparations as well as most of the enzymes, serums, toxins, vaccines and related products is expressed in terms of *units*. Officially, these units refer to U.S.P. units of activity, and they are equivalent to the corresponding international units, where such exist, and to the units of activity established by the Food and Drug Administration in the case of antibiotics, and by the National Institutes of Health in the case of biological products. There is no relationship between the unit of potency of one drug and the unit of potency of another drug.

A comparison of units of potency of some official drugs and their respective weight equivalents is given in the table which follows:

**TABLE OF DRUG UNITAGE EQUIVALENTS**

| *Drug* | *Units of Potency* | *Weight Equivalents* |
|---|---|---|
| Bacitracin | 40 to 50 Units | 1 mg of bacitracin |
| Bacitracin Zinc | 40 to 50 Units | 1 mg of bacitracin |
| Ergocalciferol | 40 U.S.P. Vitamin D Units | 1 μg of vitamin D |
| Heparin Sodium | 140 U.S.P. Heparin Units | 1 mg of heparin sodium |
| Hyaluronidase | 1 U.S.P. Hyaluronidase Unit | 0.25 μg of tyrosine |
| Insulin | 26 U.S.P. Insulin Units | 1 mg of crystallized insulin |
| Insulin Human | 26 U.S.P. Insulin Units | 1 mg of crystallized insulin |
| Nystatin | 4400 Nystatin Units | 1 mg of nystatin |
| Penicillin G Benzathine | 1211 Penicillin G Units | 1 mg of penicillin G |
| Penicillin G Potassium | 1595 Penicillin G Units | 1 mg of penicillin G potassium |
| Penicillin G Procaine | 1009 Penicillin G Units | 1 mg of penicillin G |
| Penicillin V | 1520 Penicillin V Units | 1 mg of penicillin V |
| Penicillin V Potassium | 1380 Penicillin V Units | 1 mg of penicillin V |

Just as potencies of certain drugs are designated in units, so too, the doses of these drugs and of their preparations are measured in units; and problems involving the computation of the amount of a drug or its preparation corresponding to a prescribed dose are usually solved by simple proportion.

Of the drugs whose potency is expressed in units, insulin and the antibiotics are perhaps the most commonly used. In the case of insulin, several types which may vary according to the time of onset of action and the duration of action are commercially available in different strengths. These strengths are designated as U-40, U-100 and U-500, and their potencies refer to 40, 100 and 500 U.S.P. Insulin Units per mL of solution or suspension. Special syringes are available for measuring units of insulin, but frequently a 1-mL tuberculin syringe or a regular syringe of 1 or 2 mL capacity is used, and the required dosage is then measured in milliliters, minims or directly in units, depending upon the calibration of the syringe.

**To calculate the amount of a drug or preparation equivalent to a dose expressed in units:**

*Examples:*

*How many milliliters of U-100 insulin should be used to obtain 40 units of insulin?*

U-100 insulin contains 100 units per mL

$$\frac{100 \text{ (units)}}{40 \text{ (units)}} = \frac{1 \text{ (mL)}}{x \text{ (mL)}}$$

x = 0.4 mL, *answer.*

*How many minims of U-40 insulin zinc suspension should be used to obtain 17 units of insulin?*

U-40 insulin zinc suspension contains 40 units per mL

Using 16 minims as the equivalent for 1 mL,

$$\frac{40 \text{ (units)}}{17 \text{ (units)}} = \frac{16 \text{ (minims)}}{x \text{ (minims)}}$$

x = 6.8 or 7 minims, *answer.*

*How many milliliters of a heparin sodium injection containing 200,000 units in 10 mL should be used to obtain 5,000 heparin sodium units which are to be added to an intravenous dextrose solution?*

$$\frac{200{,}000 \text{ (units)}}{5{,}000 \text{ (units)}} = \frac{10 \text{ (mL)}}{x \text{ (mL)}}$$

$$x = 0.25 \text{ mL, } \textit{answer.}$$

## Practice Problems

1. How many milliliters of U-40 insulin zinc suspension should be used to obtain 18 units of insulin?

2. A patient is required to take 9 units of U-40 isophane insulin suspension and 16 units of U-100 protamine zinc insulin. What volume, in minims, of each type will provide the desired dosage?

3. How many minims of U-100 insulin injection should be used to obtain 60 units?

4. How many milliliters of U-40 isophane insulin suspension should be used to provide 28 units of insulin?

5. A physician prescribes 60 mL of phenoxymethyl penicillin for oral suspension containing 4,800,000 units. How many penicillin units will be represented in each teaspoonful dose of the prepared suspension?

6. The contents of a vial of penicillin G potassium weigh 600 mg and represent one million units. How many milligrams are needed to prepare 15 g of an ointment which is to contain 15,000 units of penicillin G potassium per g?

7. If 10 μg of ergocalciferol represent 400 units of vitamin D, how many 1.25-mg ergocalciferol capsules will provide a dose of 200,000 units of vitamin D?

8. A physician prescribes 2.5 million units of penicillin G potassium daily for one week. If 1 unit of penicillin G potassium equals 0.6 μg, how many tablets, each containing 250 mg, will provide the penicillin G potassium for the prescribed dosage regimen?

9. ℞ Penicillin G Potassium 5,000 units per mL
Isotonic Sodium Chloride Solution ad 15 mL
Sig. Nose drops.

Using soluble penicillin tablets, each containing 200,000 units of crystalline penicillin G potassium, explain how you would obtain the penicillin G potassium needed in compounding the prescription.

10. If 1 mg of penicillin V represents 1520 penicillin V units, how many micrograms represent 1 unit?

11. Corticotropin injection is available in a concentration of 40 units per mL. How many milliliters of the injection should be administered to provide 0.4 unit per kg for a child weighing 66 lb?

12. If 1 mg of heparin sodium is equivalent to 140 U.S.P. Heparin Units, how many micrograms of heparin sodium represent 1 unit?

13. A physician's hospital medication order calls for a patient to receive 1 unit of insulin injection subcutaneously for every 10 mg% of blood sugar over 175 mg%, with blood sugar levels and injections performed twice daily in the morning and evening. The patient's blood sugar was 200 mg% in the morning and 320 mg% in the evening. How many total units of insulin injection were administered?

14. A physician's hospital medication order calls for isophane insulin suspension to be administered to a 136-lb patient on the basis of 1 unit per kilogram per 24 hours. How many units of isophane insulin suspension should be administered daily?

15. A physician's hospital medication order calls for 0.5 mL of U-500 insulin injection to be placed in a 500-mL bottle of 5% dextrose injection for infusion into a patient. If the rate of infusion was set to run for eight hours, how many units of insulin did the patient receive in the first 90 minutes of infusion?

APPENDIX

# H

# Some Calculations Involving the Use of Dry Powders for Reconstitution

Many drugs which are unstable for prolonged periods of time in solution, notably the penicillins and other antibiotics, are usually packaged and marketed in the dry form. The dry powder is dissolved in water or other aqueous diluent when the dosage form is dispensed or when it is to be used by the pharmacist as the source of a prescribed quantity of the drug. In the case of most antibiotics the reconstituted product retains its potency for the period of its use, particularly when it is kept refrigerated.

If the quantity of the dry drug powder is small and does not contribute significantly to the final volume of the reconstituted solution, the volume of diluent used will approximate the final volume of solution. For example, if 1000 units of a certain antibiotic in dry form are to be dissolved and if the powder does not account for any significant portion of the final volume, the addition of 5 mL of diluent will produce a solution containing 200 units per mL.

But if the dry powder, because of its bulk, contributes to the final volume of the reconstituted solution, the increase in volume produced by the drug must be taken into consideration, and this factor must then be used in calculating the amount of diluent to be used in preparing a solution of a desired concentration. For example, the package directions for making solutions of streptomycin sulfate specify that 4.2 mL of sterile diluent be added to 1 g of the dry powder to produce 5.0 mL of a solution which is to contain 200 mg per mL. The drug, in this case, accounts for 0.8 mL of the final volume. And again, in dissolving 20,000,000 units of penicillin G potassium, the addition of 32 mL of sterile diluent provides a total volume of 40 mL of a solution which contains 500,000 units per mL. The dry powder now accounts for 8 mL of the final volume.

Information concerning this increase in volume is particularly useful to the pharmacist when he prepares solutions of these drugs in concentrations other than those which are specifically mentioned in the package literature. The reconstituted solutions of the dry powders are most frequently prescribed alone, but they may also be used as a source for obtaining desired quantities of the drugs in solution.

**To calculate the amount of diluent to be used for a given vial content of a dry powder to produce a desired concentration when the solid material does not significantly account for any portion of the reconstituted solution:**

*Examples:*

*Using a vial containing 200,000 units of penicillin G potassium, how many milliliters of diluent should be added to the dry powder in preparing a solution having a concentration of 25,000 units per mL?*

$$\frac{25{,}000 \text{ (units)}}{200{,}000 \text{ (units)}} = \frac{1 \text{ (mL)}}{x \text{ (mL)}}$$

$x = 8$ mL, *answer.*

*Using a vial containing 200,000 units of penicillin G sodium and sodium chloride injection as the diluent, explain how you would obtain the penicillin G sodium needed in compounding the following prescription.*

℞ Penicillin G Sodium 15,000 units per mL
Sodium Chloride Injection ad 10 mL
Sig. For IM Injection.

15,000 units × 10 = 150,000 units of penicillin G sodium needed

Since the dry powder represents 200,000 units of penicillin G sodium or $\frac{4}{3}$ *times* the number of units desired, $\frac{3}{4}$ of the powder will contain the required number of units.

*Step 1.* Dissolve the dry powder in 4 mL of sodium chloride injection.

*Step 2.* Use 3 mL of the reconstituted solution, *answer.*

**To calculate the amount of diluent to be used for a given vial content of a dry powder to produce a desired concentration when the solid material accounts for a definite volume of the reconstituted solution:**

*Examples:*

*The package information enclosed with a vial containing 5,000,000 units of penicillin G potassium (buffered) specifies that when 23 mL of a sterile diluent are added to the dry powder the resulting concentration is 200,000*

*units per mL. On the basis of this information, how many milliliters of water for injection should be used in preparing the following solution?*

> ℞ Penicillin G Potassium (buffered) 5,000,000 units
> Water for Injection q.s.
> Make solution containing 500,000 units per mL
> Sig. One mL = 500,000 units of Penicillin G Potassium.

It should be noted from the package information that the reconstituted solution prepared by dissolving 5,000,000 units of the dry powder in 23 mL of sterile diluent has a final volume of 25 mL. The dry powder, then, accounts for 2 mL of this volume.

*Step 1.* The final volume of the prescription is determined as follows:

$$\frac{500{,}000 \text{ (units)}}{5{,}000{,}000 \text{ (units)}} = \frac{1 \text{ (mL)}}{x \text{ (mL)}}$$

$$x = 10 \text{ mL}$$

*Step 2.* 10 mL − 2 mL (dry powder accounts for this volume) = 8 mL, *answer.*

*Streptomycin sulfate is available in 1-g vials, and the dry powder accounts for 0.8 mL of the volume of the reconstituted solution. Using a 1-g vial of streptomycin sulfate and sodium chloride injection as the diluent, explain how you would obtain the streptomycin sulfate needed for the following prescription.*

> ℞ Streptomycin Sulfate 250 mg
> Sodium Chloride Injection ad 15 mL
> Sig. For IM Injection.

*Step 1.* Dissolve the dry powder in 9.2 mL of sodium chloride injection. The reconstituted solution will measure 10 mL and will contain 100 mg of streptomycin sulfate per mL.

*Step 2.* Use 2.5 mL of the reconstituted solution, *answer.*

## Practice Problems

1. ℞ Penicillin G Potassium 5,000,000 units
   Water for Injection q.s.
   M. et. ft. sol. 250,000 units per ½ mL
   Sig. One-half mL (250,000 units) by aerosol inhalation every 3 hours.

The package information enclosed with a vial containing 5,000,000 units of penicillin G potassium specifies that when 23 mL of a sterile diluent are added to the powder the resulting concentration is 200,000 units per mL. On the basis of this information, how many milliliters of water for injection should be used in compounding the prescription?

2. ℞ Bacitracin 1000 units per g
Distilled Water q.s.
Hydrophilic Ointment ad 30 g
Sig. Apply as directed. Store in the refrigerator.

The only source of bacitracin is a vial containing 50,000 units of the dry powder. Using distilled water as the diluent, explain how you would obtain the bacitracin needed in compounding the prescription.

3. ℞ Polymyxin B Sulfate 10,000 units per mL
Sterile Distilled Water ad 15 mL
Sig. Use topically.

Using the contents of a vial (500,000 units) of polymyxin B sulfate and sterile distilled water as the diluent, explain how you would obtain the polymyxin B sulfate needed in compounding the prescription.

4. A medication order calls for 400 mg of cefazolin sodium to be administered IM to a patient every 12 hours. Vials containing 250 mg, 500 mg and 1 g of cefazolin sodium are available. According to the manufacturer's directions, dilutions may be made as follows:

| *Vial Size* | *Diluent to Be Added* | *Final Volume* |
|---|---|---|
| 250 mg | 2 mL | 2 mL |
| 500 mg | 2 mL | 2.2 mL |
| 1 g | 2.5 mL | 3 mL |

Explain how the prescribed amount of cefazolin sodium could be obtained.

5. Using the vial sizes in problem #4 as the source of cefazolin sodium, how many milliliters of the diluted 500 mg vial should be administered to a 40-lb child who is to receive 8 mg of cefazolin sodium per kilogram of body weight?

6. Using cefazolin sodium injection in a concentration of 125 mg/mL, complete the following table representing a *Pediatric Dosage Guide:*

| *Weight* | | *Dose—25 mg/kg/day divided into 3 doses* | |
|---|---|---|---|
| *lb* | *kg* | *Approximate single dose (mg/q8h)* | *mL of dilution (125 mg/mL) needed* |
| 10 | 4.5 | 37.5 or 38 mg | 0.3 mL |
| 20 | ____ | ________ | ________ |
| 30 | ____ | ________ | ________ |
| 40 | ____ | ________ | ________ |
| 50 | ____ | ________ | ________ |

7. A pharmacist receives a medication order for 300,000 units of penicillin G potassium to be added to 500 mL of $D_5W$. The directions on the 1,000,000-unit package state that if 1.6 mL of diluent are added the reconstituted solution will measure 2 mL. How many milliliters of the reconstituted solution must be withdrawn and added to the $D_5W$?

APPENDIX

# I

# Exponential and Logarithmic Notation

## EXPONENTIAL NOTATION

Many physical and chemical measurements deal with either very large or very small numbers. Since it is difficult, in many instances, to handle conveniently numbers of such magnitude in performing even the simplest arithmetic operations in the usual manner, it is best to use exponential notation or *powers of 10* to express them. Thus, we may express *121* as $1.21 \times 10^2$, *1210* as $1.21 \times 10^3$, and *1,210,000* as $1.21 \times 10^6$. Likewise, we may express *0.0121* as $1.21 \times 10^{-2}$, *0.00121* as $1.21 \times 10^{-3}$, and *0.00000121* as $1.21 \times 10^{-6}$.

When numbers are written in this manner, the first part is called the *coefficient*, customarily written with one figure to the left of the decimal point. The second part is the *exponential factor* or *power of ten.*

The exponent represents the number of places that the decimal point has been moved—positive to the left and negative to the right—to form the exponential. Thus, when we convert *19000* to $1.9 \times 10^4$, we move the decimal point 4 places to the left; hence the exponent$^4$. And when we convert *0.0000019* to $1.9 \times 10^{-6}$, we move the decimal point 6 places to the right; hence the *negative* exponent$^{-6}$.

## FUNDAMENTAL ARITHMETIC OPERATIONS WITH EXPONENTIALS

In the *multiplication* of exponentials, the exponents are *added*. For example, $10^2 \times 10^4 = 10^6$. In the multiplication of numbers that are expressed in exponential form, the *coefficients* are multiplied together in the usual manner and this product is then multiplied by the power of *10* found by algebraically *adding* the exponents.

*Examples:*

$$(2.5 \times 10^2) \times (2.5 \times 10^4) = 6.25 \times 10^6, \text{ or } 6.3 \times 10^6$$
$$(2.5 \times 10^2) \times (2.5 \times 10^{-4}) = 6.25 \times 10^{-2}, \text{ or } 6.3 \times 10^{-2}$$
$$(5.4 \times 10^2) \times (4.5 \times 10^3) = 24.3 \times 10^5 = 2.4 \times 10^6$$

In the *division* of exponentials, the exponents are *subtracted*. For example, $10^2 \div 10^5 = 10^{-3}$. And in the division of numbers that are expressed in exponential form, the *coefficients* are divided in the usual way and the result is multiplied by the power of *10* found by algebraically *subtracting* the exponents.

*Examples:*

$$(7.5 \times 10^5) \div (2.5 \times 10^3) = 3.0 \times 10^2$$
$$(7.5 \times 10^{-4}) \div (2.5 \times 10^6) = 3.0 \times 10^{-10}$$
$$(2.8 \times 10^{-2}) \div (8.0 \times 10^{-6}) = 0.35 \times 10^4 = 3.5 \times 10^3$$

Note that in each of the examples above the result is rounded off to the number of *significant figures* contained in the *least* accurate factor, and it is expressed with only one figure to the left of the decimal point.

In the *addition* and *subtraction* of exponentials, the expressions must be changed (by moving the decimal points) to forms having any common power of 10 and then the coefficients only are added or subtracted. The result should be rounded off to the number of *decimal places* contained in the *least* precise component, and it should be expressed with only one figure to the left of the decimal point.

*Examples:*

$$(1.4 \times 10^4) + (5.1 \times 10^3)$$
$$
\begin{array}{rl}
 & 1.4 \times 10^4 \\
5.1 \times 10^3 = & \underline{0.51} \times 10^4 \\
\text{Total:} & 1.91 \times 10^4, \text{ or } 1.9 \times 10^4, \textit{ answer.}
\end{array}
$$

$$(1.4 \times 10^4) - (5.1 \times 10^3)$$
$$
\begin{array}{rl}
1.4 \times 10^4 = & 14.0 \times 10^3 \\
 & \underline{-5.1} \times 10^3 \\
\text{Difference:} & 8.9 \times 10^3, \textit{ answer.}
\end{array}
$$

$$(9.83 \times 10^3) + (4.1 \times 10^1) + (2.6 \times 10^3)$$
$$
\begin{array}{rl}
 & 9.83 \times 10^3 \\
4.1 \times 10^1 = & 0.041 \times 10^3 \\
 & \underline{2.6 \times 10^3} \\
\text{Total:} & 12.471 \times 10^3, \text{ or} \\
 & 12.5 \times 10^3 = 1.25 \times 10^4, \textit{ answer.}
\end{array}
$$

### Practice Problems

1. Write each of the following in exponential form:

   (a) 12,650
   (b) 0.0000000055
   (c) 451
   (d) 0.065
   (e) 625,000,000

2. Write each of the following in the usual numerical form:

   (a) $4.1 \times 10^6$
   (b) $3.65 \times 10^{-2}$
   (c) $5.13 \times 10^{-6}$
   (d) $2.5 \times 10^5$
   (e) $8.6956 \times 10^3$

3. Find the product:

   (a) $(3.5 \times 10^3) \times (5.0 \times 10^4)$
   (b) $(8.2 \times 10^2) \times (2.0 \times 10^{-6})$
   (c) $(1.5 \times 10^{-6}) \times (4.0 \times 10^6)$
   (d) $(1.5 \times 10^3) \times (8.0 \times 10^4)$
   (e) $(7.2 \times 10^5) \times (5.0 \times 10^{-3})$

4. Find the quotient:

   (a) $(9.3 \times 10^5) \div (3.1 \times 10^2)$
   (b) $(3.6 \times 10^{-4}) \div (1.2 \times 10^6)$
   (c) $(3.3 \times 10^7) \div (1.1 \times 10^{-2})$

5. Find the sum:

   (a) $(9.2 \times 10^3) + (7.6 \times 10^4)$
   (b) $(1.8 \times 10^{-6}) + (3.4 \times 10^{-5})$
   (c) $(4.9 \times 10^2) + (2.5 \times 10^3)$

6. Find the difference:

   (a) $(6.5 \times 10^6) - (5.9 \times 10^4)$
   (b) $(8.2 \times 10^{-3}) - (1.6 \times 10^{-3})$
   (c) $(7.4 \times 10^3) - (4.6 \times 10^2)$

## COMMON LOGARITHMIC NOTATION

We have seen that exponential notation allows us to express any number as a *coefficient times a whole-number power of 10*—as when we interpret *150* to mean $1.5 \times 10^2$—and that this system of notation offers us a convenient shorthand, as it were, for expressing and manipulating very large or very small numbers.

Still another system, called *common logarithmic notation,* goes the exponential system one better. In common logarithmic notation *every number is expressed simply as a power of 10*—not with absolute precision, but with sufficient accuracy for any given purpose—and we may multiply any two numbers so expressed, or divide one by the other, by the simple process of adding or subtracting their exponents.

The *exponent* that indicates *to what power 10 must be raised to equal approximately a given number* is called the *common logarithm* of that number.

It follows that the logarithm of *10* or of any integral power of *10* is always a positive or negative integer:

$$\log 10 \text{ (or } 1 \times 10^1) = 1$$
$$\log 100 \text{ (or } 1 \times 10^2) = 2$$
$$\log 1000 \text{ (or } 1 \times 10^3) = 3$$

and so on; and

$$\log 1 \text{ (or } 1 \times 10^0) = 0$$
$$\log 0.1 \text{ (or } 1 \times 10^{-1}) = -1$$
$$\log 0.01 \text{ (or } 1 \times 10^{-2}) = -2$$

and so on. And if these were the only numbers in existence, no table of logarithms should be needed; for, given a number, say *1,000,000* (or $1 \times 10^6$) if we know the system we can readily supply its logarithm: 6; or, given the logarithm *6,* we can readily reconstruct the number it represents: *1,000,000.*

But any number *not* in the *10's* series must contain a certain *excess* over some power of *10*—as *150* contains $10^2$ plus an excess of *50.* Therefore, the logarithm of such a number always consists of a positive or negative whole-numbered exponent *plus* a positive decimal-fraction exponent (carried to as many decimal places as suit our purpose). As it turns out, the power of *10* that approximates *150* (or $1.5 \times 10^2$) is $10^{2.1761}$, and therefore $\log 150 = 2.1761$.

The *whole-number exponent* is called the *characteristic.* It accounts for the integral power of *10* contained in the given number and hence serves to locate the *decimal point* in that number. If a number is given in ordinary notation, you can find the characteristic by converting it to exponential notation, in which the characteristic appears as a power of *10.*

The *decimal-fraction exponent* is called the *mantissa.* You can find the mantissa in a table of logarithms. The mantissa represents the *significant figures* in a given number, regardless of the location of the decimal point. In other words, given the sequence *610,* a four-place table will tell you the mantissa is *7853,* whether the number be *61.0,* or *6.10,* or *0.00610.*

Compare this series of logarithms with the logarithms of the 10's series given above:

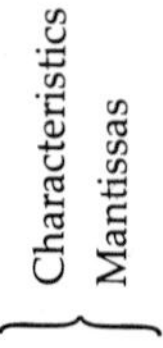


$$\begin{aligned}
\log\ 6.10\ (\text{or } 6.10 \times 10^{0}) &= 0.7853 \\
\log\ 61.0\ (\text{or } 6.10 \times 10^{1}) &= 1.7853 \\
\log\ 610\ (\text{or } 6.10 \times 10^{2}) &= 2.7853 \\
\log\ 6100\ (\text{or } 6.10 \times 10^{3}) &= 3.7853
\end{aligned}$$

and so on; and

$$\begin{aligned}
\log 0.610\ (\text{or } 6.10 \times 10^{-1}) &= \bar{1}.7853 \\
\log 0.0610\ (\text{or } 6.10 \times 10^{-2}) &= \bar{2}.7853 \\
\log 0.00610\ (\text{or } 6.10 \times 10^{-3}) &= \bar{3}.7853
\end{aligned}$$

and so on. Note that by putting the minus sign *over* the characteristic we indicate that it alone is negative, and that the mantissa, as always, is positive.

## NATURAL LOGARITHMS

The base of the *natural* or *Naperian* system of logarithms is *e* which is the irrational number 2.71828. . . . When it becomes necessary to change from a natural logarithm to a common logarithm, the computation may be performed by using the following relationship:

$$\log_e n = 2.303 \log_{10} n$$

where 2.303 is the logarithm of 10 to the base 2.71828.

## USE OF LOGARITHM TABLES

Logarithm tables give mantissas calculated to four-place, five-place accuracy, and upwards, depending on the table and its purpose. A four-place table insures an accuracy within 0.5% when we work with three figure numbers.

The Table (pp. 306–307) has typical features. It contains (1) a column to the left and a row at the top to guide us in locating the mantissas of 3-figure numbers, (2) the 4-place mantissas of all 3-figure numbers, and (3) columns of proportional parts providing us with a quick means of calculating more accurate mantissas when given numbers of 4-figure accuracy—a process called *interpolation*.

**To find the logarithm of a number:**

First, determine the characteristic, then find the mantissa in the log table.

*Examples:*

*Find the log of 262.*

$262 = 2.62 \times 10^2$
By inspection of the ten factor, the characteristic = 2.
To find the mantissa, focus attention on the digits *262*.
If the left-hand column in the log table find *26;* opposite it and in the column numbered *2* is the desired mantissa 0.4183. (The table omits the 0.)

Therefore, log 262 = 2.4183, *answer.*

*Find the log of 2627.*

$2627 = 2.627 \times 10^3$
By inspection of the ten factor, the characteristic = 3.
In the left-hand column in the table find *26;* opposite it and in the column numbered *2* find the mantissa 0.4183; opposite *26* and in column 7 under proportional parts find 11 (meaning 0.0011 but written without zeros) and add it to 0.4183 to obtain the desired mantissa 0.4194.

Therefore, log 2627 = 3.4194, *answer.*

*Find the log of 0.002627.*

$0.002627 = 2.627 \times 10^{-3}$
By inspection of the ten factor, the characteristic = $\bar{3}$.
The mantissa is determined as in the preceding example.

Therefore, log 0.002627 = $\bar{3}.4194$, *answer.*

**To find the antilogarithm of a logarithm:**

When a problem is solved by logarithms, the result is expressed as the *logarithm* of the answer. This necessitates the finding of the *antilogarithm* or *the number corresponding to the logarithm.* If the mantissa of a logarithm is known, its antilogarithm can be found by a *reverse reading* of the log table.

*Examples:*

*Find the antilogarithm of the logarithm 1.7604.*

The mantissa 0.7604 is found in the column numbered *6* opposite *57*, and the resulting figure is 576.
The characteristic is 1 and, the required number is

$5.76 \times 10^1$ or 57.6, *answer.*

*Find the antilogarithm of the logarithm 3.7607.*

Since the mantissa 0.7607 is not found in the log table, interpolation must be used. In the log table, 0.7607 falls *between 0.7604* and *0.7612;* therefore, the resulting figure must be between *576* and *577.*
The *given* mantissa is 0.0003 (or 3 units) more than the mantissa 0.7604. Therefore opposite 0.7604 find 3 in column *4* of proportional parts. Then the required figure is *5764.*
The characteristic is 3 and the required number is

$5.764 \times 10^3 = 5764$, *answer.*

## SOME LOGARITHMIC COMPUTATIONS

As shown in the first example below, when a negative number is "added" it is actually *subtracted;* and as shown in the third example, when a negative number is "subtracted" it is actually *added.*

The fourth example shows the curious but consistent fact that, in subtracting one logarithm from another, if you *borrow* from a negative characteristic (as 1 is borrowed from the $-1$ of the minuend) you *increase* the value of the negative characteristic (as the $-1$ becomes $-2$, which is canceled out when the *2* of the subtrahend is "subtracted" from it).

*Examples:*

*Multiply* $(5.25 \times 10^3)$ *by* $(8.92 \times 10^{-6})$ *by* $(7.56 \times 10^5)$.

$$\begin{aligned} \log (5.25 \times 10^3) &= 3.7202 \\ \log (8.92 \times 10^{-6}) &= \bar{6}.9504 \\ \log (7.56 \times 10^5) &= \underline{5.8785} \\ \text{Total:} \quad & \phantom{=} 4.5491 \end{aligned}$$

Antilogarithm of $4.5491 = 3.541 \times 10^4 = 35410$, or (retaining only 3 significant figures), 35400, *answer.*

*Divide 29600 by 5.544.*

$29600 = 2.96 \times 10^4$
$5.544 = 5.544 \times 10^0$
$\log(2.96 \times 10^4) = 4.4713$
$\log(5.544 \times 10^0) = 0.7438$
Difference: 3.7275

Antilogarithm of 3.7275 = $5.34 \times 10^3$ = 5340, *answer.*

*Divide 7500 by 0.627.*

$7500 = 7.50 \times 10^3$
$0.627 = 6.27 \times 10^{-1}$
$\log(7.50 \times 10^3) = 3.8751$
$\log(6.27 \times 10^{-1}) = \bar{1}.7973$
Difference: 4.0778

Antilogarithm of 4.0778 = $1.196 \times 10^4$ = 11960, or (retaining only 3 significant figures), 12000, *answer.*

*Divide 0.191 by 0.0452.*

$0.191 = 1.91 \times 10^{-1}$
$0.0452 = 4.52 \times 10^{-2}$
$\log(1.91 \times 10^{-1}) = \bar{1}.2810$
$\log(4.52 \times 10^{-2}) = \bar{2}.6551$
Difference: 0.6259

Antilogarithm of 0.6259 = $4.226 \times 10^0$ = 4.226, or (retaining only 3 significant figures), 4.23, *answer.*

*Find the value of* $\dfrac{(4.54 \times 10^6) \times (3.25 \times 10^3)}{(1.21 \times 10^8)}$

$\log(4.54 \times 10^6) = 6.6571$
$\log(3.25 \times 10^3) = 3.5119$
Total: 10.1690 = *log of numerator*

$\log(1.21 \times 10^8) = 8.0828$ = *log of denominator*
Difference: 2.0862

Antilogarithm of 2.0862 = 1.219 or $1.22 \times 10^2$ = 122, *answer.*

## LOGARITHMS

| Natural Numbers | 0 | 1 | 2 | 3 | 4 | 5 | 6 | 7 | 8 | 9 | Proportional Parts | | | | | | | | |
|---|---|---|---|---|---|---|---|---|---|---|---|---|---|---|---|---|---|---|---|
| | | | | | | | | | | | 1 | 2 | 3 | 4 | 5 | 6 | 7 | 8 | 9 |
| 10 | 0000 | 0043 | 0086 | 0128 | 0170 | 0212 | 0253 | 0294 | 0334 | 0374 | 4 | 8 | 12 | 17 | 21 | 25 | 29 | 33 | 37 |
| 11 | 0414 | 0453 | 0492 | 0531 | 0569 | 0607 | 0645 | 0682 | 0719 | 0755 | 4 | 8 | 11 | 15 | 19 | 23 | 26 | 30 | 34 |
| 12 | 0792 | 0828 | 0864 | 0899 | 0934 | 0969 | 1004 | 1038 | 1072 | 1106 | 3 | 7 | 10 | 14 | 17 | 21 | 24 | 28 | 31 |
| 13 | 1139 | 1173 | 1206 | 1239 | 1271 | 1303 | 1335 | 1367 | 1399 | 1430 | 3 | 6 | 10 | 13 | 16 | 19 | 23 | 26 | 29 |
| 14 | 1461 | 1492 | 1523 | 1553 | 1584 | 1614 | 1644 | 1673 | 1703 | 1732 | 3 | 6 | 9 | 12 | 15 | 18 | 21 | 24 | 27 |
| 15 | 1761 | 1790 | 1818 | 1847 | 1875 | 1903 | 1931 | 1959 | 1987 | 2014 | 3 | 6 | 8 | 11 | 14 | 17 | 20 | 22 | 25 |
| 16 | 2041 | 2068 | 2095 | 2122 | 2148 | 2175 | 2201 | 2227 | 2253 | 2279 | 3 | 5 | 8 | 11 | 13 | 16 | 18 | 21 | 24 |
| 17 | 2304 | 2330 | 2355 | 2380 | 2405 | 2430 | 2455 | 2480 | 2504 | 2529 | 2 | 5 | 7 | 10 | 12 | 15 | 17 | 20 | 22 |
| 18 | 2553 | 2577 | 2601 | 2625 | 2648 | 2672 | 2695 | 2718 | 2742 | 2765 | 2 | 5 | 7 | 9 | 12 | 14 | 16 | 19 | 21 |
| 19 | 2788 | 2810 | 2833 | 2856 | 2878 | 2900 | 2923 | 2945 | 2967 | 2989 | 2 | 4 | 7 | 9 | 11 | 13 | 16 | 18 | 20 |
| 20 | 3010 | 3032 | 3054 | 3075 | 3096 | 3118 | 3139 | 3160 | 3181 | 3201 | 2 | 4 | 6 | 8 | 11 | 13 | 15 | 17 | 19 |
| 21 | 3222 | 3243 | 3263 | 3284 | 3304 | 3324 | 3345 | 3365 | 3385 | 3404 | 2 | 4 | 6 | 8 | 10 | 12 | 14 | 16 | 18 |
| 22 | 3424 | 3444 | 3464 | 3483 | 3502 | 3522 | 3541 | 3560 | 3579 | 3598 | 2 | 4 | 6 | 8 | 10 | 12 | 14 | 15 | 17 |
| 23 | 3617 | 3636 | 3655 | 3674 | 3692 | 3711 | 3729 | 3747 | 3766 | 3784 | 2 | 4 | 6 | 7 | 9 | 11 | 13 | 15 | 17 |
| 24 | 3802 | 3820 | 3838 | 3856 | 3874 | 3892 | 3909 | 3927 | 3945 | 3962 | 2 | 4 | 5 | 7 | 9 | 11 | 12 | 14 | 16 |
| 25 | 3979 | 3997 | 4014 | 4031 | 4048 | 4065 | 4082 | 4099 | 4116 | 4133 | 2 | 3 | 5 | 7 | 9 | 10 | 12 | 14 | 15 |
| 26 | 4150 | 4166 | 4183 | 4200 | 4216 | 4232 | 4249 | 4265 | 4281 | 4298 | 2 | 3 | 5 | 7 | 8 | 10 | 11 | 13 | 15 |
| 27 | 4314 | 4330 | 4346 | 4362 | 4378 | 4393 | 4409 | 4425 | 4440 | 4456 | 2 | 3 | 5 | 6 | 8 | 9 | 11 | 13 | 14 |
| 28 | 4472 | 4487 | 4502 | 4518 | 4533 | 4548 | 4564 | 4579 | 4594 | 4609 | 2 | 3 | 5 | 6 | 8 | 9 | 11 | 12 | 14 |
| 29 | 4624 | 4639 | 4654 | 4669 | 4683 | 4698 | 4713 | 4728 | 4742 | 4757 | 1 | 3 | 4 | 6 | 7 | 9 | 10 | 12 | 13 |
| 30 | 4771 | 4786 | 4800 | 4814 | 4829 | 4843 | 4857 | 4871 | 4886 | 4900 | 1 | 3 | 4 | 6 | 7 | 9 | 10 | 11 | 13 |
| 31 | 4914 | 4928 | 4942 | 4955 | 4969 | 4983 | 4997 | 5011 | 5024 | 5038 | 1 | 3 | 4 | 6 | 7 | 8 | 10 | 11 | 12 |
| 32 | 5051 | 5065 | 5079 | 5092 | 5105 | 5119 | 5132 | 5145 | 5159 | 5172 | 1 | 3 | 4 | 5 | 7 | 8 | 9 | 11 | 12 |
| 33 | 5185 | 5198 | 5211 | 5224 | 5237 | 5250 | 5263 | 5276 | 5289 | 5302 | 1 | 3 | 4 | 5 | 6 | 8 | 9 | 10 | 12 |
| 34 | 5315 | 5328 | 5340 | 5353 | 5366 | 5378 | 5391 | 5403 | 5416 | 5428 | 1 | 3 | 4 | 5 | 6 | 8 | 9 | 10 | 11 |
| 35 | 5441 | 5453 | 5465 | 5478 | 5490 | 5502 | 5514 | 5527 | 5539 | 5551 | 1 | 2 | 4 | 5 | 6 | 7 | 9 | 10 | 11 |
| 36 | 5563 | 5575 | 5587 | 5599 | 5611 | 5623 | 5635 | 5647 | 5658 | 5670 | 1 | 2 | 4 | 5 | 6 | 7 | 8 | 10 | 11 |
| 37 | 5682 | 5694 | 5705 | 5717 | 5729 | 5740 | 5752 | 5763 | 5775 | 5786 | 1 | 2 | 3 | 5 | 6 | 7 | 8 | 9 | 10 |
| 38 | 5798 | 5809 | 5821 | 5832 | 5843 | 5855 | 5866 | 5877 | 5888 | 5899 | 1 | 2 | 3 | 5 | 6 | 7 | 8 | 9 | 10 |
| 39 | 5911 | 5922 | 5933 | 5944 | 5955 | 5966 | 5977 | 5988 | 5999 | 6010 | 1 | 2 | 3 | 4 | 5 | 7 | 8 | 9 | 10 |
| 40 | 6021 | 6031 | 6042 | 6053 | 6064 | 6075 | 6085 | 6096 | 6107 | 6117 | 1 | 2 | 3 | 4 | 5 | 6 | 8 | 9 | 10 |
| 41 | 6128 | 6138 | 6149 | 6160 | 6170 | 6180 | 6191 | 6201 | 6212 | 6222 | 1 | 2 | 3 | 4 | 5 | 6 | 7 | 8 | 9 |
| 42 | 6232 | 6243 | 6253 | 6263 | 6274 | 6284 | 6294 | 6304 | 6314 | 6325 | 1 | 2 | 3 | 4 | 5 | 6 | 7 | 8 | 9 |
| 43 | 6335 | 6345 | 6355 | 6365 | 6375 | 6385 | 6395 | 6405 | 6415 | 6425 | 1 | 2 | 3 | 4 | 5 | 6 | 7 | 8 | 9 |
| 44 | 6435 | 6444 | 6454 | 6464 | 6474 | 6484 | 6493 | 6503 | 6513 | 6522 | 1 | 2 | 3 | 4 | 5 | 6 | 7 | 8 | 9 |
| 45 | 6532 | 6542 | 6551 | 6561 | 6571 | 6580 | 6590 | 6599 | 6609 | 6618 | 1 | 2 | 3 | 4 | 5 | 6 | 7 | 8 | 9 |
| 46 | 6628 | 6637 | 6646 | 6656 | 6665 | 6675 | 6684 | 6693 | 6702 | 6712 | 1 | 2 | 3 | 4 | 5 | 6 | 7 | 7 | 8 |
| 47 | 6721 | 6730 | 6739 | 6749 | 6758 | 6767 | 6776 | 6785 | 6794 | 6803 | 1 | 2 | 3 | 4 | 5 | 5 | 6 | 7 | 8 |
| 48 | 6812 | 6821 | 6830 | 6839 | 6848 | 6857 | 6866 | 6875 | 6884 | 6893 | 1 | 2 | 3 | 4 | 4 | 5 | 6 | 7 | 8 |
| 49 | 6902 | 6911 | 6920 | 6928 | 6937 | 6946 | 6955 | 6964 | 6972 | 6981 | 1 | 2 | 3 | 4 | 4 | 5 | 6 | 7 | 8 |
| 50 | 6990 | 6998 | 7007 | 7016 | 7024 | 7033 | 7042 | 7050 | 7059 | 7067 | 1 | 2 | 3 | 3 | 4 | 5 | 6 | 7 | 8 |
| 51 | 7076 | 7084 | 7093 | 7101 | 7110 | 7118 | 7126 | 7135 | 7143 | 7152 | 1 | 2 | 3 | 3 | 4 | 5 | 6 | 7 | 8 |
| 52 | 7160 | 7168 | 7177 | 7185 | 7193 | 7202 | 7210 | 7218 | 7226 | 7235 | 1 | 2 | 2 | 3 | 4 | 5 | 6 | 7 | 7 |
| 53 | 7243 | 7251 | 7259 | 7267 | 7275 | 7284 | 7292 | 7300 | 7308 | 7316 | 1 | 2 | 2 | 3 | 4 | 5 | 6 | 6 | 7 |
| 54 | 7324 | 7332 | 7340 | 7348 | 7356 | 7364 | 7372 | 7380 | 7388 | 7396 | 1 | 2 | 2 | 3 | 4 | 5 | 6 | 6 | 7 |

## LOGARITHMS

| Natural Numbers | 0 | 1 | 2 | 3 | 4 | 5 | 6 | 7 | 8 | 9 | Proportional Parts | | | | | | | | |
|---|---|---|---|---|---|---|---|---|---|---|---|---|---|---|---|---|---|---|---|
| | | | | | | | | | | | 1 | 2 | 3 | 4 | 5 | 6 | 7 | 8 | 9 |
| 55 | 7404 | 7412 | 7419 | 7427 | 7435 | 7443 | 7451 | 7459 | 7466 | 7474 | 1 | 2 | 2 | 3 | 4 | 5 | 5 | 6 | 7 |
| 56 | 7482 | 7490 | 7497 | 7505 | 7513 | 7520 | 7528 | 7536 | 7543 | 7551 | 1 | 2 | 2 | 3 | 4 | 5 | 5 | 6 | 7 |
| 57 | 7559 | 7566 | 7574 | 7582 | 7589 | 7597 | 7604 | 7612 | 7619 | 7627 | 1 | 2 | 2 | 3 | 4 | 5 | 5 | 6 | 7 |
| 58 | 7634 | 7642 | 7649 | 7657 | 7664 | 7672 | 7679 | 7686 | 7694 | 7701 | 1 | 1 | 2 | 3 | 4 | 4 | 5 | 6 | 7 |
| 59 | 7709 | 7716 | 7723 | 7731 | 7738 | 7745 | 7752 | 7760 | 7767 | 7774 | 1 | 1 | 2 | 3 | 4 | 4 | 5 | 6 | 7 |
| 60 | 7782 | 7789 | 7796 | 7803 | 7810 | 7818 | 7825 | 7832 | 7839 | 7846 | 1 | 1 | 2 | 3 | 4 | 4 | 5 | 6 | 6 |
| 61 | 7853 | 7860 | 7868 | 7875 | 7882 | 7889 | 7896 | 7903 | 7910 | 7917 | 1 | 1 | 2 | 3 | 4 | 4 | 5 | 6 | 6 |
| 62 | 7924 | 7931 | 7938 | 7945 | 7952 | 7959 | 7966 | 7973 | 7980 | 7987 | 1 | 1 | 2 | 3 | 3 | 4 | 5 | 6 | 6 |
| 63 | 7993 | 8000 | 8007 | 8014 | 8021 | 8028 | 8035 | 8041 | 8048 | 8055 | 1 | 1 | 2 | 3 | 3 | 4 | 5 | 5 | 6 |
| 64 | 8062 | 8069 | 8075 | 8082 | 8089 | 8096 | 8102 | 8109 | 8116 | 8122 | 1 | 1 | 2 | 3 | 3 | 4 | 5 | 5 | 6 |
| 65 | 8129 | 8136 | 8142 | 8149 | 8156 | 8162 | 8169 | 8176 | 8182 | 8189 | 1 | 1 | 2 | 3 | 3 | 4 | 5 | 5 | 6 |
| 66 | 8195 | 8202 | 8209 | 8215 | 8222 | 8228 | 8235 | 8241 | 8248 | 8254 | 1 | 1 | 2 | 3 | 3 | 4 | 5 | 5 | 6 |
| 67 | 8261 | 8267 | 8274 | 8280 | 8287 | 8293 | 8299 | 8306 | 8312 | 8319 | 1 | 1 | 2 | 3 | 3 | 4 | 5 | 5 | 6 |
| 68 | 8325 | 8331 | 8338 | 8344 | 8351 | 8357 | 8363 | 8370 | 8376 | 8382 | 1 | 1 | 2 | 3 | 3 | 4 | 4 | 5 | 6 |
| 69 | 8388 | 8395 | 8401 | 8407 | 8414 | 8420 | 8426 | 8432 | 8439 | 8445 | 1 | 1 | 2 | 2 | 3 | 4 | 4 | 5 | 6 |
| 70 | 8451 | 8457 | 8463 | 8470 | 8476 | 8482 | 8488 | 8494 | 8500 | 8506 | 1 | 1 | 2 | 2 | 3 | 4 | 4 | 5 | 6 |
| 71 | 8513 | 8519 | 8525 | 8531 | 8537 | 8543 | 8549 | 8555 | 8561 | 8567 | 1 | 1 | 2 | 2 | 3 | 4 | 4 | 5 | 5 |
| 72 | 8573 | 8579 | 8585 | 8591 | 8597 | 8603 | 8609 | 8615 | 8621 | 8627 | 1 | 1 | 2 | 2 | 3 | 4 | 4 | 5 | 5 |
| 73 | 8633 | 8639 | 8645 | 8651 | 8657 | 8663 | 8669 | 8675 | 8681 | 8686 | 1 | 1 | 2 | 2 | 3 | 4 | 4 | 5 | 5 |
| 74 | 8692 | 8698 | 8704 | 8710 | 8716 | 8722 | 8727 | 8733 | 8739 | 8745 | 1 | 1 | 2 | 2 | 3 | 4 | 4 | 5 | 5 |
| 75 | 8751 | 8756 | 8762 | 8768 | 8774 | 8779 | 8785 | 8791 | 8797 | 8802 | 1 | 1 | 2 | 2 | 3 | 3 | 4 | 5 | 5 |
| 76 | 8808 | 8814 | 8820 | 8825 | 8831 | 8837 | 8842 | 8848 | 8854 | 8859 | 1 | 1 | 2 | 2 | 3 | 3 | 4 | 5 | 5 |
| 77 | 8865 | 8871 | 8876 | 8882 | 8887 | 8893 | 8899 | 8904 | 8910 | 8915 | 1 | 1 | 2 | 2 | 3 | 3 | 4 | 4 | 5 |
| 78 | 8921 | 8927 | 8932 | 8938 | 8943 | 8949 | 8954 | 8960 | 8965 | 8971 | 1 | 1 | 2 | 2 | 3 | 3 | 4 | 4 | 5 |
| 79 | 8976 | 8982 | 8987 | 8993 | 8998 | 9004 | 9009 | 9015 | 9020 | 9026 | 1 | 1 | 2 | 2 | 3 | 3 | 4 | 4 | 5 |
| 80 | 9031 | 9036 | 9042 | 9047 | 9053 | 9058 | 9063 | 9069 | 9074 | 9079 | 1 | 1 | 2 | 2 | 3 | 3 | 4 | 4 | 5 |
| 81 | 9085 | 9090 | 9096 | 9101 | 9106 | 9112 | 9117 | 9122 | 9128 | 9133 | 1 | 1 | 2 | 2 | 3 | 3 | 4 | 4 | 5 |
| 82 | 9138 | 9143 | 9149 | 9154 | 9159 | 9165 | 9170 | 9175 | 9180 | 9186 | 1 | 1 | 2 | 2 | 3 | 3 | 4 | 4 | 5 |
| 83 | 9191 | 9196 | 9201 | 9206 | 9212 | 9217 | 9222 | 9227 | 9232 | 9238 | 1 | 1 | 2 | 2 | 3 | 3 | 4 | 4 | 5 |
| 84 | 9243 | 9248 | 9253 | 9258 | 9263 | 9269 | 9274 | 9279 | 9284 | 9289 | 1 | 1 | 2 | 2 | 3 | 3 | 4 | 4 | 5 |
| 85 | 9294 | 9299 | 9304 | 9309 | 9315 | 9320 | 9325 | 9330 | 9335 | 9340 | 1 | 1 | 2 | 2 | 3 | 3 | 4 | 4 | 5 |
| 86 | 9345 | 9350 | 9355 | 9360 | 9365 | 9370 | 9375 | 9380 | 9385 | 9390 | 1 | 1 | 2 | 2 | 3 | 3 | 4 | 4 | 5 |
| 87 | 9395 | 9400 | 9405 | 9410 | 9415 | 9420 | 9425 | 9430 | 9435 | 9440 | 0 | 1 | 1 | 2 | 2 | 3 | 3 | 4 | 4 |
| 88 | 9445 | 9450 | 9455 | 9460 | 9465 | 9469 | 9474 | 9479 | 9484 | 9489 | 0 | 1 | 1 | 2 | 2 | 3 | 3 | 4 | 4 |
| 89 | 9494 | 9499 | 9504 | 9509 | 9513 | 9518 | 9523 | 9528 | 9533 | 9538 | 0 | 1 | 1 | 2 | 2 | 3 | 3 | 4 | 4 |
| 90 | 9542 | 9547 | 9552 | 9557 | 9562 | 9566 | 9571 | 9576 | 9581 | 9586 | 0 | 1 | 1 | 2 | 2 | 3 | 3 | 4 | 4 |
| 91 | 9590 | 9595 | 9600 | 9605 | 9609 | 9614 | 9619 | 9624 | 9628 | 9633 | 0 | 1 | 1 | 2 | 2 | 3 | 3 | 4 | 4 |
| 92 | 9638 | 9643 | 9647 | 9652 | 9657 | 9661 | 9666 | 9671 | 9675 | 9680 | 0 | 1 | 1 | 2 | 2 | 3 | 3 | 4 | 4 |
| 93 | 9685 | 9689 | 9694 | 9699 | 9703 | 9708 | 9713 | 9717 | 9722 | 9727 | 0 | 1 | 1 | 2 | 2 | 3 | 3 | 4 | 4 |
| 94 | 9731 | 9736 | 9741 | 9745 | 9750 | 9754 | 9759 | 9763 | 9768 | 9773 | 0 | 1 | 1 | 2 | 2 | 3 | 3 | 4 | 4 |
| 95 | 9777 | 9782 | 9786 | 9791 | 9795 | 9800 | 9805 | 9809 | 9814 | 9818 | 0 | 1 | 1 | 2 | 2 | 3 | 3 | 4 | 4 |
| 96 | 9823 | 9827 | 9832 | 9836 | 9841 | 9845 | 9850 | 9854 | 9859 | 9863 | 0 | 1 | 1 | 2 | 2 | 3 | 3 | 4 | 4 |
| 97 | 9868 | 9872 | 9877 | 9881 | 9886 | 9890 | 9894 | 9899 | 9903 | 9908 | 0 | 1 | 1 | 2 | 2 | 3 | 3 | 4 | 4 |
| 98 | 9912 | 9917 | 9921 | 9926 | 9930 | 9934 | 9939 | 9943 | 9948 | 9952 | 0 | 1 | 1 | 2 | 2 | 3 | 3 | 4 | 4 |
| 99 | 9956 | 9961 | 9965 | 9969 | 9974 | 9978 | 9983 | 9987 | 9991 | 9996 | 0 | 1 | 1 | 2 | 2 | 3 | 3 | 3 | 4 |

## Practice Problems

1. Find the logarithm of each of the following numbers.

(a) 2245
(b) 5.265
(c) 7000
(d) 187.9
(e) 0.002934
(f) 0.7245
(g) 215000
(h) 0.0001372
(i) 63.78
(j) $6.2 \times 10^6$

2. Find the antilogarithm corresponding to each of the following logarithms.

(a) 4.4512
(b) 1.1523
(c) 0.3302
(d) $\bar{1}.1105$
(e) 2.7892
(f) 2.1668
(g) 0.0261
(h) $\bar{3}.8902$
(i) 1.9234
(j) $\bar{2}.1234$

3. Compute each of the following by means of logarithms.

(a) $23.87 \times 954.6$
(b) $8542 \times 0.8562$
(c) $655.7 \times 0.02253$
(d) $(8.235 \times 10^2) \times (4.296 \times 10^{-4}) \times (2.325 \times 10^3)$
(e) $26.74 \times 5.987 \times 106.7$

4. Compute each of the following by means of logarithms.

(a) $9525 \div 1.267$
(b) $2500 \div 12.65$
(c) $0.2925 \div 56.85$
(d) $(1.658 \times 10^4) \div (4.689 \times 10^2)$
(e) $0.491 \div 0.0357$

5. Find the value of each of the following by means of logarithms.

(a) $\dfrac{(6.29 \times 10^2) \times (1.23 \times 10^4)}{(9.75 \times 10^4)} =$

(b) $\dfrac{1{,}667{,}000 \times 0.4101}{(6.31 \times 10^3)} =$

(c) $\dfrac{(7.32 \times 10^2)}{(4.315 \times 10^{-4}) \times (5.795 \times 10^3)} =$

APPENDIX

# J
# Chemical Problems

## ATOMIC AND MOLECULAR WEIGHTS

Most chemical problems involve the use of *atomic* or *combining weights* of the elements, and the validity of their solutions depends upon the *Law of Definite Proportions.*

The *atomic weight* of an element is the ratio of the weight of its atom to the weight of an atom of another element taken as a standard. Long ago, hydrogen, with a weight taken as 1, was used as the standard. For many years, the weight of oxygen, taken as 16, has proved a more convenient standard. In August 1961, however, the International Union of Pure and Applied Chemistry (following similar action by the International Union of Pure and Applied Physics) officially released the most up-to-date table of atomic weights based on carbon, taking 12 as the relative nuclidic mass of the isotope $^{12}C$. It should be noted that the rounded-off *approximate* atomic weights in the table given on the inside back cover and those based on the long-familiar oxygen table are identical and continue to be sufficiently accurate for most chemical calculations likely to be encountered by pharmacists.

The *combining* or *equivalent weight* of an *element* is that weight of the element which will combine with (or displace) one gram atomic weight of hydrogen (or the equivalent weight of some other element). For example, when hydrogen and chlorine react to form HCl, 1.008 g of hydrogen react with 35.45 g of chlorine; therefore the equivalent weight of chlorine is 35.45.

The *equivalent weight* of a *compound* is that weight of a compound which is chemically equivalent to 1.008 g of hydrogen. Thus, one mole or 36.46 g of HCl contains 1.008 g of hydrogen and this is displaceable by one equivalent weight of a metal; hence its equivalent weight is 36.46. Also, one mole or 40.00 g of NaOH is capable of neutralizing 1.008 g of hydrogen; therefore its equivalent weight is 40.00. But one mole or 98.08 of $H_2SO_4$ contains 2.016 g of hydrogen and this is displaceable by *two* equivalent weights of a metal; consequently its equivalent weight is $\frac{98.08}{2}$ or 49.04.

The *Law of Definite Proportions* states that elements invariably combine in the same proportion by weight to form a given compound.

## PERCENTAGE COMPOSITION

**To calculate the percentage composition of a compound:**

*Example:*

*Calculate the percentage composition of anhydrous dextrose, $C_6H_{12}O_6$.*

$$\begin{array}{ccccccc} C_6 & & H_{12} & & O_6 & & \\ (6 \times 12.01) & + & (12 \times 1.008) & + & (6 \times 16.00) & = & \\ 72.06 & + & 12.096 & + & 96.00 & = & 180.16 \end{array}$$

$$\frac{180.16}{72.06} = \frac{100\ (\%)}{x\ (\%)}$$

$x = 40.00\%$ of carbon, *and*

$$\frac{180.16}{12.096} = \frac{100\ (\%)}{y\ (\%)}$$

$y = 6.71\%$ of hydrogen, *and*

$$\frac{180.16}{96.00} = \frac{100\ (\%)}{z\ (\%)}$$

$z = 53.29\%$ of oxygen, *answer.*

Check: $40.00\% + 6.71\% + 53.29\% = 100\%$

**To calculate the percentage of a constituent in a compound:**

Approximate atomic weights may ordinarily be used in solving problems of this kind.

*Example:*

*Calculate the percentage of lithium (Li) in lithium carbonate, $Li_2CO_3$.*

Molecular weight of lithium carbonate = 74

Atomic weight of lithium = 7

$$\frac{74}{2 \times 7} = \frac{100\ (\%)}{x\ (\%)}$$

x = 18.9%, *answer.*

**To calculate the weight of a constituent, given the weight of a compound:**

Approximate atomic weights may ordinarily be used in solving problems of this kind.

*Example:*

*A ferrous sulfate elixir contains 220 mg of ferrous sulfate ($FeSO_4 \cdot 7H_2O$) per teaspoonful dose. How many milligrams of elemental iron are represented in the dose?*

Molecular weight of $FeSO_4 \cdot 7H_2O$ = 278

Atomic weight of Fe = 56

$$\frac{278}{56} = \frac{220\ (mg)}{x\ (mg)}$$

x = 44.3 or 44 mg, *answer.*

**To calculate the weight of a compound, given the weight of a constituent:**

Approximate atomic weights may ordinarily be used in solving problems of this kind.

*Example:*

*How many milligrams of sodium fluoride will provide 500 μg of fluoride ion?*

Na F
23 + 19 = 42

$$\frac{19}{42} = \frac{500\ (\mu g)}{x\ (\mu g)}$$

x = 1105 μg or 1.1 mg, *answer.*

## CHEMICALS IN REACTIONS

**To calculate the weights of pure chemicals involved in reactions:**

Approximate atomic weights may ordinarily be used in solving problems of this kind.

*Examples:*

*How many grams of iron are required to react with 100 g of iodine?*

$$\begin{array}{lll} Fe + & I_2 & = FeI_2 \\ 56 & 2(127) & \\ & \text{or } 254 & \end{array}$$

$$\frac{254}{56} = \frac{100 \text{ (g)}}{x \text{ (g)}}$$

$x = 22.1$ g, *answer.*

*How many grams of p-aminobenzoic acid and how many grams of sodium bicarbonate should be used to prepare 100 g of sodium p-aminobenzoate?*

$$\begin{array}{ccccc} NH_2C_6H_4COOH + & NaHCO_3 = & NH_2C_6H_4COONa & + H_2O & + CO_2 \\ 137 & 84 & 159 & & \end{array}$$

$$\frac{159}{137} = \frac{100 \text{ (g)}}{x \text{ (g)}}$$

$x = 86.2$ g of p-aminobenzoic acid, *and*

$$\frac{159}{84} = \frac{100 \text{ (g)}}{y \text{ (g)}}$$

$y = 52.8$ of sodium bicarbonate, *answers.*

**To calculate the weights of chemicals involved in reactions, with consideration of percentage strengths:**

In solving problems of this type, it is important to remember that proportions based upon atomic and molecular weights apply only to *pure* (absolute) or *100%* chemicals. If *volume-in-volume* or *weight-in-volume* strength is specified, *it must be converted to weight-in-weight strength.*

*Example:*

*How many grams of potassium bicarbonate and how many milliliters of 36% acetic acid, sp. gr. 1.045, are required to prepare 200 g of potassium acetate?*

$$KHCO_3 + HC_2H_3O_2 = KC_2H_3O_2 + CO_2 + H_2O$$

$$100 \qquad 60 \qquad 98$$

$$\frac{98}{100} = \frac{200\ (g)}{x\ (g)}$$

x = 204 g of potassium bicarbonate, *and*

If

$$\frac{98}{60} = \frac{200\ (g)}{y\ (g)}$$

y = 122 g of 100% acetic acid,

then

$$\frac{36\ (\%)}{100\ (\%)} = \frac{122\ (g)}{z\ (g)}$$

z = 339 g of 36% acetic acid

339 g of water measure 339 mL

$$\frac{339\ mL}{1.045} = 324\ mL \text{ of 36\% acetic acid, } \textit{answers.}$$

**To solve problems involving chemically equivalent quantities:**

*Example:*

*The formula for Magnesium Citrate Oral Solution calls for 27.4 g of anhydrous citric acid ($C_6H_8O_7$) in 350 mL of the product. How many grams of citric acid monohydrate ($C_6H_8O_7 \cdot H_2O$) may be used in place of the anhydrous salt?*

Molecular weights:

$C_6H_8O_7 \cdot H_2O = 210$ $\qquad$ $C_6H_8O_7 = 192$

$$\frac{192}{210} = \frac{27.4 \text{ (g)}}{x \text{ (g)}}$$

x = 29.97 or 30 g, *answer.*

## SAPONIFICATION VALUE

**To solve chemical problems based upon saponification value:**

*Saponification value* refers to the number of milligrams of 100% potassium hydroxide required to saponify the free acids and esters in 1 g of a fat or oil. For example, when we say that olive oil has a saponification value of 190, we means that 190 mg of 100% KOH are required to saponify completely 1 g of olive oil.

*Examples:*

*How many grams of 85% potassium hydroxide are required to saponify completely 100 g of coconut oil having a saponification value of 260?*

260 = 260 mg = 0.260 g

If

$$\frac{1 \text{ (g)}}{100 \text{ (g)}} = \frac{0.260 \text{ (g)}}{x \text{ (g)}}$$

x = 26 g of 100% KOH,

then

$$\frac{85 \text{ (\%)}}{100 \text{ (\%)}} = \frac{26 \text{ (g)}}{y \text{ (g)}}$$

y = 30.6 g, *answer.*

*In a formula for soft soap, 100 g of 88% potassium hydroxide are used to saponify 400 g of a vegetable oil. Calculate the saponification value of the oil.*

If

$$\frac{100 \text{ (\%)}}{88 \text{ (\%)}} = \frac{100 \text{ (g)}}{x \text{ (g)}}$$

x = 88 g of 100% KOH, required to saponify 400 g of the oil, then

$$\frac{400\ (g)}{1\ (g)} = \frac{88\ (g)}{y\ (g)}$$

$y = 0.220$ g = 220 mg = 220, *answer.*

## ACID VALUE

**To solve chemical problems based on acid value:**

*Acid value* refers to the number of milligrams of 100% potassium hydroxide required to neutralize the free fatty acids in 1 g of a substance. For example, if a wax has an acid value of 22, 1 g of it will require 22 mg of 100% KOH (or the equivalent weight of some other alkali) for the neutralization of the free fatty acids.

In the formulation of cold creams and other emulsions containing waxes, the amount of alkali depends upon the acid value of the wax.

*Example:*

*A cold cream formula calls for 1000 g of white wax having an acid value of 20.* (a) *How many grams of 85% potassium hydroxide (KOH) should be used in formulating the cream?* (b) *If sodium borate ($Na_2B_4O_7 \cdot 10H_2O$) is used in formulating the cream, how many grams are required?*

*(a)* 20 = 20 mg = 0.020 g

If

$$\frac{1\ (g)}{1000\ (g)} = \frac{0.020\ (g)}{x\ (g)}$$

$x = 20$ g of 100% KOH,

then

$$\frac{85\ (\%)}{100\ (\%)} = \frac{20\ (g)}{y\ (g)}$$

$y = 23.5$ g of 85% KOH, *answer.*

*(b)* Since one molecule of sodium borate (mol. wt. 382) gives two molecules of sodium hydroxide that can react with two atoms of hydrogen, its equivalent weight is ½ of its molecular weight (382 ÷ 2) or 191, and therefore 191 g are chemically equivalent to 56 g of KOH (mol. wt. 56).

In *(a)* it was calculated that 20 g of 100% KOH are required.

Therefore,

$$\frac{56}{191} = \frac{20\ (g)}{x\ (g)}$$

$x = 68.2$ g of sodium borate, *answer.*

## WEIGHTS AND VOLUMES OF GASES

The methods by which we may calculate the volume of a given weight of any gas—or the weight of a given volume—depend on Avogadro's Law, which states that *under the same conditions of temperature and pressure, equal volumes of all gases contain the same number of molecules.*

When the molecular weight of a gas is taken to indicate a number of grams, the expression is called the *mole* or the *gram-molecular weight* of that gas. By another consequence of Avogadro's Law, the gram-molecular weights of all gases have a common volume, *22.4 liters,* under standard conditions of temperature and pressure (S.T.P.)—that is, at 0°C and a barometric pressure of 760 mm. Since under normal conditions the molecule of gas contains two atoms, this volume is shared by $2 \times 16$ or 32 g of oxygen, $2 \times 1$ or 2 g of hydrogen, $2 \times 14$ or 28 g of nitrogen, and so on. Hence, 22.4 liters (S.T.P.) of any gaseous element or compound will weigh a number of grams equal to the number expressing its molecular weight.

**To calculate the volume of a gas under standard conditions of temperature and pressure, given its weight:**

*Example:*

*What is the volume (S.T.P.) of 3.87 g of hydrogen, $H_2$?*

Molecular weight of hydrogen $= 2 \times 1 = 2$
2 g of hydrogen measure 22.4 liters.

$$\frac{2\ (g)}{3.87\ (g)} = \frac{22.4\ (liters)}{x\ (liters)}$$

$x = 43$ liters, *answers.*

**To calculate the volume of a gas when corrections for temperature and pressure must be made:**

In the problem above the gases were assumed to be measured at S.T.P. The volume of a gas measured under any conditions of temperature and pressure may be used to calculate the volume of the same gas under different conditions by application of the Laws of Boyle and Charles.

According to Boyle's Law, the *volume of a given mass of gas varies inversely with the pressure, when the temperature is constant.* Thus, an increase in pressure results in a decrease in the volume of a gas and a decrease in pressure results in an increase in its volume.

And according to Charles' Law, the *volume of a gas is proportional to its absolute temperature, when the pressure is constant.* A gas, under constant pressure, will expand, therefore, $\frac{1}{273}$ of its volume when heated through 1°C.

*Examples:*

*The volume of a gas measured at a pressure of 750 mm is 380 mL. What is its volume at 760 mm, if the temperature remains constant?*

$$\frac{760\ (\text{mm})}{750\ (\text{mm})} = \frac{380\ (\text{mL})}{x\ (\text{mL})}$$

$$x = 380\ \text{mL} \times \frac{750}{760} = 375\ \text{mL},\ \textit{answer}.$$

*The volume of a gas is 686 mL at 70°C. What is its volume at 27°C, if the pressure remains constant?*

70°C = 343° Absolute
27°C = 300° Absolute

$$\frac{343\ (°\text{A})}{300\ (°\text{A})} = \frac{686\ (\text{mL})}{x\ (\text{mL})}$$

$$x = 686\ \text{mL} \times \frac{300}{343} = 600\ \text{mL},\ \textit{answer}.$$

Since the changes in the volume of a gas due to variations in pressure and temperature are *independent* of one another, the corrections may be conveniently made together by combining the proportions used in the preceding examples.

*Example:*

*A sample of gas measured 300 mL at 27°C and 740 mm. Calculate its volume at S.T.P.*

27°C = 300° Absolute
0°C = 273° Absolute

$$\text{Volume at S.T.P.} = 300\ \text{mL} \times \frac{273}{300} \times \frac{740}{760} = 266\ \text{mL},\ \textit{answer}.$$

**Practice Problems**

1. Calculate the percentage composition of ether, $(C_2H_5)_2O$.

2. What is the percentage composition of Dibasic Sodium Phosphate, U.S.P., $Na_2HPO_4 \cdot 7H_2O$?

3. What is the percentage composition of Monobasic Sodium Phosphate, U.S.P., $NaH_2PO_4 \cdot H_2O$?

4. Calculate the percentage of water in dextrose, $C_6H_{12}O_6 \cdot H_2O$.

5. How many grams of water are represented in 2000 g of magnesium sulfate, $MgSO_4 \cdot 7H_2O$?

6. What is the percentage of calcium in calcium gluconate, $C_{12}H_{22}CaO_{14}$?

7. A commercially available tablet contains 0.2 g of $FeSO_4 \cdot 2H_2O$. How many milligrams of elemental iron are represented in a daily dose of three tablets?

8. A certain solution contains 110 mg of sodium fluoride, NaF, in each 1000 mL. How many milligrams of fluoride ion are represented in each 2 mL of the solution?

9. ℞ Sodium Fluoride q.s.
Distilled Water ad 500 mL
Sig. 2 mL diluted to 100 mL will give a 1:1,000,000 solution of fluoride ion.

How many milligrams of sodium fluoride, NaF, should be used in compounding the prescription?

10. How many milliliters of a solution containing 0.275 mg of histamine acid phosphate (mol. wt. 307) per mL should be used in preparing 30 mL of a solution which is to contain the equivalent of 1:10,000 of histamine (mol. wt. 111)?

11. ℞ Sodium Fluoride q.s.
Multiple Vitamin Drops ad 60.0 mL
(Five drops = 1 mg of fluoride ion)
Sig. Five drops in orange juice daily.

The dispensing dropper calibrates 20 drops per mL. How many milligrams of sodium fluoride should be used in compounding the prescription?

12. How many grams of potassium bicarbonate (mol. wt. 100) and how many grams of citric acid (mol. wt. 210) should be used in preparing 10 liters of a solution which is to contain 0.3 g of potassium citrate (mol. wt. 324) per teaspoonful?

$$3KHCO_3 + H_3C_6H_5O_7 = K_3C_6H_5O_7 + 3H_2O + 3CO_2$$

13. In preparing magnesium citrate oral solution, 2.5 g of potassium bicarbonate ($KHCO_3$) are needed to charge each bottle. If no potassium

bicarbonate is available, how much sodium bicarbonate ($NaHCO_3$) should be used?

14. How many grams of potassium bicarbonate (mol. wt. 100) and how many milliliters of 36% acetic acid (mol. wt. 60), specific gravity 1.050, are required to prepare 1 gallon of a 10% solution of potassium acetate (mol. wt. 98)?

$$KHCO_3 + HC_2H_3O_2 = KC_2H_3O_2 + CO_2 + H_2O$$

15. In preparing Benedict's solution, you are directed to use 100 g of anhydrous sodium carbonate ($Na_2CO_3$) in 1000 mL of the reagent. Calculate the amount of monohydrated sodium carbonate ($Na_2CO_3 \cdot H_2O$) that should be used in preparing 5 liters of the solution.

16. The formula for Albright's solution "M" calls for 8.84 g of anhydrous sodium carbonate ($Na_2CO_3$) per 1000 mL. How many grams of 95% sodium hydroxide (NaOH) should be used to replace the anhydrous sodium carbonate in preparing 5 liters of the solution?

17.

| | |
|---|---|
| Precipitated Sulfur | 50.0 g |
| Potassium Hydroxide | 10.0 g |
| Stearic Acid | 200.0 g |
| Glycerin | 40.0 g |
| Water, to make | 1000.0 g |

Label: Sulfur cream.

If potassium carbonate ($K_2CO_3 \cdot 1\frac{1}{2}H_2O$) were to be used in formulating 10 lb (avoir.) of the cream, how many grams should be used to replace the potassium hydroxide (KOH)?

18. Ferrous sulfate syrup contains 40 g of ferrous sulfate ($FeSO_4 \cdot 7H_2O$) per 1000 mL. How many milligrams of iron (Fe) are represented in the usual dose of 10 mL of the syrup?

19. How many grams of 42% (MgO equivalent) magnesium carbonate are required to prepare 14 liters of magnesium citrate oral solution so that 350 mL contain the equivalent of 6.0 g of MgO?

20. Five hundred grams of effervescent sodium phosphate contain 100 g of anhydrous dibasic sodium phosphate ($Na_2HPO_4$). How much Dibasic Sodium Phosphate, U.S.P., ($Na_2HPO_4 \cdot 7H_2O$) is represented in each 10-g dose of effervescent sodium phosphate?

21. How many grams of epinephrine bitartrate (mol. wt. 333) should be used in preparing 500 mL of an ophthalmic solution containing the equivalent of 2% of epinephrine (mol. wt. 183)?

22. Coconut oil has a saponification value of 255. How much 85%

potassium hydroxide should be used to saponify completely 750 g of coconut oil?

23. The saponification value of stearic acid is 208. In a vanishing cream formula containing 250 g of stearic acid, how much 88% potassium hydroxide is required to saponify 20% of the stearic acid?

24. How many grams of 85% potassium hydroxide should be used to saponify completely 2000 mL of a vegetable oil (sp. gr. 0.90) having a saponification value of 190?

25.

| | |
|---|---|
| Stearic Acid | 120 g |
| Potassium Hydroxide | q.s. |
| Propylene Glycol | 50 g |
| Water, to make | 1000 g |

*(a)* If the saponificiation value of stearic acid is 210, how many grams of 88% potassium hydroxide should be used to saponify 30% of the stearic acid?

*(b)* The equivalent weight of triethanolamine is 149. How many grams of triethanolamine could be used to replace the quantity of potassium hydroxide needed to saponify 30% of the stearic acid in the formula?

26.

| | |
|---|---|
| Stearic Acid | 20.0 |
| Liquid Petrolatum | 5.0 |
| Triethanolamine | 5.0 |
| Coconut Oil Soap | 40.0 |
| Glycerin | 5.0 |
| Water | 25.0 |

Coconut oil soap contains 40% of coconut oil. How many grams of 85% potassium hydroxide are required to saponify the coconut oil (saponification value 255) needed to prepare the soap for 5 lb (avoir.) of this formula?

27. A formula for a cold cream calls for 500 g of white wax. If the sample of white wax used has an acid value of 20, how much 88% potassium hydroxide is required to neutralize the free acids contained in the wax?

28. A cold cream formula contains 1500 g of white wax. The acid value of the wax is 21.

(a) How many grams of pure KOH are needed?
(b) How many grams of 85% KOH should be used?
(c) The equivalent weight of sodium borate is 191. How many grams of sodium borate should be used?

29.

| | |
|---|---|
| Stearic Acid | 200 g |
| Potassium Carbonate | q.s. |
| Propylene Glycol | 100 g |
| Lanolin | 50 g |
| Distilled Water, to make | 1000 g |

How many grams of potassium carbonate ($K_2CO_3 \cdot 1\frac{1}{2}H_2O$) should be used to saponify 25% of the stearic acid ($C_{17}H_{35}COOH$)? Assume the stearic acid (saponification value 210) to be 100% pure.

30. What is the volume (S.T.P.) of 28.46 g of oxygen, $O_2$?

31. The volume of a gas measured at 780 mm is 475 mL. What is its volume at 760 mm, if the temperature remains constant?

32. Calculate the volume of 10 g of hydrogen measured under standard conditions. What would be its volume if the pressure upon the gas were diminished to 750 mm, the temperature remaining constant?

33. Calculate the volume of 10 g of oxygen under standard conditions. What would be its volume if the temperature of the gas were increased to 27°C, the pressure remaining constant?

34. The volume of a gas measured at 25°C is 540 mL. What is its volume at 0°C, if the pressure remains constant?

35. Calculate the volume (S.T.P.) of a sample of oxygen that occupies 1000 mL at 30°C and 745 mm pressure.

APPENDIX

# K

# Some Commercial Problems

## DISCOUNTS

One of the more important discounts that the community pharmacist encounters in everyday practice is the *trade discount* which is a deduction from the list price (manufacturer's suggested retail price) of merchandise. Published guides to products and prices provide, in many instances, a minimum selling price to the consumer which is 10% less than the suggested retail price. It should be noted, however, that the manufacturer usually bills merchandise to the buyer on the basis of the suggested retail price less the trade discount.

Other discounts allowable by manufacturers under certain conditions are based on (1) quantity buying, (2) selected promotional deals, (3) bonuses in terms of free merchandise, (4) off invoice allowances, (5) advertising and display allowances, and (6) payment of invoices within a designated time (cash discount). These deductions may be offered singly or in combination by certain manufacturers and provide the buyer with a means of increasing the percent of gross profit on selected merchandise.

**To compute the net cost of merchandise, given the list price and allowable discount:**

*Example:*

*The list price of an antihistamine elixir is $6.50 per pint, less 40%. What is the net cost per pint of the elixir?*

| List price | | Discount | | Net cost |
|---|---|---|---|---|
| 100% | − | 40% | = | 60% |
| $6.50 | × | 0.60 | = | $3.90, *answer.* |

Several discounts may be allowed on promotional deals. For example, the list price on some merchandise may be subject to a trade discount of 33.5%, plus a quantity discount of 12% and a cash discount of 2% for prompt payment of the invoice. This chain of deductions, sometimes referred to as a *series discount,* may be converted to a single discount equivalent. In such cases, the discounts in the series cannot be figured by adding them; rather, the first discount is deducted from the list price and each successive discount is taken upon the balance remaining after the preceding discount has been deducted. The order in which the discounts in a series discount are taken is immaterial.

**To compute the net cost of merchandise, given the list price and a series of allowable discounts:**

*Example:*

*The list price of 12 bottles (100's) of analgesic tablets is $36.00, less a trade discount of 33⅓%. If purchased in quantities of 12 dozens, an additional discount of 10% is allowed by the manufacturer, plus a 2% cash discount for payment of the invoice within ten days of the billing. Calculate the net cost of 144 bottles (100's) of the analgesic tablets when purchased under the terms of the offer.*

List price of 12 (100's) = $36.00
List price of 144 (100's) = $432.00

100% − 33⅓% = 66⅔% 100% − 10% = 90% 100% − 2% = 98%

$432.00 × 66⅔% = $288.00, cost after 33⅓% is deducted
$288.00 × 90% = $259.20, cost after 10% is deducted
$259.20 × 98% = $254.02, net cost, *answer.*

**To compute a single discount equivalent to a series of discounts:**

This is done by subtracting each discount in the series from 100% and multiplying together the net percentages. The product thus obtained is subtracted from 100% to give the single discount equivalent to the series of discounts.

*Example:*

*A promotional deal provides a trade discount of 33.5%, an off invoice allowance of 12% and a display allowance of 5%. Calculate the single discount equivalent to these deductions.*

100% − 33.5% = 66.5% 100% − 12% = 88% 100% − 5% = 95%

0.665 × 0.88 × 0.95 = 0.556 or 55.6% = % to be paid

Discount = 100% − 55.6% = 44.4%, *answer.*

## MARKUP

The term *markup,* sometimes used interchangeably with the term *margin of profit (gross profit),* refers to the difference between the cost of merchandise and its selling price. For example, if a pharmacist buys an article for \$1.50 and sells it for \$2.50, the markup (or gross profit) as a dollars-and-cents item is \$1.00.

*Markup percentage (percentage of gross profit)* refers to the markup (gross profit) divided by the selling price. The expression of the percent of markup may be somewhat ambiguous since it may be based on either the cost or the selling price of merchandise. In modern retail practice, this percentage is invariably based on selling price, and when reference is made to markup percentage (or % of gross profit), it means the % that the markup is of the selling price. However, if a pharmacist chooses, for the sake of convenience, to base percentage markup on the cost of merchandise, he may do so providing he does not overlook the fact that the markup on cost must yield the desired percentage of gross profit on the selling price.

**To calculate the selling price of merchandise to yield a given % of gross profit on the cost:**

*Example:*

*The cost of 100 antacid tablets is \$2.10. What should be the selling price per hundred tablets to yield a 66⅔% gross profit on the cost?*

Cost × % of gross profit = Gross profit

\$2.10 × 66⅔% = \$1.40

Cost + Gross profit = Selling price

\$2.10 + \$1.40 = \$3.50, *answer.*

**To calculate the selling price of merchandise to yield a given % of gross profit on the selling price:**

*Example:*

*The cost of 100 antacid tablets is \$2.10. What should be the selling price per hundred tablets to yield a 40% gross profit on the selling price?*

Selling price = 100%

Selling price − Gross profit = Cost

$$100\% \quad - \quad 40\% \quad = 60\%$$

$$\frac{60\ (\%)}{100\ (\%)} = \frac{(\$)\ 2.10}{(\$)\ x}$$

$x = \$3.50$, *answer.*

**To calculate the cost of merchandise given the selling price and % of gross profit on the cost:**

*Example:*

*A bottle of headache tablets is sold for $2.25, thereby yielding a gross profit of 60% on the cost. What was the cost of the bottle of tablets?*

$$\text{Cost} + \text{Gross Profit} = \text{Selling Price}$$
$$x + 0.6x = \$2.25$$
$$1.6x = \$2.25$$
$$x = \$1.40, \textit{ answer.}$$

**To calculate the percentage markup on the cost that will yield a desired % of gross profit on the selling price:**

*Example:*

*What should the percentage markup on the cost of an item be to yield a 40% gross profit on the selling price?*

$$\text{Selling price} = 100\%$$
$$\text{Selling price} - \text{Gross profit} = \text{Cost}$$
$$100\% \quad - \quad 40\% \quad = 60\%$$

$$\frac{\text{Cost as \% of selling price}}{\text{Selling price as \%}} = \frac{\text{Gross profit as \% of selling price}}{x\ (\%)}$$

$x = \%$ gross profit on the cost

$$\frac{60\ (\%)}{100\ (\%)} = \frac{40\ (\%)}{x\ (\%)}$$

$x = 66\frac{2}{3}\%$, *answer.*

## Practice Problems

1. Calculate the single discount equivalent to each of the series of deductions listed below.

(*a*) A trade discount of 40%, a quantity discount of 5% and a cash discount of 2%.

(*b*) A trade discount of 33⅓%, a 10% off invoice allowance and a 6% display allowance.

(*c*) A trade discount of 30%, a display allowance of 5% and a cash discount of 2%.

2. If an ointment is listed at $5.40 per pound, less 33⅓%, what is the net cost of 10 pounds?

3. A pain relief lotion is listed at $41.88 per dozen 6-oz bottles, less a discount of 33.5%. The manufacturer offers 2 bottles free with the purchase of 10 on a promotional deal. What is the net cost per bottle when the lotion is purchased on the deal?

4. A cough syrup is listed at $54.00 per gallon, less 40%. What is the net cost of 1 pint of the cough syrup?

5. A pharmacist receives a bill of goods amounting to $1,200.00, less a 5% discount for quantity buying and a 2% cash discount for paying the invoice within 10 days. What is the net amount of the bill?

6. If a cough syrup is listed at $24.00 per dozen 4-oz bottles, less a discount of 33.4%, and the manufacturer provides 1 unit free with 11 on an order for 1 gross, what is the net cost per bottle of the cough syrup?

7. A decongestant spray lists at $42.24 per dozen units, less a discount of 33⅓%, plus an additional promotional discount of 10%. Calculate the net cost per unit.

8. The list price of an antacid tablet is $112.50 per 5000, less 40%. What is the net cost of 100 tablets?

9. Calculate the difference in the net cost of a bill of goods amounting to $2,500 if the bill is discounted at 45%, and if it is discounted at 33% and 12%.

10. ℞ Glycerin 120.0
Boric Acid Solution
Witch Hazel aa ad 500.0
Sig. Apply to affected areas.

Witch hazel is listed at $4.00 per half gallon, less 34.5%. What is the net cost of the amount needed in filling the prescription?

11. ℞ Belladonna Tincture 30.0
Phenobarbital Elixir ad 240.0
Sig. 5 mL in water a.c.

Belladonna tincture costs $7.50 per pint, and the phenobarbital elixir was bought on a special deal at $17.50 per gallon, less 15%. Calculate the net cost of the ingredients in the prescription.

12. Zinc oxide ointment in 1-oz tubes is purchased at $7.20 per 12 tubes. At what price per tube must it be sold to yield a gross profit of 66⅔% on the cost?

13. A jar of cleansing cream is sold for $5.00, thereby yielding a gross profit of 60% on the cost. What did it cost?

14. A bottle of mouth wash costs $1.35. At what price must it be sold to yield a gross profit of 40% on the selling price?

15. If a surgical lubricating jelly is listed at $11.60 per dozen tubes, with discounts of 15% and 5% when purchased in gross lots, what is the net cost per tube?

16. A topical antibacterial ointment is listed at $1.85 per tube, less 35% and the manufacturer allows 6 tubes free with the purchase of 66 tubes. *(a)* What is the net cost per tube? *(b)* At what price per tube must the ointment be sold to yield a gross profit of 45% on the selling price?

17. Twelve (12) bottles of 100 analgesic tablets cost $18.96 when bought on a promotional deal. If the tablets sell for $2.69 per 100, what percent of gross profit is realized on the selling price?

18. If chloroform (specific gravity 1.475) costs $2.50 per pound, at what price per pint must it be sold to yield a gross profit of 50% on the selling price?

19. A pharmacist buys 20,000 tablets for $400.00 with discounts of 16% and 2%. At what price per hundred must the tablets be sold in order to yield a gross profit of 40% on the selling price?

20. A pharmacist buys glycerin (specific gravity 1.25) for $2.00 per pound. At what price must 8 fluidounces be sold in order to realize a gross profit of 50% on the selling price?

21. A pharmacist sells a bottle of tablets for $3.75, thereby realizing a gross profit of 60% on the cost. Calculate the cost of the tablets.

22. An oil is purchased for $7.00 per liter. If a pint is sold for $8.00, what percent of gross profit on the selling price is realized?

23. Calculate the difference between a single discount of 40% and successive discounts of 33.5% and 6.5%.

24. A pharmacist finds that a gross profit of 40% on the selling price is realized if a medicine is sold for $3.75 per bottle. What percentage of gross profit does this represent if based on the cost of the medicine?

25. A pharmacist sells a jar of a cosmetic cream for $7.50, thereby realizing a profit of 60% on the selling price. Calculate the cost of the cosmetic cream.

26. A pharmacist bought 5 gallons of an elixir for $100.00, which was 20% off the list price. Four (4) gallons of the elixir were sold at 10% off the list and the balance at 10% above list. What was the percentage of gross profit, the basis of the calculation to be the selling price?

27. A pharmacist purchased one dozen bottles of an ophthalmic solution listed at $30.00 per dozen. A discount of 35% was allowed on the purchase plus a 2% discount for paying the bill before the 10th of the month. At what price per unit must the solution be sold in order to yield a gross profit of 50% on the selling price?

28. At what price must a pharmacist mark an item that costs $2.60 so that the selling price can be reduced 25% for a special sale and still yield a gross profit of 35% on the cost price?

APPENDIX

# L

# Graphical Methods

In pharmacy, as in other sciences, the study of the influence of one variable on another is common. Curves, and the equations they represent, give a clear picture of tabulated data and the relationship between variables. Pharmacists are often called on to plot experimental data, interpret graphical material and equations, and manipulate the relationship between curves and their equations.

For simple first degree equations, where the variable contains no exponent greater than one, a straight line will result when the two variables are plotted on rectangular graph paper (rectangular coordinates). Pharmaceutical phenomena as the influence of temperature on solubility, decomposition of drug suspensions, influence of drug dose on pharmacological response, and standard assay curves usually give straight line relationships when plotted on rectangular graph paper.

Exponential or logarithmic relationships are a common occurrence in pharmaceutical studies. Drug degradation in solution, chemical equilibria and vapor pressure changes are some examples of exponential phenomena. If a logarithmic or exponential relationship occurs between the two variables, a straight line usually can be obtained by plotting the logarithm of one variable against the other variable or plotting the data on semilogarithmic graph paper.

## LINEAR RELATIONSHIPS ON RECTANGULAR GRAPH PAPER

Several straight lines and their corresponding equations on rectangular graph paper are presented in Figure 1. The plotting of data on rectangular coordinates should be familiar to all students. The horizontal axis is called the $X$ axis, and the magnitude of the independent variable is plotted along this horizontal scale. The other variable, the dependent variable, is measured along the vertical or $Y$ axis. A point on any of the curves in Figure 1 is defined by two coordinates. The $x$ value, or abscissa, is the distance from the $Y$ axis, and the $y$ value, or ordinate, is the distance from the $X$ axis. By convention the $x$ value is designated first and the $y$ value second. For example, the point 1, 3 when substituted into the equation $y = -2x + 5$ gives $3 = -2 + 5$ and, as expected, satisfies the equation. The point 0, 4.5 satisfies the equation $y = 4.5$ whereas the point 2.5, 0 satisfies the equation $x = 2.5$ since both of these curves run parallel to the $X$ or $Y$ axis respectively.

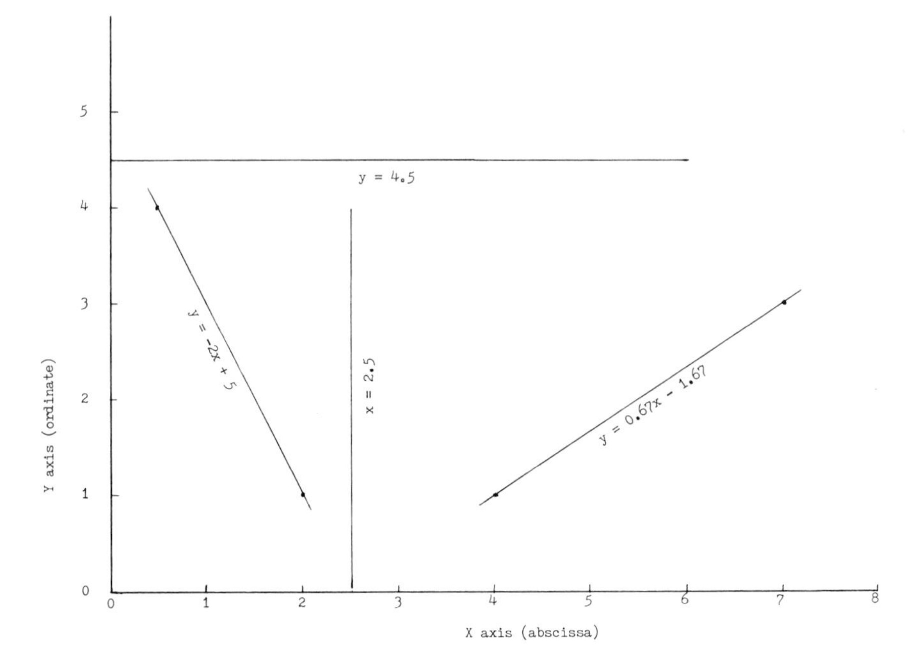


Figure 1. Straight lines and their first degree equations.

The fundamental algebraic equation that describes first degree or straight line equations is:

$$y = mx + b$$

where $m$ and $b$ are constants. The constant $m$ is the slope of the line. It is a ratio of a change in $y$ with a corresponding change in $x$ and is expressed as $m = \Delta y/\Delta x$. The constant $b$ is the $y$ intercept when $x = 0$ and can usually be determined by extrapolating the straight line to the $Y$ axis.

The most convenient equation for determining the equation for the straight line which passes through two given points is the two-point form of the straight line equation,

$$y - y_1 = \frac{y_2 - y_1}{x_2 - x_1}(x - x_1)$$

The results of measuring the ultraviolet absorbance (UV) of various concentrations of Drug A and Drug B in solutions are shown in Table 1.

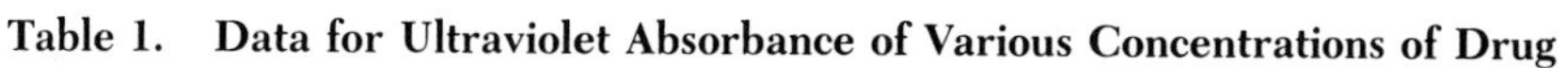
**Table 1. Data for Ultraviolet Absorbance of Various Concentrations of Drug**

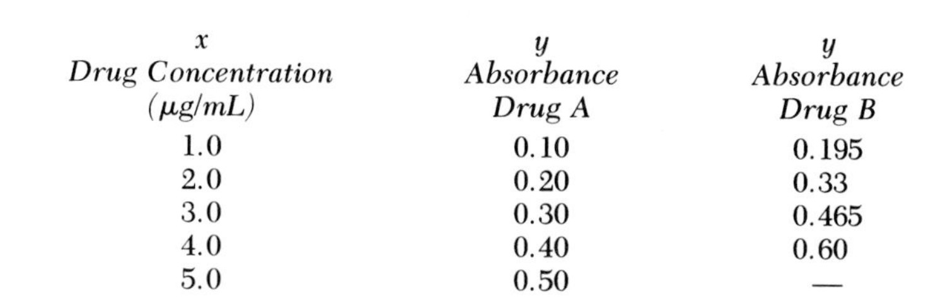

| $x$ Drug Concentration ($\mu g/mL$) | $y$ Absorbance Drug A | $y$ Absorbance Drug B |
|---|---|---|
| 1.0 | 0.10 | 0.195 |
| 2.0 | 0.20 | 0.33 |
| 3.0 | 0.30 | 0.465 |
| 4.0 | 0.40 | 0.60 |
| 5.0 | 0.50 | — |

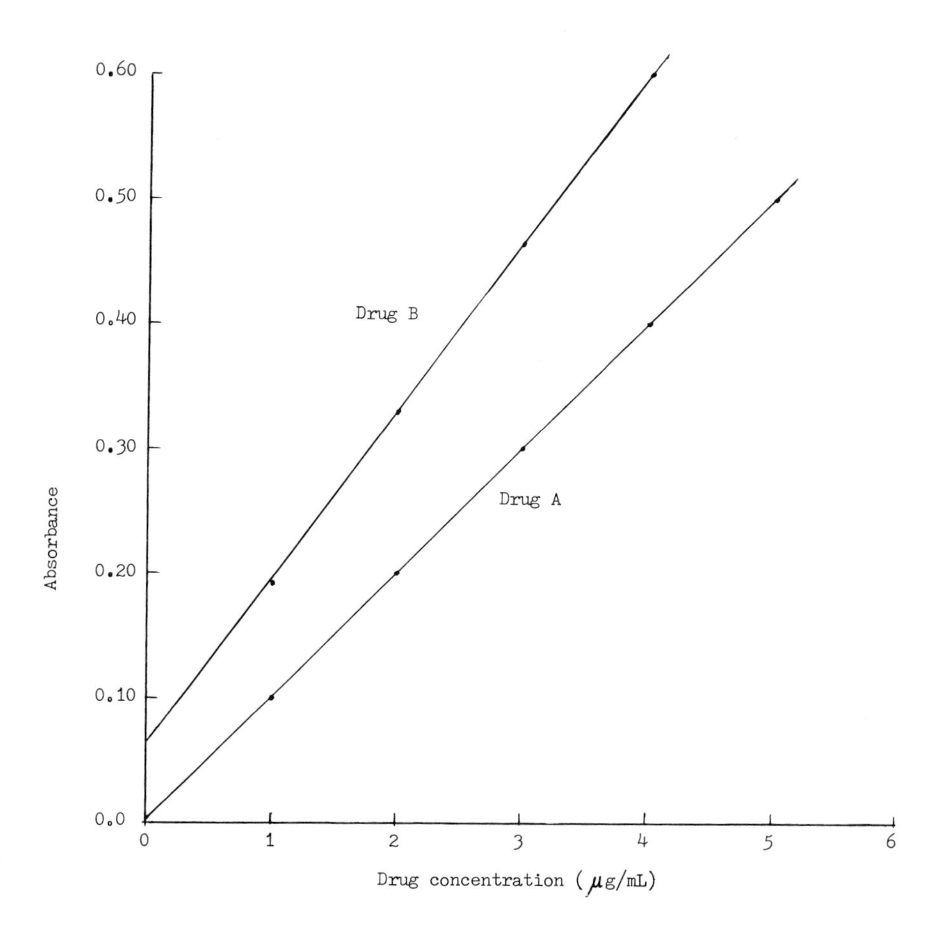


Figure 2. Plot of absorbance against drug concentration

The data of Table 1 are plotted in Figure 2 and the results are two straight lines with positive slopes. By selecting two widely separated points (1, 0.1) and (5, 0.5) on the Drug A curve and substituting the values into the two-point equation as follows,

$$y - 0.1 = \frac{0.5 - 0.1}{5 - 1}(x - 1)$$

the equation for the straight line becomes

$$y - 0.1 = \frac{0.4}{4.0}(x - 1)$$

$$y - 0.1 = 0.1\,(x - 1)$$

$$y - 0.1 = 0.1x - 0.1$$

$$y = 0.1x$$

Since the line passes through the origin, the constant *b* in the straight line equation is 0.

The equation of the line for Drug B is obtained the same way using the points (1, 0.195) and (4, 0.60), and substituting into the two-point equation to give:

$$y - 0.195 = \frac{0.6 - 0.195}{4 - 1}(x - 1)$$

$$y - 0.195 = \frac{0.405}{3}(x - 1)$$

$$y - 0.195 = 0.135x - 0.135$$

$$y = 0.135x + 0.06$$

This equation can now be used to calculate one variable given a value for the other. For example, what is the concentration of Drug B in solution when the absorbance reading is 0.30? Substituting into the equation gives $0.30 = 0.135x + 0.06$ and solving for x gives 1.78 μg/mL. The same value can also be determined directly from the curve in Figure 2.

## LINEAR RELATIONSHIPS ON SEMILOGARITHMIC GRAPH PAPER

Data for the degradation of an antibiotic in aqueous solution over a period of time at two different temperatures are presented in Table 2.

**Table 2. Decrease of Antibiotic in Solution at 30° and 40°C**

| *Time (Days)* | *Concentration (mg/mL) (y) and Logarithm of Concentration (Log y)* | | | |
|---|---|---|---|---|
| | *at 30°C* | | *at 40°C* | |
| *x* | *y* | *Log y* | *y* | *Log y* |
| 0 | 80.0 | 1.903 | 80 | 1.903 |
| 2 | 72.1 | 1.858 | 63 | 1.799 |
| 3 | 69.0 | 1.839 | 56.2 | 1.750 |
| 5 | 62.0 | 1.792 | 44.8 | 1.651 |
| 10 | 49.0 | 1.690 | 25.2 | 1.401 |
| 15 | 38.5 | 1.586 | 14.2 | 1.152 |
| 20 | 30.5 | 1.480 | — | — |
| 25 | 24.0 | 1.380 | — | — |

Three different ways of plotting the above data are shown in Figures 3, 4 and 5. In Figure 3 the experimental measurements are plotted directly on rectangular graph paper to give curvilinear lines typical of exponential phenomena. In Figure 4 the logarithms of the concentrations are plotted against time on rectangular coordinate paper and the resulting curves are straight lines. In Figure 5 the concentration values are plotted on semilogarithmic paper and the curves are straight lines equivalent to those in Figure 4. Figure 5 is convenient for reading the concentration values directly from the graph, whereas Figure 4 is more convenient for obtaining the straight line equation of each curve.

The straight line equation that describes the degradation of antibiotic in solution at 40°C is determined by using the two-point equation.

$$\log y - \log y_1 = \frac{\log y_2 - \log y_1}{x_2 - x_1}(x - x_1)$$

$$\log y - 1.903 = \frac{1.152 - 1.903}{15 - 0}(x - 0)$$

$$\log y - 1.903 = -0.05x$$

$$\log y = -0.05x + 1.903$$

Figures 3 to 5. Three different ways of plotting the concentration of antibiotic (y) as a function of time (x).

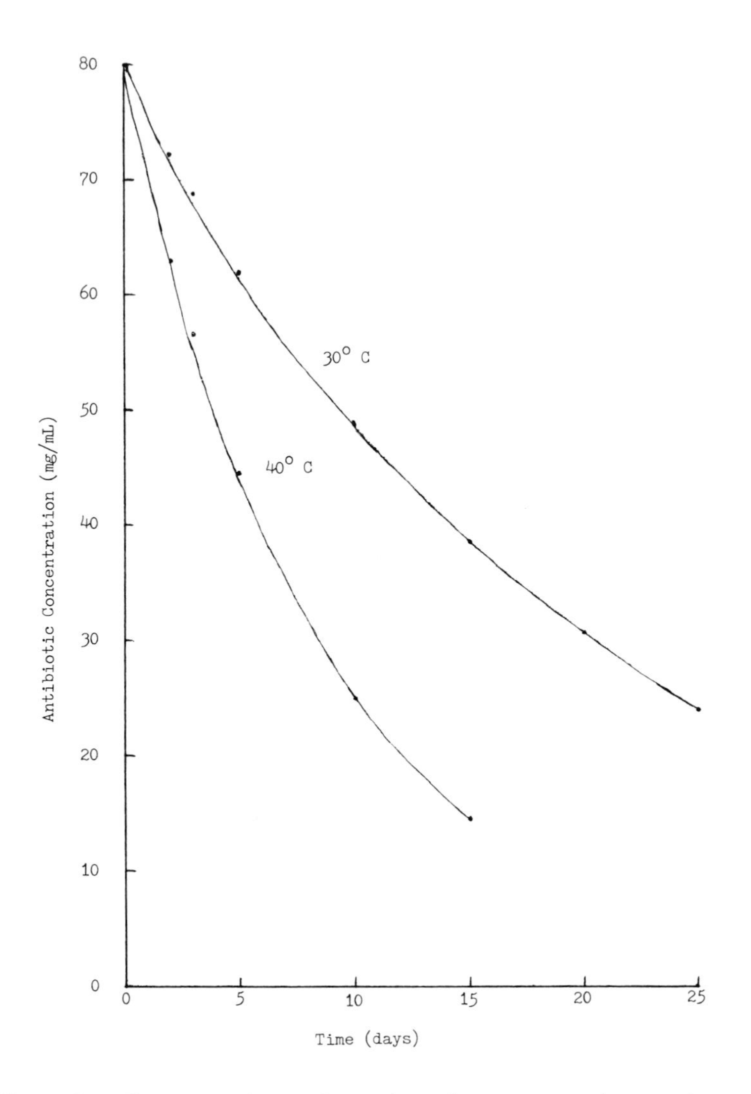


Figure 3. Concentration values plotted on rectangular graph paper.

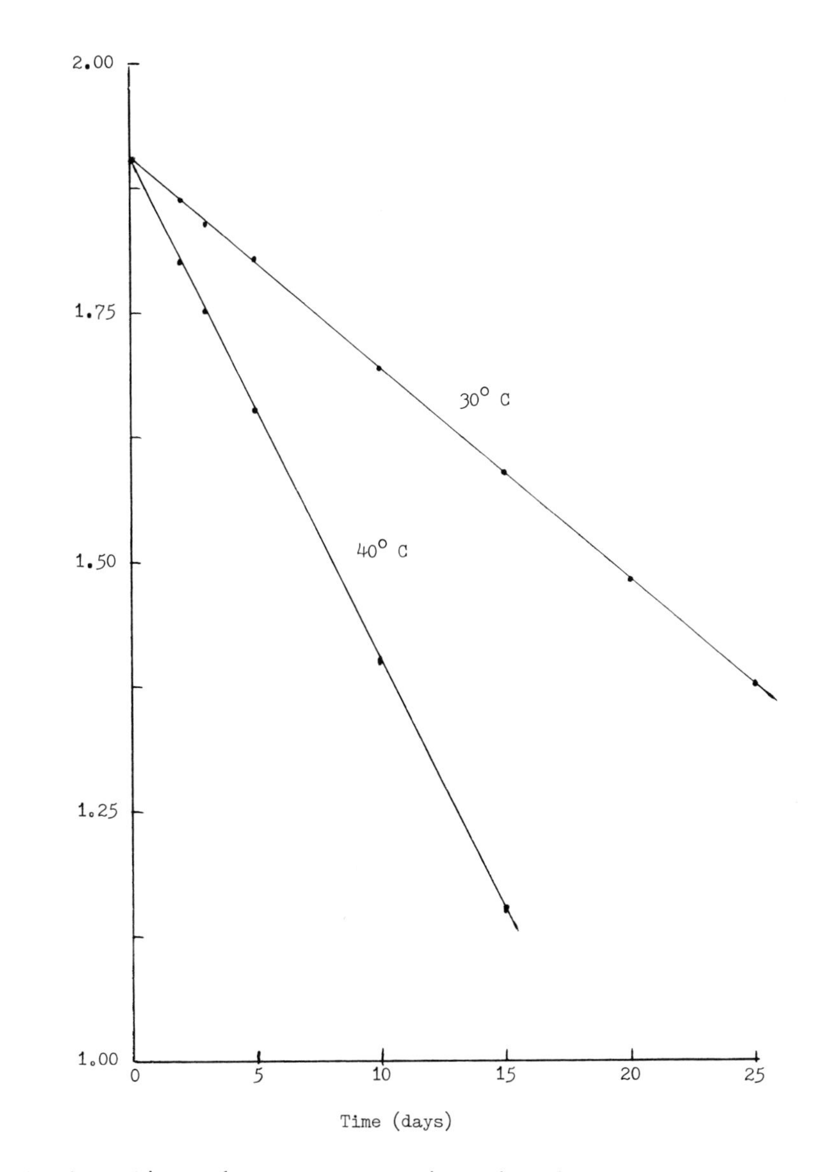


Figure 4. Logarithms of concentration values plotted against time on rectangular coordinate paper.

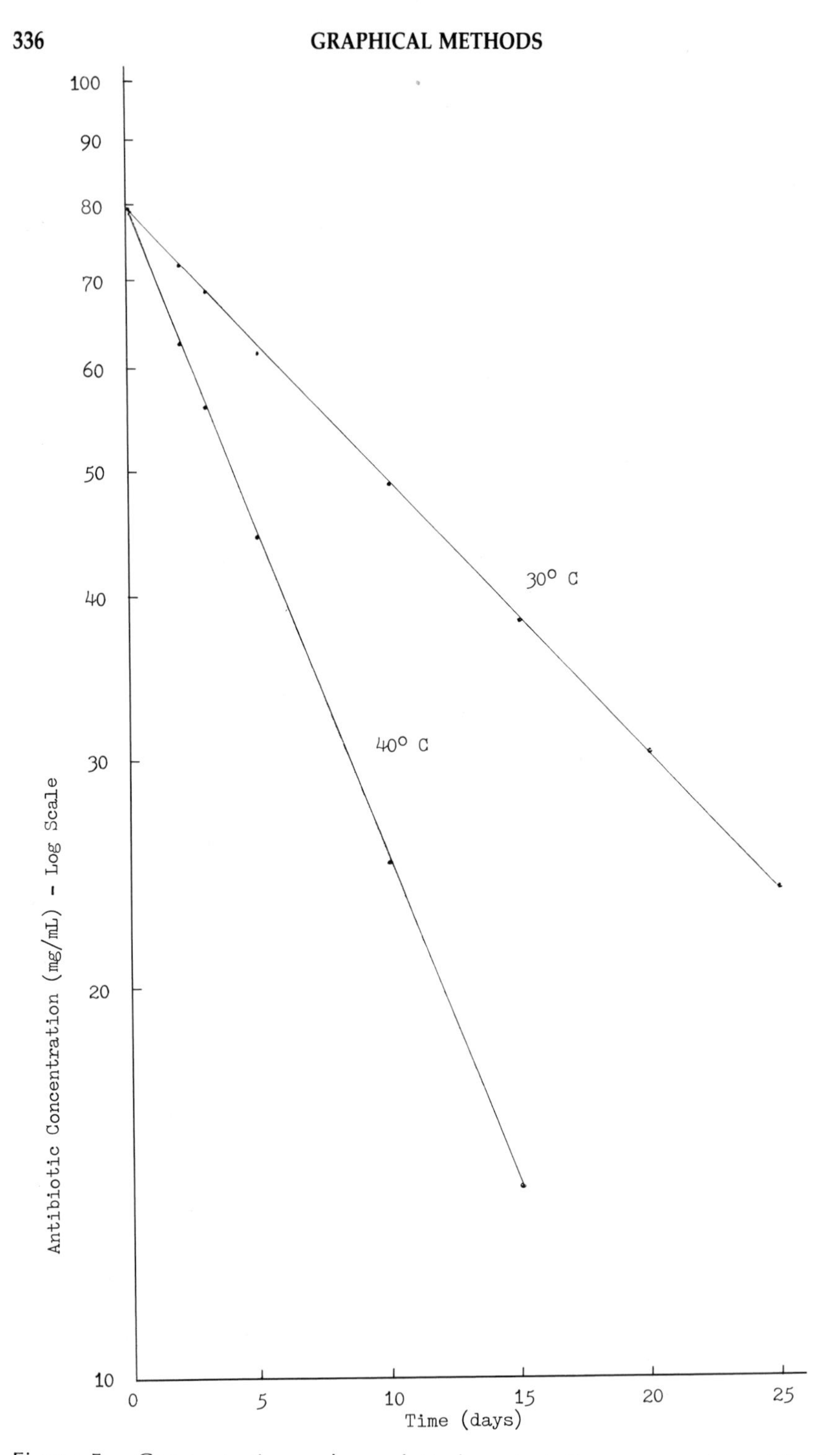


Figure 5. Concentration values plotted against time on semilogarithmic graph paper.

## Practice Problems

1. In Figure 1, what is the $y$ intercept for the equation $y = -2x + 5$? For $y = 0.67x - 1.67$?

2. On regular coordinate graph paper, plot the curves for the following equations.

   (a) $y = -4.0 \times 10^{-2}x + 1.5$
   (b) $y = 500x + 3$
   (c) $3y = 9x + 21$

3. A drug suspension containing 250 mg of drug per 5 mL was placed in a 50°C storage oven, and samples removed periodically and assayed for drug content. The following results were obtained.

| Time (Days) | 5 | 10 | 20 | 30 | 40 | 50 |
|---|---|---|---|---|---|---|
| Drug Concentration (mg/5 mL) | 232 | 213 | 175 | 133 | 102 | 65 |

   (a) Plot the data on rectangular coordinate paper.
   (b) Calculate the straight line equation.
   (c) What is the concentration after 15 days?
   (d) The rate of decomposition K is equal to the slope of the curve. What is this rate of decomposition?

4. From Figure 4, calculate the straight line equation for the degradation of antibiotic solution at 30°C. How much antibiotic would be left in solution after 30 days?

5. An area of a wound was determined every four days by drawing the outline of the wound on a sterile sheet of transparent plastic. After applying an antibiotic cream on the initial day (0), the following results were obtained:

| Time (Days) | 0 | 4 | 8 | 12 | 16 | 20 |
|---|---|---|---|---|---|---|
| Area ($cm^2$) | 60 | 46.5 | 36 | 28 | 21.5 | 16.7 |

   (a) Plot the data on regular coordinate graph paper.
   (b) Plot the data on semilogarithmic graph paper.
   (c) Plot the log area versus time on regular coordinate graph paper.
   (d) Calculate the straight line equation.
   (e) How much time would elapse before the wound reduced to 50% of the original size? to 5 $cm^2$?
   (f) If the rate constant of this equation is defined as $k = 2.3m$, calculate $k$.

APPENDIX

# M

# Some Calculations Associated with Drug Availability and Pharmacokinetics

The availability to the biologic system of a drug substance formulated into a pharmaceutical product is integral to the goals of dosage form design and paramount to the effectiveness of the medication.

Before a drug substance can be absorbed by the biologic system, it must be released from its dosage form (e.g., tablet) or drug delivery system (e.g., transdermal patch) and dissolved in the physiologic fluids. A number of factors play a role in a drug's biologic availability, including the physical and chemical characteristics of the drug itself, as its particle size and solubility, and the features of the dosage form or delivery system, as the nature of the formulative ingredients and the method of manufacture. The area of study which deals with the properties of drug substances and dosage forms which influence the release of the drug for biologic activity is termed *biopharmaceutics.* The term *bioavailability* refers to the *relative amount* of drug from an administered dosage form which enters the systemic circulation.

*Pharmacokinetics* is the study and characterization of the time course of the absorption, distribution, metabolism and excretion of drugs. *Drug absorption* is the process of uptake of the compound from the site of administration into the systemic circulation. *Drug distribution* refers to the transfer of drug from the blood to extravascular fluids and tissues. *Drug metabolism* is the enzymatic or biochemical transformation of the drug substance to (usually less-toxic) metabolic products which may be more readily eliminated from the body. *Drug excretion* is the final elimination of the drug substance or its metabolites from the body as through the kidney (urine), intestines (feces), skin (sweat), saliva and/or milk.

The relationship between the processes of absorption, distribution, metabolism and excretion influences the therapeutic and toxicologic effects of drugs. The application of pharmacokinetic principles in the treatment of individual patients in optimizing drug therapy is referred to as *clinical pharmacokinetics.*

## DRUG AVAILABILITY FROM DOSAGE FORMS AND DELIVERY SYSTEMS

The availability of a drug from a dosage form or delivery system is determined by measuring its dissolution characteristics *in vitro* and/or its absorption patterns *in vivo*. Generally, data are collected which provide information on both *rate* and *extent* of drug dissolution and/or absorption. The data collected may be plotted on graph paper to depict concentration vs. time curves for the drug's dissolution and/or absorption.

### To plot and interpret drug dissolution data:

Drug dissolution data are obtained in vitro for tablets or capsules using the U.S.P. Dissolution Test which defines the apparatus to be used and methods employed.[1] The data obtained may be presented in tabular form and depicted graphically as in the following example.

*Example:*

*The following dissolution data were obtained from a 250-mg capsule of ampicillin. Plot the data on graph paper and determine the approximate percentage of ampicillin dissolved following 15, 30 and 45 minutes of the study.*

| *time period, minutes* | *ampicillin dissolved, mg* |
|---|---|
| 5 | 12 |
| 10 | 30 |
| 20 | 75 |
| 40 | 120 |
| 60 | 150 |

Plotting the data:

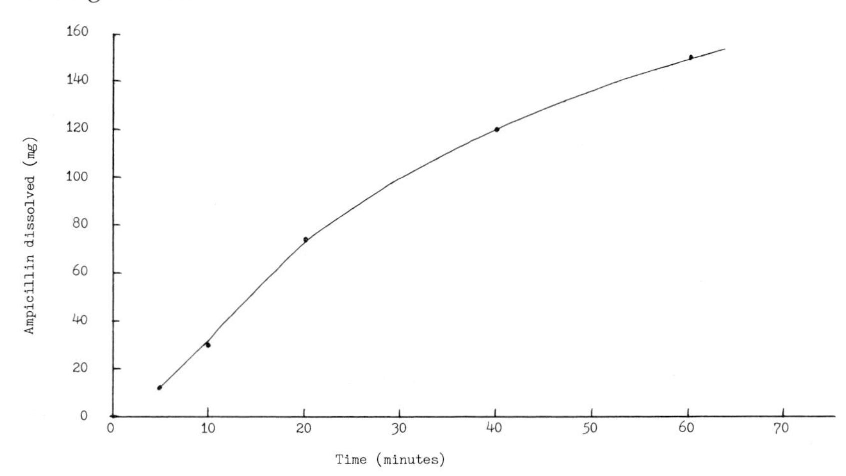


[1]United States Pharmacopeia XXI, pp. 1243–1244, United States Pharmacopeial Convention, Inc., Washington, D.C., 1985.

Determining the intercepts at 15, 30 and 45 minutes:

At 15 minutes, approximately 50 mg or 20% of the ampicillin,
At 30 minutes, approximately 100 mg or 40% of the ampicillin,
At 45 minutes, approximately 125 mg or 50% of the ampicillin, *answers.*

**To calculate the amount of drug which is bioavailable from a dosage form:**

If drug dissolution or drug absorption studies demonstrate consistently that only a portion of a drug substance in a dosage form is "available" for biologic absorption, the drug's bioavailability factor (F) which represents the decimal percent of a drug substance available may be used to calculate bioavailability.

*Example:*

*If the bioavailability factor (F) for a drug substance in a dosage form is 0.60, how many milligrams of drug would be available for absorption from a 100-mg tablet of the drug?*

The bioavailability factor (F) indicates that only 60% of the drug present in the dosage form is available for absorption, thus:

100 mg × 0.60 = 60 mg, *answer.*

**To calculate the "bioequivalent" amounts of "bio*in*equivalent" dosage forms:**

The bioavailability of a drug substance may vary in different dosage forms, or in the same dosage form, but of a different manufacturer. Thus, it may be desired to calculate the equivalent doses for two *bioinequivalent* products.

*Example:*

*If the bioavailability (F) of digoxin in a 0.25-mg tablet is 0.60 compared to the bioavailability (F) of 0.75 in a digoxin elixir (0.05 mg/mL), calculate the dose of the elixir equivalent to the tablet.*

First, calculate the amount of "bioavailable" digoxin in the tablet:

0.25 mg × 0.60 = 0.15 mg, bioavailable amount of digoxin in the tablet.

Next, calculate the amount of "bioavailable" digoxin per mL of the elixir:

0.05 mg × 0.75 = 0.0375 mg, bioavailable amount of digoxin per mL of the elixir.

Finally, determine the quantity of elixir which will provide 0.15 mg of bioavailable digoxin:

By proportion:

$$\frac{0.0375 \text{ (mg)}}{0.15 \text{ (mg)}} = \frac{1 \text{ (mL)}}{\text{x (mL)}}$$

x = 4 mL, *answer.*

**To plot and interpret a blood drug concentration-time curve:**

Following the administration of a medication, if blood samples are drawn from the patient at specific time intervals and analyzed for drug content, the resulting data may be plotted on ordinary graph paper to prepare a blood drug concentration-time curve. The vertical axis of this type of plot characteristically presents the concentration of drug present in the blood (or serum or plasma) and the horizontal axis presents the times the samples were obtained following the administration of the drug. When the drug is first administered (time zero), the blood concentration of the drug should also be zero. As an orally administered drug passes into the stomach and/or intestine, it is released from the dosage form, eventually dissolves, and is absorbed. As the sampling and analysis continue, the blood samples reveal increasing concentrations of drug until the maximum (peak) concentration ($C_{max}$) is reached. Then, the blood level of the drug progressively decreases and, if no additional dose is given, eventually falls to zero.

For conventional dosage forms, as tablets and capsules, the $C_{max}$ will usually occur at only a single time point, referred to as $T_{max}$. The amount of drug is usually expressed in terms of its concentration in relation to a specific volume of blood, serum, or plasma. For example, the concentration may be expressed as g/100 mL, μg/mL or mg% (mg/100 mL). The size of the dose administered influences the blood level concentration for a drug substance. The rate or speed of drug absorption greatly affects the $T_{max}$, the time of greatest blood drug concentration following administration, the faster the rate of absorption, the sooner the $T_{max}$.

In a blood drug concentration-time curve, the area-under-the-curve (AUC) is considered representative of the *total* amount of drug absorbed into the systemic circulation. The area under the curve may be measured mathematically, using a technique known as the trapezoidal rule. The procedure may be found in other texts and references including the one cited below.[1]

[1]Gibaldi, M.: *Biopharmaceutics and Clinical Pharmacokinetics.* 3rd Ed., Philadelphia, Lea & Febiger, 1983, p. 315.

*Example:*

*From the following data, plot a serum concentration-time curve and determine (a) the peak height concentration ($C_{max}$) and (b) the time of the peak height concentration ($T_{max}$).*

| *time period, hours* | *serum drug conc., μg/mL* |
|---|---|
| 0.5 | 1.0 |
| 1.0 | 2.0 |
| 2.0 | 4.0 |
| 3.0 | 3.8 |
| 4.0 | 2.9 |
| 6.0 | 1.9 |
| 8.0 | 1.0 |
| 10.0 | 0.3 |
| 12.0 | 0.2 |

Plotting the data and interpretation of the curve:

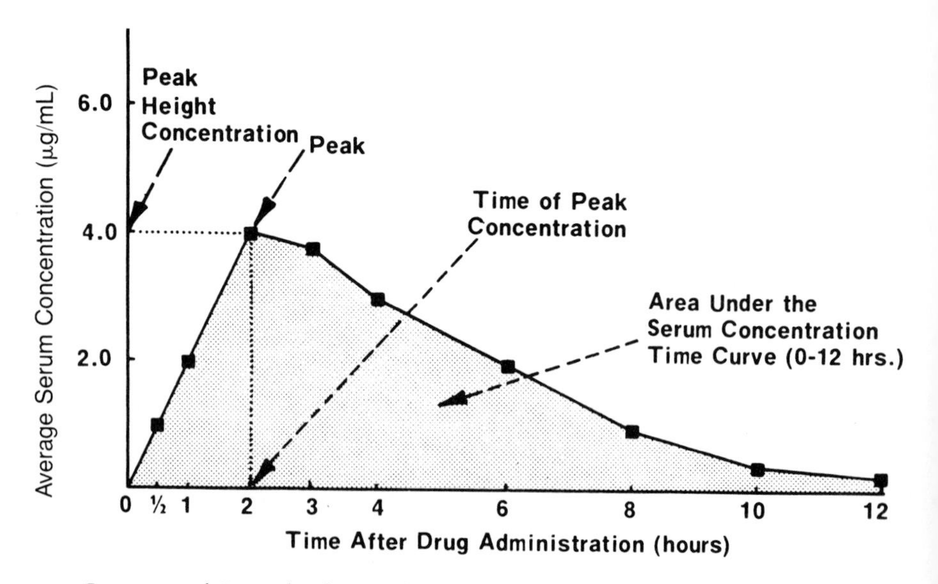


*Courtesy of D.J. Chodos and A.R. DiSanto, The Upjohn Company.*

Determining the intercept for $C_{max}$ and $T_{max}$:

$C_{max}$ = 4.0 μg/mL

$T_{max}$ = 2 hours, *answers*.

## SOME INTRODUCTORY CONCEPTS AND CALCULATIONS INVOLVED IN PHARMACOKINETICS

As defined previously, pharmacokinetics is the study and characterization of the time course of absorption, distribution, metabolism and excretion of drugs. Many of the calculations involved in pharmacokinetics are complex and the subject of advanced textbooks devoted to this important field. It is the intention here to define and describe some of the more introductory concepts and calculations.

### To calculate the plasma concentration of unbound vs. bound drugs:

Once absorbed into the bloodstream, a portion of the total drug plasma concentration ($C_T$) is bound to plasma proteins (usually albumin) and a portion remains unbound or free in the circulation. It is the unbound drug ($C_U$) which is available for further transport to its site of action in the body. The fraction of unbound drug compared to bound drug ($C_B$) is primarily a function of the affinity of the drug molecules for binding to the plasma proteins and the concentration of the latter (some patients may have a reduced or an elevated serum albumin concentration). Some drug molecules may be over 90% bound to plasma proteins, whereas others may be only slightly bound. Any change in the degree of binding of a given drug substance can alter its distribution and elimination, and thus its clinical effects.

The fraction of unbound drug in the plasma compared to the total plasma drug concentration, bound and unbound, is termed *alpha* (or $\alpha$). Thus,

$$\alpha = \frac{C_U}{C_U + C_B} = \frac{C_U}{C_T}$$

If one knows the value of $\alpha$ for a drug and the total plasma concentration ($C_T$), the concentration of free drug in the plasma may be determined by a rearranged equation:

$$C_U = (\alpha) \times (C_T)$$

*Example:*

*If the alpha ($\alpha$) value for the drug digoxin is 0.70, what would be the concentration of free drug in the plasma if the total plasma concentration of the drug were determined to be 0.7 ng/mL?*

$$C_U = (0.70) \times (0.7 \text{ ng/mL})$$
$$= 0.49 \text{ ng/mL, } \textit{answer}.$$

**To calculate the apparent volume of distribution of a drug substance:**

The apparent volume of distribution for a drug is not a "real" volume, but rather a hypothetical volume of body fluid that would be required to dissolve the total amount of drug at the same concentration as that found in the blood. The volume of distribution is an indicator of the extent of a drug's distribution in the body. The minimum volume of distribution must be at least equal to the plasma volume, about 4.3% of body weight.

If in an adult the volume of distribution is 5 liters, the drug is considered confined to the circulatory system, as it would be immediately following a rapid intravenous injection (IV bolus). If the volume of distribution is between 10 and 20 liters, or between 15 and 27% of the body weight, it is assumed that the drug has been distributed into the extracellular fluids; if it is between 25 and 30 liters, or between 35 and 42% of body weight, it is assumed that the drug has been distributed into the intracellular fluid; if it is about 40 liters, or 60% of the body weight, the assumption is that the drug has been distributed in the whole body fluid.[1] If the apparent volume of distribution actually exceeds the body weight, it is assumed that the drug is being stored in body fat, bound to body tissues, or is distributed in peripheral compartments.

The equation for determining the volume of distribution (Vd) is:

$$Vd = \frac{D}{C_p}$$

in which D is the total amount of drug in the body, and $C_p$ is the drug's plasma concentration. The apparent volume of distribution may be expressed as a simple volume or as a percent of body weight.

*Example:*

*A patient was administered a single intravenous dose of 300 mg of a drug substance which produced an immediate blood concentration of 8.2 µg of drug per mL. Calculate the apparent volume of distribution.*

$$Vd = \frac{D}{C_p}$$

$$= \frac{300 \text{ mg}}{8.2 \text{ µg/mL}} = \frac{300 \text{ mg}}{8.2 \text{ mg/L}}$$

$$= 36.6 \text{ L}, \textit{answer}.$$

[1]W.A. Ritschel, *Handbook of Basic Pharmacokinetics*, 2nd Ed., Drug Intelligence Publications, Inc., Hamilton, Illinois, 1982, p. 219.

**To calculate the total amount of drug in a body, given the volume of distribution and the plasma drug concentration:**

*Example:*

*Four hours following the intravenous administration of a drug, a patient weighing 70 kg was found to have a drug blood level concentration of 10 μg/mL. Assuming the apparent volume of distribution is 10% of body weight, calculate the total amount of drug present in body fluids four hours after the drug was administered.*

$$Vd = \frac{D}{C_p} \qquad D = (Vd) \times (C_p)$$

$$Vd = 10\% \text{ of } 70 \text{ kg} = 7 \text{ kg} = 7 \text{ L}$$

$$C_p = 10 \ \mu\text{g/mL} = 10 \text{ mg/L}$$

$$7 \text{ L} = \frac{D}{10 \text{ mg/L}}$$

$$D = (7 \text{ L}) \times (10 \text{ mg/L})$$

$$= 70 \text{ mg, } \textit{answer.}$$

**To determine the elimination half-life and elimination rate constant:**

The elimination phase of a drug from the body is reflected by a decline in the drug's plasma concentration. The *elimination half-life* ($t_{1/2}$) is the time it takes for the plasma drug concentration (as well as the amount of drug in the body) to fall by one half. For example, if it takes 3 hours for the plasma concentration of a drug to fall from 6 mg/L to 3 mg/L, its half-life would be 3 hours. It would take the same period of time (3 hours) for the concentration to fall from 3 mg/L to 1.5 mg/L, or from 1.5 mg/L to 0.75 mg/L. Many drug substances follow first-order kinetics in their elimination from the body, meaning that the rate of drug elimination per unit of time is proportional to the amount present at that time. As demonstrated above, the elimination half-life is independent of the amount of drug in the body and the amount of drug eliminated is less in each succeeding half-life. After 5 elimination half-lives it may be expected that virtually all of a drug (97%) originally present will have been eliminated. The student might wish to examine this point, starting with a 100-mg dose of a drug (after first half-life, 50 mg, etc.).

Blood level data from a drug may be plotted against time on regular graph paper to obtain an exponential curve, or it may be plotted on semilogarithmic graph paper to obtain a straight line. From the latter, the elimination half-life may be determined as shown in the example which follows in this section.

The elimination rate constant ($K_e$) characterizes the elimination process and may simply be regarded as the *fractional rate of drug removal per unit time, expressed as a decimal fraction* (e.g., 0.01 $min^{-1}$, meaning 1% per minute). The elimination rate constant for a first order process may be calculated using the equation:

$$K_e = \frac{0.693}{t_{1/2}}$$

The derivation of this equation is like that previously described for the exponential decay of radioisotopes (p. 240).

*Examples:*

*A patient is administered 12 mg of a drug intravenously and blood samples are drawn and analyzed at specific time intervals resulting in the following data. Plot the data on semilogarithmic graph paper and determine the elimination half-life of the drug.*

| *Plasma drug level concentration* $\mu$*g/100 mL* | *Time hours* |
|---|---|
| 26.5 | 1 |
| 17.5 | 2 |
| 11.5 | 3 |
| 7.6 | 4 |
| 5.0 | 5 |
| 3.3 | 6 |

Plotting the data:

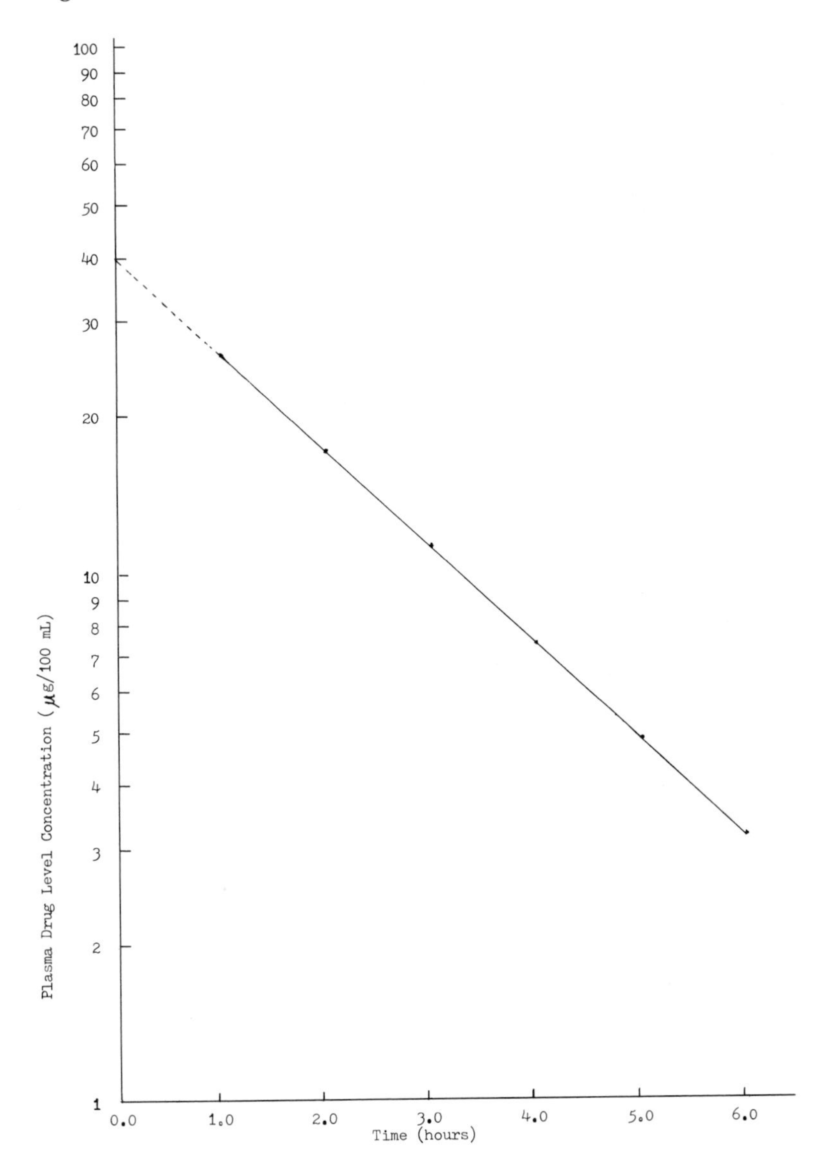


From the plotted data the straight line may by extrapolated to time zero to determine the initial plasma drug concentration. If this is done, the concentration is found to be 40 μg/100 mL. The time it takes to reduce that level to one-half, or 20 μg/100 mL, is the elimination half-life. The 20 μg/100 mL concentration intersects the straight line at 1.7 hours.

Therefore, the elimination half-life is 1.7 hours, *answer.*

*Note:* The same answer may be obtained by selecting any plasma drug concentration (for example, 10 μg/100 mL), determining the time of that plasma level from the intercept, repeating the process for one-half of that drug level (5 μg/100 mL) and determining the elapsed time by subtraction to obtain the elimination half-life.

*Calculate the elimination rate constant for a drug which has an elimination half-life of 50 minutes.*

$$K_e = \frac{0.693}{t_{1/2}}$$

$$= \frac{0.693}{50 \text{ min}}$$

$$= 0.0139 \text{ min}^{-1}, \textit{ answer.}$$

## DOSAGE CALCULATIONS BASED ON CREATININE CLEARANCE

**To calculate the dose of a drug based on creatinine clearance:**

The two major mechanisms by which drugs are eliminated from the body are through hepatic (liver) metabolism and renal (kidney) excretion. When renal excretion is the major route of elimination of a drug, a loss of kidney function will dramatically affect the rate at which the drug is cleared from the body. Polar drugs are eliminated predominately by renal excretion and are generally affected by decreased kidney function.

With many drugs it is important that a specific drug concentration be reached in the blood and maintained to realize proper therapeutic effect. The initial blood concentration attained from a specific dose is dependent, in part, on the weight of the patient and the volume of body fluids in which the drug is distributed.

The lean body mass (LBM) provides an excellent estimation of the distribution volume, particularly for some polar drugs which are not well distributed in adipose (fat) tissue. LBM calculations have been utilized clinically with the aminoglycoside antibiotics and with digoxin to dose and predict blood levels. The lean body mass may be calculated readily through the use of the following formulas based on the patient's height and sex.

*For males:*

LBM = 50 kg + 2.3 kg for each inch of patient's height over 5 feet

*or, in pounds*

110 lb + 5 lb for each inch over 5 feet

*For females:*

LBM = 45.5 kg + 2.3 kg for each inch of patient height over 5 feet

*or, in pounds*

100 lb + 5 lb for each inch over 5 feet

*Examples:*

*Calculate the lean body mass for a male patient weighing 164 pounds and measuring 5 feet 8 inches in height.*

LBM = 110 lb + (8 × 5 lb)

110 lb + 40 lb = 150 lb, *answer.*

*Calculate the lean body mass for a female patient weighing 60 kilograms and measuring 160 centimeters in height.*

160 cm = 63 inches = 5 feet 3 inches

LBM = 45.5 kg + (3 × 2.3 kg)

45.5 kg + 6.9 kg = 52.4 kg, *answer.*

NOTE: In instances in which the LBM is determined to be greater than the actual body weight, the latter is employed in dosage calculations.

The kidneys receive about 20% of the cardiac output (blood flow) and filter approximately 125 milliliters per minute of plasma. As kidney function is lost, the quantity of plasma filtered per minute decreases, with an accompanying decrease in drug clearance. The filtration rate of the kidney can be estimated by a number of methods. However, one of the most useful is the estimation of the creatinine clearance rate (Ccr) through the use of the following empirical formulas based on the patient's age and serum creatinine value.[1] The creatinine clearance rate represents the volume of blood plasma which is cleared of creatinine by kidney filtration per minute. It is expressed in milliliters per minute.

---

[1]Creatinine, which is a break-down product of muscle metabolism, is generally produced at a constant rate and in quantities dependent upon the muscle mass of the patient. Since creatinine is eliminated from the body essentially through renal filtration, reduced kidney performance results in a reduced creatinine clearance rate.

*For males:*

$$\text{Creatinine Clearance Rate (Ccr)} = \frac{98 - 0.8 \times (\text{patient's age in years} - 20)}{\text{Serum Creatinine as mg\% (mg/100 mL)}}$$

*For females:*

$$\text{Creatinine Clearance Rate (Ccr)} = 0.9 \times \text{Ccr determined using formula for males}$$

*Example:*

*Determine the creatinine clearance rate for an 80-year-old male patient having a serum creatinine of 2 mg%.*

$$\text{Ccr} = \frac{98 - 0.8 \times (80 - 20)}{2\ (\text{mg\%})}$$

$$= \frac{98 - (0.8 \times 60)}{2\ (\text{mg\%})} = \frac{98 - 48}{2\ (\text{mg\%})} = \frac{50}{2\ (\text{mg\%})}$$

$$= 25\ \text{mL/min, } \textit{answer.}$$

Normal creatinine clearance rate may be considered 100 milliliters per minute. Thus, in the example above, the patient would exhibit one fourth or 25% of normal creatinine clearance.

The creatinine clearance rate method for determining drug dose is used primarily in aminoglycoside therapy in which reduced renal function is a factor. The primary drugs involved are gentamicin, tobramycin, amikacin, and kanamycin.

Once the creatinine clearance rate and the lean body mass have been calculated, the *loading dose* (initial dose) required to reach a certain drug concentration in the patient and the *maintenance dose* needed to maintain the specified concentration can be calculated.

The loading dose is based solely on the lean body mass of the patient whereas the maintenance dose is based on the lean body mass *and* the renal clearance rate of the drug.

**To calculate the loading dose (LD):**

$$\text{LD} = \text{lean body mass (LBM) in kg or lb} \times \text{drug dose per kg or lb}$$

**To calculate the maintenance dose (MD):**

For "normal" patient:

$$MD = LBM\ (kg) \times \text{dose per kg per dosing interval}$$

For "renally-impaired" patient:

$$MD = \frac{Ccr\ (patient)}{Ccr\ (normal)} \times \text{dose for "normal" patient}$$

*Example:*

*Determine the loading dose and maintenance dose of gentamicin for a 76-year-old male patient weighing 190 lb with a height of 6 ft and having a serum creatinine of 2.4 mg%. The physician desires a loading dose of 1.5 mg per kg of lean body mass and a maintenance dose of 1.0 mg per kg of lean body mass to be administered every 8 hours following initial dose.*

$$LBM = 110\ lb + (5\ lb \times 12)$$

$$= 110\ lb + 60\ lb$$

$$= 170\ lb \text{ or } 77.3\ kg$$

$$Ccr = \frac{98 - 0.8 \times (76 - 20)}{2.4\ (mg\%)}$$

$$= \frac{98 - 44.8}{2.4\ (mg\%)} = \frac{53.2}{2.4\ (mg\%)} = 22.2\ mL \text{ per minute}$$

$$LD = 77.3\ kg \times 1.5\ mg \text{ per } kg = 116,\ mg,\ \textit{answer}.$$

MD for "normal" patient:

$$= 77.3\ kg \times 1.0\ mg \text{ per kg every 8 hr}$$

$$= 77.3\ mg \text{ every 8 hr}$$

MD for "renally-impaired" patient:

$$= \frac{22.2\ mL \text{ per minute}}{100\ mL \text{ per minute}} \times 77.3\ mg$$

$$= 17.2\ mg \text{ every 8 hr, } \textit{answer}.$$

## Practice Problems

1. If the bioavailability factor (F) for a 100-mg tablet of a drug is 0.70 compared to the bioavailability factor of 1.0 for an injection of the same

drug, how many milliliters of the injection containing 40 mg/mL would be considered bioequivalent to the tablet?

2. If 5 mL of an elixir containing 2 mg of a drug per mL is bioequivalent to a 15-mg tablet having a bioavailability factor of 0.60, what is the bioavailability factor of the elixir?

3. If at equilibrium, two-thirds of the amount of a drug substance in the blood is bound to protein, what would be the alpha ($\alpha$) value of the drug?

4. The alpha ($\alpha$) value for a drug in the blood is 0.90 equating to 0.55 ng/mL. What is the concentration of total drug in the blood?

5. A patient was administered an intravenous dose of 10 mg of a drug. A blood sample was drawn and found to contain 40 $\mu$g/100 mL. Calculate the apparent volume of distribution for the drug.

6. The volume of distribution for a drug was found to be 10 liters with a blood level concentration of 2 $\mu$g/mL. Calculate the total amount of drug present in the patient.

7. Calculate the elimination rate constant for a drug having an elimination half-life of 1.7 hours.

8. Plot the following data on semilogarithmic graph paper and determine (a) the elimination half-life of the drug and (b) the elimination rate constant.

| *Plasma drug concentration $\mu$g/100 mL* | *Time, hours* |
|---|---|
| 8.5 | 0.5 |
| 6.8 | 1.0 |
| 5.4 | 1.5 |
| 4.0 | 2.0 |
| 3.2 | 2.5 |
| 2.5 | 3.0 |

9. What percentage of an originally administered intravenous dose of a drug remains in the body following three half-lives?

10. If the half-life of a drug is 4 hours, approximately what percent of the drug administered would remain in the body 15 hours after administration?

11. Determine the loading and maintenance doses of tobramycin for a 72-year-old female patient weighing 187 lb and measuring 5′3″ in height with a serum creatinine of 2.8 mg%. The loading dose desired is 1.0 mg per kg of lean body mass and 1.66 mg per kg every 8 hours as the maintenance dose.

12. Determine the loading and maintenance doses of amikacin for a 42-year-old female patient weighing 210 lb and measuring 5 ft in height with a serum creatinine of 1.8 mg%. The physician requests a loading dose of 7.5 mg per kg of lean body mass and a maintenance dose of 5 mg per kg of lean body mass to be administered continually at intervals of 8 hours.

# Review Problems

1. A prescription for 240 mL of a liquid contains 15 mg of atropine sulfate and has a dose of 10 mL. *(a)* Calculate the fraction of a grain of atropine sulfate that is contained in each dose. *(b)* Using a torsion prescription balance having a sensitivity requirement of 6.5 mg, explain how you would obtain the 15 mg of atropine sulfate with an error not greater than 5%. Use distilled water as the diluent.

2. A pharmacist weighed 20 mg of cocaine alkaloid on a prescription balance having a sensitivity requirement of 4 mg. Calculate the maximum potential error in terms of percentage.

3. In preparing a cough syrup containing 0.030 g of hydromorphone hydrochloride, a pharmacist weighed the hydromorphone hydrochloride on a torsion balance having a sensitivity requirement of 4 mg. Calculate the percentage of error that may have been incurred by the pharmacist.

4. Using a torsion prescription balance having a sensitivity requirement of 4 mg, explain how you would weigh the atropine sulfate needed to prepare 250 mL of a solution which is to contain 120 μg of atropine sulfate in each 5-mL dose. Assume an error in weighing not greater than 5%.

5. In compounding a prescription for ℥ii of a 5% benzocaine cream, a pharmacist used 45 gr of benzocaine instead of the 48 gr that should have been used. Calculate the percentage of error that may have been incurred by the pharmacist.

6. In preparing one fluidounce of a saturated solution of potassium iodide, a pharmacist used ʒvii of potassium iodide instead of the 455 gr called for. Calculate the percentage of error on the basis of what should have been used by the pharmacist.

7. ℞ Atropine Sulfate 0.5 mg
Bismuth Subgallate 0.3 g
Carbowax Base q.s.
Make 10 such suppositories
Sig. One at night.

Using a torsion prescription balance having a sensitivity requirement of 6 mg, explain how you would obtain the correct amount of atropine sulfate with an error not greater than 5%. Use bismuth subgallate as the diluent.

8. In checking the inventory of narcotics in a hospital pharmacy, the checker found it to be kept in the metric system. The inventory showed 124.4 g (4 one-ounce original bottles) of codeine sulfate on hand at the beginning of the inventory period. The prescriptions on file showed that 96 g of codeine sulfate had been dispensed. On weighing the contents of the one-ounce bottle that remained, the checker found that only 17.4 g were left, instead of 28.4 g that apparently should have remained. What percentage of error, if any, had been made in the inventory?

9. A vitamin liquid contains, in each 0.5 mL, the following:

| | |
|---|---|
| Thiamine Hydrochloride | 1 mg |
| Riboflavin | 400 μg |
| Ascorbic Acid | 50 mg |
| Nicotinamide | 2 mg |

Calculate the quantity, expressed in grams, of each ingredient in 30 mL of the liquid.

10. A certain injectable solution contains 30 mg of a drug substance in 30 mL. How many milliliters of the solution should be administered to provide a weekly dose of 100 μg of the drug substance?

11. The prophylactic dose of riboflavin is 2 mg. How many micrograms of riboflavin are there in a capsule containing 3 times the prophylactic dose?

12. How many grams of codeine phosphate are left in an original ⅛-oz (avoir.) bottle after the amount required to prepare 100 capsules each containing ¼ gr of codeine phosphate as one of the ingredients is used?

13. How many grains of atropine sulfate are left in a ½-oz (avoir.) bottle after enough of it is used to make 10,000 tablets, each containing $^1/_{200}$ gr?

14. A pharmacist purchased 5 gallons of alcohol. At different times 0ii, 2 gallons, 8f℥, and ½ gallon were used by the pharmacist. What volume, in fluidounces, remained?

15. A prescription calls for 1.25 g of phenacaine hydrochloride. If the phenacaine hydrochloride costs $13.20 per oz (avoir.), what is the cost of the amount needed for the prescription?

16. If homatropine hydrobromide costs $12.65 per ⅛ oz (avoir.), what is the cost of 300 mg?

17. A pharmacist purchased 5 g of codeine phosphate. It was used by the pharmacist in preparing 50 capsules each containing ½ gr of codeine phosphate and in formulating 1 pt of a cough syrup containing 1 gr of codeine phosphate per fluidounce. For purposes of inventory, how many grams of codeine phosphate remained?

18. How many micrograms of nitroglycerin are contained in a $\frac{1}{200}$-gr tablet?

19. If iodine costs $30.00 a pound, and iodine tincture contains 20 g of iodine in a liter, what will be the cost of the iodine in one pint of the tincture?

20. ℞ Podophyllum Resin 25%
Compound Benzoin Tincture ad 30 mL
Sig. Apply locally for venereal warts.

At $27.25 per oz (avoir.), what is the cost of the podophyllum resin needed in compounding the prescription?

21. The dose of a certain antibiotic is 5 mg per kg of body weight. How many milligrams should be used for a person weighing 145 lb?

22. If chloral hydrate costs $11.00 per lb (avoir.), what is the cost of the amount needed to prepare a liter of a solution containing 300 mg per teaspoonful?

23. An elixir is to contain 250 μg of an alkaloid in each teaspoonful dose. How many grams of the alkaloid will be required to prepare 5 liters of the elixir?

24. The dose of a drug is 0.5 mg. How many micrograms should be given to a child 10 years old?

25. A f℥vi mixture contains, in each teaspoonful, ⅙ gr of codeine phosphate. How many grains of codeine phosphate are contained in the entire mixture?

26. The initial dose of a drug is 0.25 mg per kg of body weight. How many milligrams should be prescribed for a person weighing 154 lb?

27. ℞ Lugol's Solution 30 mL
Sig. Ten drops in water once a day.

Lugol's solution contains 5% of iodine. If the dispensing dropper calibrates 25 drops per mL, calculate the amount, in milligrams, of iodine in each dose of the solution.

28. ℞ Cyanocobalamin 10 μg per mL
Disp. 10-mL sterile vial.
Sig. 1.5 mL every other week.

*(a)* How many micrograms of cyanocobalamin will be administered in a period of 12 weeks?

*(b)* How many milligrams of cyanocobalamin are there in 10 mL of this preparation?

29. The pediatric dose of chloral hydrate may be determined on the basis of 8 mg per kg of body weight or on the basis of 250 mg per $m^2$. Calculate the dose on each basis for a child weighing 44 lb and measuring 36 in. in height.

30. The rectal dose of sodium thiopental is 45 mg per kg of body weight. How many milliliters of a 10% solution should be used for a person weighing 150 lb?

31. ℞ Penicillin G Procaine 300,000 units
Buffered Crystalline Penicillin G 100,000 units
Crystalline Dihydrostreptomycin 1 g
Water for Injection ad 3 mL
Make a multiple-dose vial containing 5 doses.
Sig. For intramuscular use only. Sterile.

To permit withdrawal of the five doses prescribed, an excess volume of 0.80 mL must be present in the 15 mL vial. How much of each of the three antibiotics should be used in compounding the prescription?

32. ℞ Sodium Fluoride q.s.
Vitamin Drops ad 50 mL
(10 drops = 2.2 mg NaF)
Sig. Ten (10) drops in orange juice.

Assuming that the dispensing dropper calibrates 25 drops per mL, how many milligrams of sodium fluoride should be used in compounding the prescription?

33. How many chloramphenicol capsules, each containing 250 mg, are needed to provide 25 mg per kg per day for 1 week for a person weighing 175 lb?

34. The dose of piperazine citrate is 50 mg per kg of body weight once daily for seven consecutive days. How many milliliters of piperazine citrate syrup containing 500 mg per teaspoonful should be prescribed for a child weighing 66 lb?

35. A physician prescribed 5 mg of a drug per kg of body weight once daily for a patient weighing 132 lb. How many 100-mg tablets of the drug are required for a dosage regimen of 2 weeks?

36. ℞ Morphine Sulfate

| | | | |
|---|---|---|---|
| Morphine Sulfate | | | |
| Cocaine Hydrochloride | | aa | 10 mg/f℥ |
| Compazine | | | 5 mg/f℥ |
| Aromatic Elixir | q.s. | ad | f℥xvi |

Sig. Tsp. ii p.r.n. pain.

*(a)* How many milligrams of morphine sulfate would be contained per dose; *(b)* how many milligrams of cocaine hydrochloride would be used in filling the prescription; *(c)* how many milliliters of a solution containing 5 mg of Compazine per mL would be used in filling the prescription?

37. ℞

| | |
|---|---|
| Coal Tar | 5 parts |
| Zinc Oxide Paste | 50 parts |

Disp. 240 g
Sig. Apply.

How many grams of coal tar should be used in compounding the prescription?

38.

| | |
|---|---|
| Coal Tar | 50 g |
| Bentonite | 80 g |
| Water | 300 mL |
| Hydrophilic Ointment | 80 g |
| Zinc Oxide Paste, to make | 1000 g |

How much of each ingredient should be used in preparing 5 lb (avoir.) of the ointment?

39.

| | |
|---|---|
| Aminophylline | 250 mg |
| Phenobarbital Sodium | 50 mg |
| Benzocaine | 20 mg |
| Carbowax Base | 2 g |

Calculate the quantity of each ingredient to be used in preparing 250 suppositories.

40.

| | |
|---|---|
| Witch Hazel | 120 mL |
| Glycerin | 50 mL |
| Boric Acid Solution, to make | 1000 mL |

How much of each ingredient should be used in preparing 5 gallons of the lotion?

41. Set up a formula for 5 lb (avoir.) of glycerogelatin containing 10

parts, by weight, of zinc oxide, 15 parts, by weight, of gelatin, 40 parts, by weight, of glycerin, and 35 parts, by weight, of water.

42.

| | | |
|---|---|---|
| Coal Tar | | 10 g |
| Polysorbate 80 | | 5 g |
| Zinc Oxide Paste | | 985 g |

Calculate the quantity of each ingredient required to prepare 10 lb (avoir.) of the ointment.

43.

| | | |
|---|---|---|
| Menthol | | 0.2 g |
| Hexachlorophene | | 0.1 g |
| Glycerin | | 10 mL |
| Isopropyl Alcohol | | 35 mL |
| Purified Water | ad | 100 mL |

Calculate the quantity of each ingredient required to prepare 1 gallon of the lotion.

44.

| | | |
|---|---|---|
| Isopropyl Alcohol | | 50 mL |
| Propylene Glycol | | 2 mL |
| Glacial Acetic Acid | | 0.1 mL |
| Purified Water | ad | 100 mL |

Calculate the quantity of each ingredient required to prepare 1 gallon of the lotion.

45.

| | |
|---|---|
| Benzoic Acid | 6 parts |
| Salicylic Acid | 3 parts |
| Polyethylene Glycol Ointment | 91 parts |

Calculate the quantity of each ingredient required to prepare 1 lb (avoir.) of the ointment.

46. If 5000 mL of a syrup weigh 6565 g, calculate *(a)* its specific gravity and *(b)* its specific volume.

47. If the specific volume of a liquid is 1.264, what is its specific gravity?

48. A saturated solution contains, in each 100 mL, 100 g of a substance. If the solubility of the substance is 1 g in 0.7 mL of water, what is the specific gravity of the saturated solution?

49. In making a certain syrup, 6800 g of sucrose were dissolved in enough water to make 8 liters. Assuming the specific gravity of the syrup to be 1.313, how many milliliters of water were used?

50. A certain liniment is prepared by mixing 2 lb of methyl salicylate (sp. gr. 1.18), 1 liter of alcohol (sp. gr. 0.8) and 1 lb of chloroform (sp. gr. 1.475). What is the volume, in milliliters, of the mixture?

51. A formula for 200 g of an ointment contains 10 g of glycerin. How many milliliters of glycerin having a specific gravity of 1.25 should be used in preparing 1 lb (avoir.) of the ointment?

52.

| | |
|---|---|
| White Wax | 12.5 g |
| Mineral Oil | 60.0 g |
| Lanolin | 2.5 g |
| Sodium Borate | 1.0 g |
| Rose Water | 24.0 g |

Label: Cold cream.

How many milliliters of mineral oil having a specific gravity of 0.900 should be used in preparing 10 lb (avoir.) of the cream?

53. How many milliliters of a commercially available 50% (v/v) solution of glycerin should be used to provide 2 g of glycerin per kilogram of body weight for a person weighing 110 lb? The specific gravity of glycerin is 1.25.

54. Given a solution of potassium permanganate prepared by dissolving sixteen 0.2-g tablets in enough distilled water to make 1600 mL,

*(a)* What is the percentage strength of the solution?
*(b)* What is the ratio strength of the solution?

55. Given a salt solution of 1:1500 concentration, what is:

*(a)* the percentage strength?
*(b)* the weight, in grains, of the salt per pint?
*(c)* the weight, in micrograms, of the salt per mL?
*(d)* the number of milliliters required to prepare 2 liters of a 1:2500 solution?

56. The manufacturer specifies that one Domeboro tablet dissolved in a pint of water makes a modified Burow's Solution approximately equivalent to a 1:40 dilution. How many tablets should be used in preparing ½ gallon of a 1:10 dilution?

57. ℞ Potassium Iodide
(50 mg per tsp)
Ephedrine Sulfate Syrup ad 240 mL
Sig. Teaspoonful as directed.

Potassium Iodide Oral Solution, U.S.P., contains 100% (w/v) of potassium iodide. How many milliliters of the solution should be used to obtain the potassium iodide required in compounding the prescription?

58. Eight hundred and seventy grams of sucrose are dissolved in 470 mL of water, and the resulting volume is 1010 mL. Calculate *(a)* the

percentage strength (w/v) of the solution, *(b)* the percentage strength (w/w) of the solution and *(c)* the specific gravity of the solution.

59. A formula for a cosmetic cream calls for 0.04% of a mixture of 65 parts of methylparaben and 35 parts of propylparaben. How many grams of each should be used in formulating 10 lb (avoir.) of the cream?

60. On June first a pharmacist purchased 1 oz (avoir.) of cocaine hydrochloride. During the month the following were dispensed:

℥i of an ointment containing 3% of cocaine hydrochloride
f℥ii of a solution containing 1% of cocaine hydrochloride
fʒiv of a solution containing 4% of cocaine hydrochloride

How many grains of cocaine hydrochloride were left in stock for the July first narcotic inventory?

61. How many grams of benzethonium chloride should be used in preparing 5 gallons of an 0.025% (w/v) solution?

62. How many grains of gentian violet should be used in preparing f℥vi of a 0.25% solution?

63. ℞

| | | |
|---|---|---|
| Clindamycin Hydrochloride | | 0.6 g |
| Propylene Glycol | | 6.0 mL |
| Purified Water | | 8.0 mL |
| Isopropyl Alcohol | ad | 60.0 mL |
| Sig. Apply b.i.d. | | |

How many capsules, each containing 150 mg of clindamycin hydrochloride, would be used in filling the prescription? Also, what would be the percentage concentration (w/v) of clindamycin hydrochloride in the prescription?

64. ℞

| | | |
|---|---|---|
| Precipitated Sulfur | | 1% |
| Isopropyl Alcohol (70%) | | 120 mL |
| Calamine Lotion | ad | 240 mL |
| Sig. Apply to affected areas. | | |

How many grams of precipitated sulfur and how many milliliters of 99% isopropyl alcohol should be used in filling the prescription?

65. ℞

| | | | |
|---|---|---|---|
| Precipitated Sulfur | | 1 | |
| Salicylic Acid | | 1 | |
| Hydrocortisone | | | 3 |
| Hydrophilic Petrolatum | ad | 30 | |
| M. ft. ungt. | | | |
| Sig. Apply to scalp h.s. | | | |

What is the percentage strength (w/w) of precipitated sulfur and of hydrocortisone in the prescription?

66. ℞ Lincomycin Hydrochloride 1.2 g
Propylene Glycol 4.0 mL
Purified Water 24.0 mL
Isopropyl Alcohol (70%) ad 60.0 mL
Sig. Apply b.i.d. for acne.

How many milliliters of a vial containing 300 mg of lincomycin hydrochloride per mL would be used in filling the prescription? Also, what would be the percentage concentration (w/v) of lincomycin hydrochloride in the prescription?

67. ℞ Triamcinolone Cream (0.1% w/w)
Aquaphor
Unibase aa 30 g
M. ft. ungt.
Sig. Apply t.i.d.

Calculate the percentage strength (w/w) of triamcinolone in the prescription.

68. Polyethylene glycol ointment contains 60% (w/w) of polyethylene glycol 400. How many milliliters of polyethylene glycol 400 having a specific gravity of 1.135 are required to make 10 lb of the ointment?

69. ℞ Precipitated Sulfur 12.5%
Zinc Oxide Ointment ad ℥ii
Sig. Apply.

How many grains of precipitated sulfur should be used in compounding the prescription?

70. Terpin hydrate elixir contains 40% (v/v) of glycerin. If glycerin (specific gravity 1.25) is bought at $18.00 for 10 lb (avoir.), what is the cost of the amount needed to prepare 5 gallons of the elixir?

71. ℞ Belladonna Tincture 60.0
Sodium Phenobarbital 1.0
Peppermint Water ad 240.0
Sig. 5 mL once a day.

Belladonna tincture contains 0.03% (w/v) of alkaloids. Express the amount, in micrograms, of alkaloids represented in each dose of the prescription.

72. Phenobarbital elixir contains 400 mg of phenobarbital in each 100 mL. A physician wants to increase the phenobarbital content to 30 mg per teaspoonful and to prescribe the dose twice a day for 24 days. How many milligrams of phenobarbital should be added to the prescribed volume of the prescription to provide the amount needed for the dosage regimen?

73. ℞ Menthol 0.25%
Magnesia Magma
Calamine Lotion
Rose Water aa ad 120 mL
Sig. Apply.

How many milligrams of menthol should be used in compounding the prescription?

74. How many grams of hydrocortisone should be used in preparing 2 lb (avoir.) of a ¼% hydrocortisone cream?

75. How many fluidounces of a commercially available 17% solution of benzalkonium chloride should be used to prepare 1 gallon of a 1:750 solution?

76. You are directed to prepare 10 liters of a 1:5000 solution of potassium permanganate. If the potassium permanganate is available only in the form of tablets, each containing 0.2 g, how many tablets should be used in preparing the solution?

77. How many milliliters of 85% (w/w) phosphoric acid having a specific gravity of 1.71 should be used in preparing 10 liters of a 1:2000 solution of phosphoric acid for bladder irrigation?

78. How many grams of coal tar should be added to 1 lb of Coal Tar Ointment, U.S.P., to increase the strength to 2%? Coal Tar Ointment, U.S.P., contains 1% of coal tar.

79. ℞ Precipitated Sulfur 4.0
Calamine 8.0
Isopropyl Alcohol 40% 200.0
Witch Hazel ad 240.0
Sig. Apply.

How many milliliters of 99% isopropyl alcohol should be used in compounding the prescription?

80. A preparation is to be made from opium tincture and must contain 0.06% of morphine. If opium tincture contains 10% of opium and if the opium contains 10% of morphine, how many milliliters of the tincture should be used to prepare a liter of the product?

81. A manufacturing pharmacist has on hand four lots of belladonna tincture, containing 25 mg, 27 mg, 33 mg, and 35 mg of alkaloids per 100 mL. How many gallons of each lot should be used to prepare 16 gallons of belladonna tincture containing 30 mg of alkaloids per 100 mL?

82. A pharmacist wishes to prepare one pint of a potent tincture (10%) and containing 64% alcohol from the corresponding fluidextract

(100%) and containing 60% of alcohol. How much 95% alcohol and how much water should be used?

83. How many grams of silver nitrate should be used in preparing 500 mL of a solution that 10 mL diluted to a liter will yield a 1:5000 solution?

84. How many milliliters of 95% (v/v) alcohol and of 30% (v/v) alcohol should be mixed to make 4000 mL of 50% (v/v) alcohol?

85. How many grams of benzethonium chloride and how many milliliters of 95% (v/v) alcohol should be used in preparing 1 gallon of a 1:1000 solution of benzethonium chloride in 70% (v/v) alcohol?

86. ℞ Resorcinol Monoacetate 10.0 mL
Castor Oil 5.0 mL
Ethyl Alcohol 85% ad 200.0 mL
Sig. Apply to scalp.

How many milliliters of 95% (v/v) ethyl alcohol and how much water should be used in compounding the prescription?

87. How many grams of talc should be added to 1 lb (avoir.) of a powder containing 20 g of zinc undecylenate per 100 g to reduce the concentration of zinc undecylenate to 3%?

88. A hospital pharmacist has on hand 14 liters of iodine tincture (2%). How many milliliters of strong iodine tincture (7%) should be mixed with it in order to get a product that will contain 3.5% of iodine?

89. How many milliliters of 36% (w/w) hydrochloric acid having a specific gravity of 1.18 are required to prepare 5 gallons of 10% (w/v) hydrochloric acid?

90. How many grams of ephedrine sulfate and of chlorobutanol should be used to make 500 mL of a solution such that 30 mL diluted to 100 mL will represent 1:500 of ephedrine sulfate and 1:3000 of chlorobutanol?

91. A formula for an ophthalmic solution calls for 500 mL of a 0.02% solution of benzalkonium chloride. How many milliliters of a 1:750 solution should be used to obtain the amount of benzalkonium chloride needed in preparing the ophthalmic solution?

92. ℞ Phenol 600 mg
Boric Acid Solution
Calamine Lotion aa ad 240 mL
Sig. Apply to affected areas.

What is the percentage of phenol in the finished product?

93. A mixture contains 60 mL of belladonna tincture (65% of alcohol), 250 mL of phenobarbital elixir (15% of alcohol) and enough peppermint water to make 500 mL. Calculate the percentage of alcohol in the mixture.

94. ℞ Potassium Permanganate q.s.
Distilled Water ad 500 mL
Sig. 5 mL diluted to a liter equals a 1:8000 solution.

How many 0.2-g tablets of potassium permanganate should be used in compounding the prescription?

95. How many millliliters of each of two liquids with specific gravities of 0.950 and 0.875 should be used to prepare 12 liters of a liquid having a specific gravity of 0.925?

96. How many milliliters of purified water must be added to 1 lb (avoir.) of wool fat to convert it to hydrous wool fat containing 25% of water?

97. ℞ Epinephrine Bitartrate 2.0 g
Sodium Bisulfite 0.1 g
Sodium Chloride 0.7 g
Distilled Water ad 100.0 mL
Sig. Use in the eyes.

How many milliliters of a 0.9% sodium chloride solution should be used to obtain the sodium chloride for the prescription?

98. ℞ Penicillin 60,000 units
Streptomycin 600 mg
Alcohol 70% 30 mL
Glycerin ad 60 mL
Sig. For the ear.

How many milliliters of 95% alcohol and how much water should be used in compounding the prescription?

99. Sorbitan Sesquioleate 6.0 g
White Petrolatum 54.0 g
Methylparaben 0.1 g
Distilled Water ad 100.0 g
Label: Hydrated petrolatum.

A mixture (1 and 9) of the first two ingredients absorbs 18 times its weight of water. How much additional water can be added to 2000 g of the above product to obtain one containing the maximum amount of water that can be absorbed.?

100. ℞ Sodium Fluoride q.s.
Distilled Water ad 60.0
Sig. Five drops added to a liter of drinking water.

The prescriber informs you that the drinking water contains 0.4 ppm of fluoride ion. How many mg of sodium fluoride should be used in preparing the solution so that five drops of it diluted to one liter with the drinking water will yield a solution containing 1 ppm of fluoride ion? The dispensing dropper calibrates 20 drops per mL.

101. ℞ Scopolamine Hydrobromide 0.25%
Phenacaine Hydrochloride 0.5%
Sodium Chloride q.s.
Sterile Distilled Water ad 50.0
Make isotonic sol.
Sig. For the eyes.

How many milliliters of a 0.9% sodium chloride solution should be used in compounding the prescription?

102. ℞ Ephedrine Sulfate 0.5%
Phenacaine Hydrochloride 0.5%
Dextrose q.s.
Distilled Water ad 30.0
Make isotonic sol.
Sig. Nasal spray.

How many grams of dextrose should be used in compounding the prescription?

103. How many milliliters of a 5% boric acid solution should be used in preparing 200 mL of a 1% isotonic solution of phenacaine hydrochloride?

104. ℞ Phenobarbital Sodium 15 mg per mL
Sodium Chloride q.s.
Sterile Distilled Water ad 20 mL
Make isotonic sol. and sterilize.
Sig. For office use.

How many grams of sodium chloride should be used in compounding the prescription?

105. Papaverine Hydrochloride 50 mg per mL
Sodium Chloride q.s.
Sterile Distilled Water ad 30.0 mL
Label: Papaverine Injection: 1 mL = 50 mg

Papaverine hydrochloride has a molecular weight of 376. Its dissociation factor is 1.8. How many grams of sodium chloride should be used to make the solution isotonic?

106. ℞ Atropine Sulfate 2%
Boric Acid q.s.
Distilled Water ad 100.0 mL
Make isotonic sol.
Sig. For the eyes.

*(a)* How many grams of boric acid should be used? *(b)* How many milliliters of a 5% boric acid solution should be used to obtain the amount of boric acid needed in the prescription? *(c)* You are directed to sterilize this prescription at a temperature not exceeding 105°C. Calculate the corresponding F temperature.

107. ℞ Epinephrine 1.0%
Sodium Bisulfite 0.2%
Chlorobutanol 0.5%
Sodium Chloride q.s.
Sterile Distilled Water ad 15.0 mL
Make isotonic sol.
Sig. For the eye.

*(a)* How many grams of epinephrine bitartrate (mol. wt.—333) should be used to obtain the amount of epinephrine (mol. wt.—183) needed in compounding the prescription?

*(b)* Starting with epinephrine bitartrate, how many milligrams of sodium chloride should be used in compounding the prescription?

108. ℞ Pontocaine 0.025 g
Zinc Sulfate 0.050 g
Epinephrine Solution 1:1000 5 mL
Boric Acid q.s.
Sterile Distilled Water ad 15 mL
Make isotonic sol.
Sig. Use in right eye.

Epinephrine solution 1:1000 is already isotonic. How many grams of boric acid should be used in compounding the prescription?

109. The formula for Albright's solution "G" calls for 4.37 g of anhydrous sodium carbonate ($Na_2CO_3$—mol. wt. 106) in 1000 mL of finished product. In preparing 5 gallons of the solution, how many grams

of monohydrated sodium carbonate ($Na_2CO_3 \cdot H_2O$—mol. wt. 124) should be used?

110.

| | |
|---|---|
| Stearic Acid | 20% |
| Potassium Hydroxide | q.s. |
| Glycerin | 10% |
| Water, to make | 1000 g |
| Label: Vanishing cream. | |

How many grams of 85% potassium hydroxide should be used to saponify 25% of the stearic acid in the formula? The saponification value of stearic acid is 208.

111. A cold cream formula calls for 350 g of white wax. The white wax to be used has an acid value of 22. How many grams of sodium borate which has an equivalent weight of 191 should be used in formulating the cream?

112. Assuming that no potassium citrate is available, how many grams of potassium bicarbonate ($KHCO_3$—mol. wt. 100) and how many grams of citric acid ($H_3C_6H_5O_7$—mol. wt. 210) are required to prepare 5 liters of a solution to contain 0.3 g of potassium citrate ($K_3C_6H_5O_7$—mol. wt. 324) in each teaspoonful?

$$3KHCO_3 + H_3C_6H_5O_7 = K_3C_6H_5O_7 + 3H_2O + 3CO_2$$

113. In the monograph on Ferrous Sulfate Tablets, the U.S.P. states that an "equivalent amount of dried ferrous sulfate may be used in place of $FeSO_4 \cdot 7H_2O$ in preparing Ferrous Sulfate Tablets." How many grams of dried ferrous sulfate (mol. wt.—179) could be used to replace the $FeSO_4 \cdot 7H_2O$ (mol. wt.—278) in preparing 10,000 tablets, each containing 0.3 g of the hydrated salt?

114. Sodium Phosphates Oral Solution contains, in each 100 mL, 18 g of dibasic sodium phosphate ($Na_2HPO_4 \cdot 7H_2O$—mol. wt. 268) and 48 g of monobasic sodium phosphate ($NaH_2PO_4 \cdot H_2O$—mol. wt. 138). How many grams of dried dibasic sodium phosphate ($Na_2PO_4$—mol. wt. 142) and of anhydrous monobasic sodium phosphate ($NaH_2PO_4$—mol. wt. 120) should be used in preparing 1 gallon of the solution?

115.

| | |
|---|---|
| Stearic Acid | 20% |
| Liquid Petrolatum | 5% |
| Triethanolamine | 5% |
| Coconut Oil Soap | 40% |
| Distilled Water | 25% |
| Glycerin | 5% |

How many grams of 85% potassium hydroxide should be used in preparing the coconut oil soap required for making 10 lb of this cream?

Coconut oil soap contains 40% (w/w) of coconut oil, and the saponification value of coconut oil is 260.

116. It is estimated that an adult with an average daily diet has a salt (sodium chloride) intake of 15 g per day.

*(a)* How many milliequivalents of sodium ($Na^+$) are represented in the daily salt intake?

*(b)* How many millimoles of sodium chloride (NaCl—mol. wt. 58.5) are represented in the daily salt intake?

117. How many grams of potassium chloride should be used in making a liter of a solution containing 5 mEq of potassium per mL?

118. What is the percent (w/v) concentration of a solution containing 100 mEq of ammonium chloride per liter?

119. Convert 20 mg% of calcium to mEq of calcium.

120. One liter of blood plasma contains 5 mEq of $Ca^{++}$. How many millimoles of calcium are represented in this concentration?

121. One hundred (100) mL of blood plasma normally contain 3 mg% of $Mg^{++}$. Express this concentration in terms of mEq per liter.

122. How many mEq of potassium are contained in each 10-mL dose of a 5% (w/v) solution of potassium chloride (KCl)?

123. ℞ Potassium Chloride 125 g
Peppermint Water ad 500 mL
Sig. 5 mL as directed.

How many mEq of potassium are represented in the prescribed dose?

124. A patient has been using one 1-g tablet of potassium chloride twice a day. His physician now wishes to change the medication to a liquid dosage form containing 134 mEq of potassium per 100 mL. What dose of the liquid preparation should be prescribed to provide the same amount of potassium as that represented by the tablets?

125. How many grams of sodium bicarbonate should be used in preparing a liter of a solution which is to contain 8 mEq of sodium bicarbonate in each 10 mL?

126. How many mEq of potassium are represented in 5 million units of penicillin G potassium ($C_{16}H_{17}KN_2O_4S$—mol. wt. 372)? One mg of penicillin G potassium represents 1595 Penicillin G Units.

127. The formula for a potassium ion elixir is as follows:

| | |
|---|---|
| Potassium Chloride | 5 mEq/tsp |
| Elixir Base | q.s. |

How many grams of potassium chloride are needed to prepare 5 gallons of the elixir?

128. An iron complex with vitamin D tablet contains 540 mg of calcium gluconate ($C_{12}H_{22}CaO_{14} \cdot H_2O$—mol. wt. 448) and 500 mg of calcium carbonate ($CaCO_3$—mol. wt. 100). How many mEq of calcium are supplied in the daily prophylactic dose of three tablets?

129. How many grams of calcium chloride ($CaCl_2 \cdot 2H_2O$—mol. wt. 147) are required to prepare half a liter of a solution containing 5 mEq of calcium chloride per mL?

130. How many milliosmoles of sodium chloride are represented in 1 liter of a 3% hypertonic sodium chloride solution? Assume complete dissociation.

131. Calculate the pH of a solution in which the hydrogen-ion concentration is $5.9 \times 10^{-6}$.

132. A certain elixir has a pH value of 4.1. Calculate the hydrogen-ion concentration of the elixir.

133. The pH value of a certain buffer solution is 9.2. Calculate the hydrogen-ion concentration of the solution.

134. Calculate the pH of a solution in which the hydrogen-ion concentration is 0.000000092 gram-ion per liter.

135. The dissociation constant of benzoic acid is $6.30 \times 10^{-5}$ at 25°C. Calculate the $pK_a$ value of benzoic acid.

136. Calculate the pH of a buffer solution containing 0.8 mole of sodium acetate and 0.5 mole of acetic acid per liter. The $pK_a$ value of acetic acid is 4.76 at 25°C.

137. What molar ratio of sodium acetate to acetic acid is required to prepare an acetate buffer solution having a pH of 5.0? The $K_a$ value of acetic acid is $1.75 \times 10^{-5}$ at 25°C.

138. Calculate the molar ratio of dibasic sodium phosphate and monobasic sodium phosphate required to prepare a buffer system having a pH of 7.9. The $pK_a$ value of monobasic sodium phosphate is 7.21 at 25°C.

139. What molar ratio of sodium borate to boric acid should be used in preparing a borate buffer having a pH of 8.8? The $K_a$ value of boric acid is $6.4 \times 10^{-10}$ at 25°C.

140. Calculate the half-life (years) of $^{60}Co$ which has a disintegration constant of 0.01096 month$^{-1}$.

141. A sodium iodide I 131 solution has a labeled activity of 1 millicurie per mL as of 12:00 noon on November 17. How many milliliters of the solution should be administered at 12:00 noon on December 1 to provide an activity of 250 microcuries? The half-life of $^{131}I$ is 8.08 days.

142. The blood hemoglobin levels, in grams per 100 mL, for a group of 25 individuals were recorded as follows:

| | | | | |
|---|---|---|---|---|
| 14.0 | 14.6 | 15.8 | 14.5 | 16.0 |
| 16.2 | 15.0 | 15.7 | 15.4 | 13.5 |
| 13.3 | 13.4 | 16.1 | 14.8 | 14.8 |
| 14.7 | 14.5 | 15.6 | 13.9 | 15.1 |
| 15.9 | 13.3 | 13.2 | 15.7 | 14.5 |

Prepare an array of the data, calculate the mean, and find the median and the mode from the array.

143. In determining the refractive index of a volatile oil, 15 observations were made at 20°C and the following values were recorded:

| | | |
|---|---|---|
| 1.4590 | 1.4650 | 1.4602 |
| 1.4645 | 1.4595 | 1.4599 |
| 1.4623 | 1.4637 | 1.4605 |
| 1.4642 | 1.4597 | 1.4593 |
| 1.4639 | 1.4645 | 1.4643 |

Calculate the mean, the range, and the average deviation for the recorded values.

144. In determining the weight variation of 20 tablets taken at random from a manufacturer's lot, the following weights, in milligrams, were recorded:

| | | | |
|---|---|---|---|
| 325 mg | 320 mg | 317 mg | 315 mg |
| 315 mg | 335 mg | 340 mg | 325 mg |
| 324 mg | 340 mg | 325 mg | 330 mg |
| 330 mg | 325 mg | 318 mg | 323 mg |
| 328 mg | 322 mg | 322 mg | 325 mg |

Calculate the mean, the average deviation, and the standard deviation for the recorded weights.

145. The diameter of oil globules in a certain emulsion was measured in micrometers (μm) and recorded as follows:

| | | | |
|---|---|---|---|
| 5.0 μm | 6.75 μm | 3.75 μm | 3.5 μm |
| 4.5 μm | 3.0 μm | 3.25 μm | 3.75 μm |
| 2.5 μm | 6.0 μm | 4.5 μm | 5.5 μm |
| 6.5 μm | 4.5 μm | 5.0 μm | 6.25 μm |
| 4.0 μm | 7.0 μm | 5.25 μm | 5.75 μm |

Calculate the mean, and find the median and the mode for the recorded measurements.

146. In checking the melting point of a new chemical compound, analyst A made 64 determinations with an average deviation of 1.5°C. Analyst B made 36 determinations with an average deviation of 0.5°C. Compare the reliability of their results and indicate which analyst probably found a truer average.

147. A volume of gas was collected at a barometric pressure of 762 mm and a temperature of 25°C. Calculate *(a)* the corresponding temperature on the F scale and *(b)* the equivalent pressure in inches.

148. A manufacturer recommends that his product be stored at a temperature not exceeding 40°F. Express this temperature on the centigrade scale.

149. A table of specifications states that a certain substance must congeal at $-30 \pm 5$°C. A sample of the substance was found to congeal at $-37$°F. Did the sample conform to specifications?

150. A hospital pharmacist has in stock 24 pints of 90 proof brandy and 10 fifths of 88 proof whisky. How many proof gallons are represented by this inventory?

151. A manufacturing pharmacist bought 50 proof gallons of spirits. How many wine gallons does this represent if the purchase was 70% (v/v) alcohol?

152. An alcohol inventory shows 27 gallons of 95% alcohol and 8 pints of absolute (100%) alcohol. How many proof gallons of alcohol are represented by this inventory?

153. If alcohol is taxed at $12.50 per proof gallon, what is the tax on 30 wine gallons of 95% (v/v) alcohol?

154. A blood sample is taken from a 150-lb person. Chemical examination shows the sample to contain 0.2% of ethyl alcohol. Assuming that the alcohol is carried in the body fluids and that 70% of the body weight consists of fluids, how many fluidounces of 100 proof whisky would have to be absorbed to produce this blood level?

155. A medication order calls for a 1-liter bottle of acetic acid irrigation solution 0.25% (w/v). How many grams of acetic acid are contained in each irrigation dose of 30 mL?

156. A medication order calls for 500 mL of an intravenous solution to contain 0.25 mg of isoproterenol in each 100 mL. How many milliliters of a 1:5000 isoproterenol solution should be used in preparing the intravenous solution?

157. The solubility of magnesium sulfate is 1 g in 1 mL of water at 25°C, and the volume of the resulting solution is 1.5 mL. How many grams of magnesium sulfate and how many milliliters of water should be used in preparing 1 gallon of a saturated solution of magnesium sulfate?

158. The solubility of salicylic acid in water is 1 g in 460 mL. Calculate the percentage strength (w/w) of a saturated solution of salicylic acid.

159. What is the solubility of a chemical if 1200 g of a saturated alcoholic solution yield a residue of 75 g upon evaporation? The specific gravity of alcohol is 0.8.

160. You are directed to prepare 5 liters of a 50% emulsion of mineral oil. How many grams of acacia and how many milliliters of water should be used in preparing the primary of the emulsion?

161. The formula for a castor oil emulsion calls for 25% of castor oil. In formulating 1 gallon of the emulsion, how many grams of acacia and how many milliliters of water should be used in preparing the nucleus or primary emulsion?

162.

| | |
|---|---|
| Mineral Oil | 30% |
| Cetyl Alcohol | 2% |
| Lanolin, Anhydrous | 3% |
| Emulsifier | 5% |
| Propylene Glycol | 10% |
| Preserved Water | ad 100% |

(*a*) Calculate the "required HLB" of the oil phase.

(*b*) How many grams of Span 60 and how many grams of Tween 20 should be used in formulating 5 lb (avoir.) of the product?

163.

| | |
|---|---|
| Stearic Acid | 10.0% |
| Lanolin | 2.0% |
| Mineral Oil | 3.0% |
| Emulsifier | 5.0% |
| Propylene Glycol | 10.0% |
| Purified Water | ad 100.0% |

The emulsifier blend is to consist of Span 80 and Tween 20. How many grams of each should be used in formulating 5 lb of the product?

164. A hospital pharmacist purchased 1 pt of belladonna fluidextract containing 60% (v/v) of alcohol from which belladonna tincture containing 70% (v/v) of alcohol is to be prepared.

*(a)* If belladonna fluidextract is ten times stronger than the tincture, how many milliliters of the tincture can be prepared from 1 pt of the fluidextract?

*(b)* How many milliliters of 95% (v/v) alcohol and how much water should be used in preparing the calculated volume of the tincture in (a)?

165. A medication order calls for triamcinolone acetonide suspension to be diluted with normal saline solution to provide 3 mg/mL of triamcinolone acetonide for injection into a lesion. If each 5 mL of the suspension contains 125 mg of triamcinolone acetonide, how many milliliters should be used to prepare 10 mL of the prescribed dilution?

166. ℞ Belladonna Extract 10 mg
Phenobarbital 30 mg
Meperidine Hydrochloride 75 mg
Make 20 such capsules
Sig. One for pain.

How many tablets, each containing 100 mg of meperidine hydrochloride, should be used to provide the meperidine hydrochloride needed in compounding the prescription?

167. ℞ Atropine Sulfate gr $\frac{1}{200}$
Codeine Phosphate gr $\frac{1}{4}$
Aspirin gr v
Make 24 such capsules
Sig. One capsule p.r.n.

The atropine sulfate is available only in the form of $\frac{1}{150}$-gr tablets. Explain how you would obtain the correct amount of atropine sulfate.

168. ℞ Sodium Phenobarbital gr $\frac{1}{8}$ per tsp.
Atropine Sulfate gr $\frac{1}{150}$ per tsp.
Syrup ad ℥iv
Sig. Teaspoonful in each feeding.

The atropine sulfate is available only in the form of $\frac{1}{150}$-gr tablets. Explain how you would obtain the correct amount of atropine sulfate.

169. ℞ Atropine Sulfate 300 μg
Phenobarbital 30 mg
Dextroamphetamine Sulfate 3 mg
Make 20 such capsules
Sig. One capsule as directed.

If the dextroamphetamine sulfate is available only in the form of tablets, each containing 15 mg, how many tablets should be used to obtain the dextroamphetamine sulfate needed in compounding the prescription?

170. ℞ Hycodan 2 mg
Colchicine gr $\frac{1}{100}$
Aspirin 300 mg
Make 24 such capsules
Sig. One capsule t.i.d.

Only colchicine granules, each containing $\frac{1}{120}$ grain, are available. Explain how you would obtain the colchicine needed in compounding the prescription.

171. ℞ Hydrocortisone 1.5%
Neomycin Ointment
Emulsion Base aa ad 30 g
Sig. Apply.

If the hydrocortisone is available only in the form of 20-mg tablets, how many tablets should be used to obtain the hydrocortisone needed in compounding the prescription?

172. ℞ Penicillin G Potassium 10,000 units per mL
Isotonic Sodium Chloride Solution ad 15 mL
Sig. For the nose. Store in the refrigerator.

Only soluble penicillin tablets, each containing 400,000 units of penicillin G potassium, are available. Explain how you would obtain the penicillin G potassium needed in compounding the prescription?

173. A certain hyperalimentation solution contains 600 mL of a 5% protein hydrolysate, 400 mL of 50% dextrose injection, 35 mL of a 20% sterile potassium chloride solution, 100 mL of sodium chloride injection, and 10 mL of a 10% calcium gluconate injection. The solution is to be administered over a period of six hours. If the dropper in the venoclysis set calibrates 20 drops per mL, at what rate, in drops per minute, should the flow be adjusted in order to administer the solution during the designated time interval?

174. A phosphate solution for intravenous infusion contains 40 millimoles of sodium phosphate ($Na_2HPO_4$) and 10 millimoles of potassium

acid phosphate ($KH_2PO_4$) per liter. Calculate *(a)* the amount, expressed as mEq, of sodium ion, *(b)* the amount, expressed as mEq, of potassium ion, and *(c)* the amount, in grams, of phosphate represented in the infusion.

175. A solution prepared by dissolving 500,000 units of polymyxin B sulfate in 10 mL of water for injection is added to 250 mL of 5% dextrose injection. The infusion is to be administered over a period of 2 hours. If the dropper in the venoclysis set calibrates 25 drops per mL, at what rate, in drops per minute, should the flow be adjusted in order to administer the total volume over the designated time interval?

176. A physician orders an intravenous solution to contain 10,000 units of heparin in 1 liter of 5% dextrose solution to be infused at such a rate that the patient will receive 500 units per hour. If the intravenous set delivers 10 drops per mL, how many drops per minute should be infused in order to deliver the desired dose?

177. An Isuprel Mistometer contains 15 mL of a 1:400 solution of isoproterenol hydrochloride and permits the delivery of 300 single oral inhalations. If each actuation delivers 0.05 mL, how many micrograms of the active ingredient are received in a single oral inhalation?

178. A physician orders 20 mL of 10% magnesium sulfate ($MgSO_4 \cdot 7H_2O$—mol. wt. 262) to be given as an anticonvulsant. How many milliosmoles of magnesium sulfate will the patient receive?

179. A medication order calls for 20 mEq of potassium chloride in 500 mL of D5/0.45 NSS to be administered at the rate of 125 mL per hour. If the intravenous set is calibrated at 12 drops per mL, what should be the infusion rate in drops per minute?

180. Calculate the net amount of a bill of goods for $3500, with a trade discount of 35% plus a 5% off invoice allowance and a cash discount of 2% for payment of the invoice within 10 days.

181. A certain nasal preparation is listed at $10.00 per dozen, less 40% and 10%. At what price per unit must the preparation be sold to yield a gross profit of 66⅔% on the cost?

182. A pharmacist buys a bottle of vitamin capsules at $7.50 less a discount of 40%. At what price must the capsules be sold to yield a gross profit of 40% on the selling price?

183. A pharmacist buys 10,000 capsules for $270.00, with a trade discount of 33⅓% plus a 5% discount for quantity buying. At what price per hundred must the capsules be sold in order to realize a gross profit of 50% on the selling price?

184. A prescription specialty is purchased at $14.50 per pint, less a

trade discount of 34.5%. At what price must 60 mL of the specialty be sold to yield a gross profit of 50% on the selling price?

185. Sodium cloxacillin for oral solution should be reconstituted at the time of dispensing and stored in a refrigerator for maximum stability. If stored at room temperature, however, the half-life of the sodium cloxacillin solution is only 10 days. If the original concentration of the reconstituted solution was 250 mg/5 mL, how much sodium cloxacillin will remain per 5 mL after storage at room temperature for 25 days?

# Answers to Practice and Review Problems

NOTE: *Answers are given to all problems in Chapter 1 (Some Fundamentals of Measurement and Calculation) and Appendix I (Exponential and Logarithmic Notation); elsewhere, only the answers to odd-numbered problems are given.*

## Chapter 1

### ROMAN NUMERALS

*(Page 4)*

1. *(a)* xviii
   *(b)* lxiv
   *(c)* lxxii
   *(d)* cxxvi
   *(e)* xcix
   *(f)* xxxvii
   *(g)* lxxxiv
   *(h)* xlviii
   *(i)* MCMLXXXIV
2. *(a)* Part 4
   *(b)* Chapter 19
   *(c)* 1959
   *(d)* 1814
3. *(a)* 45
   *(b)* 1000
   *(c)* 48
   *(d)* 64
   *(e)* 16
   *(f)* 84
4. *(a)* 5, 15, 80, 4
   *(b)* $1\frac{1}{2}$, 40, 6, $\frac{1}{2}$

### COMMON AND DECIMAL FRACTIONS

*(Page 11)*

1. *(a)* $\frac{37}{32}$ gr or $1\frac{5}{32}$ gr
   *(b)* $\frac{13}{600}$ gr
   *(c)* $\frac{77}{480}$ gr
2. *(a)* $\frac{209}{64}$ or $3\frac{17}{64}$ gr
   *(b)* $\frac{1}{120}$ gr
   *(c)* $\frac{5}{6}$ gr
3. *(a)* $\frac{225}{48}$ or $4\frac{11}{16}$
   *(b)* $\frac{105}{4}$ or $26\frac{1}{4}$
   *(c)* $\frac{9}{2500}$
4. *(a)* $\frac{10}{1}$ or 10
   *(b)* $\frac{3}{10}$
   *(c)* $\frac{1}{12}$
   *(d)* $\frac{2}{3}$
   *(e)* $\frac{8}{15}$
   *(f)* $\frac{64}{1}$ or 64
5. *(a)* $\frac{48}{3}$ or 16
   *(b)* $\frac{1}{60000}$
   *(c)* $\frac{25}{2}$ or $12\frac{1}{2}$

6. *(a)* $62\frac{1}{2}$
   *(b)* 15
   *(c)* 64
   *(d)* 12,500
7. *(a)* $\frac{1}{32}$
   *(b)* $\frac{4}{5}$
   *(c)* $\frac{64}{1}$
8. $\frac{189}{200}$ gr
9. 75 doses
10. $\frac{59}{160}$ gr
11. $\frac{223}{60}$ or $3\frac{43}{60}$ gr
12. $\frac{1}{90}$ gr
13. $\frac{1}{300}$ gr
14. 80 doses
15. *(a)* 0.125
    *(b)* 0.0002
    *(c)* 0.0625
16. 2.048
17. 1.565
18. 2000 doses
19. $\frac{1}{240}$ gr
20. $\frac{1}{1200}$ gr
21. $\frac{8}{75}$ gr
22. 2 gr
23. 0.0785 g
24. 4.481 g
25. *(a)* $\frac{7}{400}$ gr
    *(b)* 8,400,000 tablets

## Ratio, Proportion, Variation

*(Page 19)*

1. *(a)* $\frac{3 \text{ (gallons)}}{\frac{1}{2} \text{ (gallon)}}$ or $\frac{12 \text{ (quarts)}}{2 \text{ (quarts)}}$
   *(b)* $\frac{1 \text{ (yard)}}{\frac{2}{3} \text{ (yard)}}$ or $\frac{3 \text{ (feet)}}{2 \text{ (feet)}}$
   *(c)* $\frac{\frac{1}{2} \text{ (mile)}}{\frac{1}{3} \text{ (mile)}}$ or $\frac{2640 \text{ (feet)}}{1760 \text{ (feet)}}$
   *(d)* $\frac{4 \text{ (hours)}}{2 \text{ (hours)}}$ or $\frac{240 \text{ (minutes)}}{120 \text{ (minutes)}}$
   *(e)* $\frac{2 \text{ (feet)}}{\frac{1}{2} \text{ (foot)}}$ or $\frac{24 \text{ (inches)}}{6 \text{ (inches)}}$
2. $259.20
3. $316.67
4. 0.91 g
5. $\frac{9}{50}$ gr
6. $22.77
7. 2500 tablets
8. 40 pounds
9. $9.67
10. 25.6 g
11. 41.25 g
12. 0.6 mL
13. 115.4 liters
14. 14 gr
15. 300 minims
16. 0.3 mg
17. 0.547 g
18. 32,000 mg
19. 44 mg
20. 1333 mL
21. 0.02% or $\frac{1}{50}$%
22. 40 tablets
23. 10 minims
24. 16,000,000 units
25. 0.15 mL
26. 125,000 units
27. *(a)* 1.5 g
    *(b)* 1 milliequivalent
28. 0.25 mg
29. 18.75 mL
30. 0.4 mL
31. 2 mg

## SIGNIFICANT FIGURES

*(Page 26)*

1. *(a)* Six
   *(b)* Four
   *(c)* Three
   *(d)* Three
   *(e)* Seven
   *(f)* One
2. *(a)* Two
   *(b)* Three
   *(c)* Two
   *(d)* Four
   *(e)* Five
   *(f)* Two
   *(g)* Four
   *(h)* Three
   *(i)* Two
   *(j)* Two
3. *(a)* 32.8
   *(b)* 200
   *(c)* 0.0363
   *(d)* 21.6
   *(e)* 0.00944
   *(f)* 1.08
   *(g)* 27.1
   *(h)* 0.862
   *(i)* 3.14
   *(j)* 1.01
4. *(a)* 0.001
   *(b)* 34.795
   *(c)* 0.005
   *(d)* 6.130
   *(e)* 14.900
   *(f)* 1.006
5. 330.8 gr
6. 38 gr
7. 40 gr
8. *(a)* 6.38
   *(b)* 1.0
   *(c)* 90.2
   *(d)* 240 gr
   *(e)* 6.0 g
   *(f)* 211 g
   *(g)* 0.072 gr
   *(h)* 0.054 g
   *(i)* 628
   *(j)* 225
   *(k)* 2.6
   *(l)* 0.0266
   *(m)* 140
   *(n)* 24
9. 473 milliliters means $\pm 0.5$ mL
   473.0 milliliters means $\pm 0.05$ mL
10. 0.65 gram means $\pm 0.005$ g
    0.6500 grams means $\pm 0.00005$ g
11. *(a)* 4.0 gr
    *(b)* 0.43 gr
    *(c)* 14.819 g
    *(d)* 12 minims
    *(e)* 350 gr

## ESTIMATION

*(Page 31)*

NOTE: *Estimated answers will vary with methods used. Some calculated answers are given in parentheses for comparison.*

1. Six zeros
2. Four zeros
3. Three zeros
4. Two zeros

5. 20,500
*(19,881)*
6. 22,000
*(21,405)*
7. 14,500
*(14,320)*
8. 36,000
*(35,314)*
9. $240.00
*($253.19)*
10. $160.00
*($169.99)*
11. 20 × 20 = 400
*(374)*
12. 30 × 30 = 900
*(868)*
13. 8 × 50 = 400
*(384)*
14. 20 × 38 = 760
*(722)*
15. 30 × 60 = 1800
*(1736)*
16. 40 × 77 = 3080
*(3003)*
17. 40 × 40 = 1600
*(1638)*
18. 120 × 90 = 10,800 or 11,000
*(11,500)*
19. 360 × 100 = 36,000
*(35,700)*
20. 473 × 100 = 47,300
*(48,246)*
21. 600 × 200 = 120,000
*(121,584)*
22. 600 × 120 = 72,000
*(73,688)*
23. 650 × 20 = 13,000
*(12,825)*
24. 1000 × 13 = 13,000
*(12,974)*
25. 7000 × 800 = 5,600,000
*(5,435,670)*
26. 1000 × 1000 = 1,000,000
*(1,042,956)*
27. 8000 × 10,000 = 80,000,000
*(82,286,560)*
28. 7000 × 20 = 140,000
*(136,477)*
29. 5000 × 1000 = 5,000,000
*(4,917,078)*
30. 2300 × 6000 = 13,800,000
*(13,875,543)*
31. $2\frac{1}{2}$ × 14 = 35
*($36\frac{1}{4}$)*
32. 800 ÷ 3 = 266
*($266\frac{2}{3}$)*
33. 21 × 7 = 147
*($142\frac{2}{9}$)*
34. $\frac{3}{4}$ × 800 = 600
*(612)*
35. 840 ÷ 3 = 280
*(283.76)*
36. 6 × 7000 = 42,000
*(41,557)*
37. 2 × 700 = 1400
*(1438.812)*
38. 0.02 × 500 = 10
*(9.4304)*
39. (7 × 7000) ÷ 100 = 490
*(504.6426)*
40. 100 × 0.0031 = 0.31
*(0.3038)*
41. 6 × 70 = 420
*(411.079)*
42. 7500 ÷ 10 = 750
*(728.8947)*
43. 170 ÷ 20 = 8.5
*(9.0)*
44. ($\frac{2}{3}$ × 165) or 110 ÷ 10 = 11
*(11)*
45. 180 ÷ 100 ÷ 20 = 0.09
*(0.08)*
46. 300 ÷ 15 = 20
*(21.39)*
47. 16 ÷ 320 = $\frac{1}{20}$ or 0.05
*(0.05)*
48. 3600 ÷ 4 = 900
*(900)*

49. 8400 ÷ 7 = 1200
    *(1200.7)*
50. 1100 ÷ 100 = 11
    *(11)*
51. 9800 ÷ 5 = 1960
    *(2000)*
52. 1700 ÷ 6 = 283
    *(298.5)*
53. 0.01 ÷ 5 = 0.002
    *(0.002149)*
54. 200 ÷ 4 = 50
    *(48.6)*
55. 19 ÷ 0.25 = 19 × 4 = 76
    *(73.9)*
56. 19 ÷ 50 = 38 ÷ 100 = 0.38
    *(0.409)*
57. 460 ÷ 8 = 57.5
    *(57.3)*
58. 4500 ÷ 0.50 = 4500 × 2 = 9000
    *(9340)*
59. 90,000
60. 300
61. 3
62. 0.01 or $\frac{1}{100}$
63. 3.5
64. 100
65. 100
66. 20
67. 160
68. $3,750
69. $400
70. $450
71. $800
72. 0.9 g
73. 750 doses
74. $15
75. $10

## Percentage of Error

*(Page 35)*

1. 5%
2. 8%
3. 5%
4. 2.4%
5. 6.3%
6. 1.4%
7. 0.1%
8. 5.2%
9. 6.7%
10. 0.24 g
11. $3\frac{1}{8}$ gr
12. 0.2 g
13. 8.33%
14. 2.4 gr
15. 10%
16. *(a)* No; *(b)* Yes; *(c)* Yes; *(d)* No; *(e)* No; *(f)* Yes
17. 4.6%
18. 6%
19. 1.1%
20. 0.1%
21. 0.02 g
22. 0.1 mg

### Aliquot Method of Measuring

*(Page 42)*

1. (*a*) 100 mL
   (*b*) 3 mg
2. Weigh 120 mg
   Dilute with 1380 mg
   to make 1500 mg
   Weigh 150 mg
3. Weigh 80 mg
   Dilute with 1520 mg
   to make 1600 mg
   Weigh 100 mg
4. Weigh 2 gr
   Dilute with 38 gr
   to make 40 gr
   Weigh 2 gr
5. Weigh 400 mg
   Dilute with 7600 mg
   to make 8000 mg
   Weigh 400 mg
6. Weigh 4 gr
   Dilute with 16 gr
   to make 20 gr
   Weigh 5 gr
7. Weigh 160 mg
   Dilute with 3840 mg
   to make 4000 mg
   Weigh 200 mg
8. Weigh 3 gr
   Dilute with 13 gr
   to make 16 gr
   Weigh 4 gr
9. Measure 3 mL
   Dilute to 10 mL
   Measure 2 mL
10. Measure 2 mL
    Dilute to 10 mL
    Measure 2 mL
11. Measure 5 mL
    Dilute to 8 mL
    Measure 2 mL
12. Measure 3 mL
    Dilute to 8 mL
    Measure 2 mL
13. Weigh 150 mg
    Dilute with 450 mg
    to make 600 mg
    Weigh 200 mg

## Chapter 2

### Interpretation of the Prescription or Medication Order

*(Page 49)*

1. (*a*) Dispense twelve rectal suppositories.
   (*c*) Mix and divide into 40 powders.
   (*e*) Mix and make ointment. Dispense 10 grams.
   (*g*) Mix and make solution containing 1 gram per tablespoon.
   (*i*) Mix and make powder. Divide into 100 doses.
2. (*a*) Instill two (2) drops in each eye every four (4) hours as needed for pain.
   (*c*) Apply morning and night for pain as directed.
   (*e*) Take one (1) teaspoonful in water every 4 or 5 hours as needed for pain.
   (*g*) Take one (1) capsule with water at night. Do not repeat.

(*i*) Place one (1) tablet under the tongue, repeat if needed.

(*k*) Dilute with an equal volume of water and use as gargle every 5 hours.

3. (*a*) 1½ grains of Secobarbital Sodium by mouth every day at bedtime. Repeat if there is need.

(*b*) 1000 milliliters of 5% dextrose in water every 8 hours intravenously with 20 milliequivalents of potassium chloride added to every third bottle.

(*c*) 10 milligrams of Prochlorperazine intramuscularly every 3 hours, if there is need, for nausea and vomiting.

(*d*) One teaspoonful of Minocycline Hydrochloride Suspension by mouth four times a day. Discontinue after 5 days.

(*e*) 10 milligrams of Propranolol Hydrochloride by mouth three times a day before meals and at bedtime.

(*f*) 40 units of NPH 100-Unit Insulin subcutaneously every day in the morning.

(*g*) 250 milligrams of Cefamandole Nafate intramuscularly every 12 hours.

(*h*) 15 milliequivalents of Potassium Chloride by mouth twice a day after meals.

(*i*) 2 milligrams of Vincristine Sulfate per square meter of body surface area.

## Chapter 3

### THE METRIC SYSTEM

*(Page 58)*

1. 502.550 g, or 503 g
3. 0.000025 g
5. 114 g
7. 20,410 g per 25.4 mm
9. 160,000 capsules
11. 50,000 tablets
13. 15,384 tablets
15. 5 g of norgestrel
    0.5 g of ethinyl estriadol
17. 6.25 g
19. 5 mL
21. (*a*) 8.33 mg or 8 mg
    (*b*) 433.33 mg or 433 mg
    (*c*) 75 mg
23. 66 times
25. 2.1 mL
27. 24 mL
29. 400 μg
31. 1.538 g
33. 5000 μg
35. 125 mL

## Chapter 4

### The Common Systems

*(Page 69)*

1. *(a)* 150 gr
   *(b)* 1050 gr
   *(c)* 530 gr
   *(d)* 90 gr
   *(e)* 1ʒ ½ʒ 6 gr, or 1ʒ 1℈ ½℈ 6 gr
3. *(a)* 2ʒ ½ʒ 8 gr, or 2ʒ 1℈ ½℈ 8 gr
   *(b)* 2ʒ 2℈ ½℈ 5 gr, or 2ʒ ½ʒ 1℈ 5 gr
   *(c)* 2ʒ 1ʒ 1℈ ½℈, or 3ʒ 1½℈
   *(d)* 1ʒ ½℈ 5 gr
5. 84f℥
7. 218.75 or 218 tablets
9. 72 cents
11. 320 gr
13. *(a)* ʒv of salicylamide ʒiss, gr x of aspirin
    *(b)* 15 gr
15. 43,750 tablets

## Chapter 5

### Conversion

*(Page 77)*

1. 38.5 in
   36 in
3. 8.161 L
5. 2.92 or 3 minims
7. 6.6 lb per 1.0 in
9. 0.000098 or 1/10,000 in
11. 8.125 or 8 mg of ephedrine sulfate
    16.25 or 16 mg of theophylline
    4.06 or 4 mg of phenobarbital
13. 11.07 or 11 gr of codeine phosphate
    120 gr of acetaminophen
15. 2.6 mg (1/25 gr)
    6.5 mg (1/10 gr)
    1.3 mg (1/50 gr)
17. 8.07 or 8 gr of ferrous sulfate
    1.62 or 1.6 gr of elemental iron
19. $1.17
21. 54.95 or 55 mg
23. *(a)* 526.5 mg
    *(b)* 156 mg
    *(c)* 6 days
25. 14.6 gr

## Chapter 6

### Calculation of Doses

*(Page 94)*

NOTE: *In calculating the number of doses contained in a specified quantity of medicine, disregard any fractional remainder.*

1. 800 doses
3. 960 doses
5. 10 mg
7. 1 mg
9. 4 minims
11. 200 mL

13. 20 mL
15. 25 mg
    0.5 mL
17. 12 days
19. $\frac{2}{13}$ gr
21. 45 mg
23. 28 tablets
25. 30 mg
    200 mg
27. 0.25 mL
29. 0.6 mL
31. 2.2 mg
33. 7.2 mg
35. 12.5 mg
37. ½ teaspoonful (2.5 mL)
    10 days
39. 2 teaspoonfuls
41. 185 mL
    7 teaspoonfuls
    4½ teaspoonfuls
43. 3.825 or 3.8 mL
45. 10 tablets
47. 7.5 mL
49. 1.25 mL
51. 180 μg
53. 1.98 $m^2$
55. 8.7 mg
57. 4.5 mg
59. 201 mg
61. 125 mg
63. 0.525 g
65. 50 μg

## Chapter 7

### Reducing and Enlarging Formulas

*(Page 107)*

1. 45. mL
   0.9 g
   3.9 g
   ad 180. mL
3. 0.57 g
   0.34 g
   22.7 g
   272. g
   568. g
   568. g
   ad 2270. g, or 5 lb
5. 56.75 g
   54.48 g
   254.24 g
   2.27 g
   86.26 g
   Total: 454. g, or 1 lb
7. 87.07 g
   67.7 or 68. mL
   22.3 or 23. mL
   6. mL
   0.22 mL
   0.07 g
   ad 240. mL
9. 12.5 g
   112.5 g
   875. g
   Total: 1000. g
11. 800. mL
    200. mL
    3000. mL
    Total: 4000. mL, or 4L
13. 189 μg
    9.46 g
    8.04 g
    47 mg
    q.s.
    ad 473 mL
15. 118.3 or 118. mL
    59.1 or 59. mL
    117.4 g
    ad 2365. mL, or 5 pt
17. 57. mL
    96. g
    2.4 mL
    ad 120. mL

19. 63.1 g
94.6 mL
ad 473. mL, or 1 pt

21. 0.5 g
125. g
75. g

23. 2500 g or 2.5 kg
1250 g or 1.25 kg
1500 g or 1.5 kg
50 g
50 g
q.s.

25. 56.76 g
2.37 g
2.37 g
355. mL
355. mL
4.26 g
473. mL
ad 2365. mL, or 5 pt

27. 1250. g
62.5 g

## Chapter 8

### Density, Specific Gravity, and Specific Volume

*(Page 119)*

1. 0.812 g per mL
3. 1.83 g per mL
5. 1.285
7. 0.916
9. 1.180
11. 0.8633
13. 1.831
15. 3.237
17. 0.891
19. 1.110
21. 1.096, or 1.10
23. 0.548
25. 1.212 or 1.21

## Chapter 9

### Weights and Volumes of Liquids

*(Page 126)*

1. 116 g
3. 190.4 or 190 g
5. 9.2 kg
7. 8.12 kg
9. 7.37 or 7.4 lb
11. 99.83 g
13. 4.86 kg
15. 10.58 or 10.6 lb
17. 58.47 or 58.5 mL
19. 546.4 or 546 mL
21. 367.9 or 368 mL
23. 4348 or 4350 mL
25. 1101 or 1100 mL
27. 4.73 or $4\frac{7}{10}$ pt
29. 29.2 or $29\frac{1}{5}$ pt
31. $116.30
33. $19.20
35. $3.26
37. 1938 mL
39. 181.05 or 181.1 mL
41. 15.5 mL
120.77 or 120.8 mL

## Chapter 10

### PERCENTAGE PREPARATIONS

*(Page 145)*

1. 3.0 g
3. 7.5 g
5. 1.5 g
   0.45 g
7. 455 gr
9. 25 g
11. 5%
13. 5.4%
    1.4%
15. 50,444 or 50,400 mL
17. 500 mL
19. 681.8 or 682 mL
21. 70.95 or 71 mL
23. 378.5 or 379 mL
25. 250 mg
    7.5 mL
27. 2838 or 2840
29. 25%
31. 30 mg
33. 180 μg
35. 882.1 or 882 g
37. 200 g
39. 16.5%
41. 30.6%
43. 2.4 gr
45. 3%
    ½%
47. 600 mg
49. 0.227 g
51. 5.9%
53. 4 g
    1 g
    20 g
    10.5 g
55. 11 g
57. *(a)* 1:800
    *(b)* 1:40
    *(c)* 1:125
    *(d)* 1:166⅔
    *(e)* 1:300
    *(f)* 1:2000
59. 0.03%
    0.06%
    0.125%
    0.25%
61. 0.2%
63. 0.001%
65. 1:1250
    1:5000
    1:1000
67. 1:200
    0.0005%
69. 1:588
71. 1:4730
73. 3.785 g
75. 100 mg
    2.5 mg
77. 60 mg
    37.5 mg
79. 2 g
    2.5%
81. 0.005%
83. 0.75 g

## Chapter 11

### Dilution and Concentration

*(Page 180)*

1. 1:3200
3. 4%
5. 0.0159 or 0.016%
7. 32%
9. 20,000 mL
11. 6944 or 6940 mL
13. 4.7 mL
15. 5047 mL
17. 248 mL
19. 1.8 mL
21. 50 mL
23. 48 mL
    32 mL
25. 7.5 mL
27. 28.2 mL
29. 700 mL
31. 1667 mL
33. Enough to make 4150 mL
35. 101 mL
    Enough to make 240 mL
37. 115.7 or 116 mL
39. 770.4 or 770 mL
41. 0.002%
43. 14.5%
45. 5.36 g
47. 1 g
    9 g
49. 1000 g
51. 4.76%
53. 0.003%
55. 59.04 or 59 g
57. 0.050 g
59. 1.25%
61. 2.575 or 2.58%
63. 25.36 or 25.4%
65. 39.4%
67. 56.88 or 56.9%
69. 3:5
71. 1.5:27, or 3:54, or 1:18
73. 725 mL
75. 800 g
    1200 g
    2400 g
    400 g
77. 100 mL
79. 170 mL
81. 75 mL
83. 379 mL
    101 mL
85. 22,500 mL
87. *(a)* 8%
    *(b)* 164.7 or 165 g
89. 44.2 or 44 mL
    55.8 or 56 mL
91. 4500 mL

## Chapter 12

### Isotonic Solutions

*(Page 199)*

1. 1.73%
3. −0.52°C
5. −0.025°C
7. 3.3 gr
9. 0.500 g
11. 4.5 g
13. 0.1095 or 0.110 g
15. 0.467 g
17. 0.690 g
19. 17.8 or 18 mL
21. 0.7 gr
23. 0.290 g
25. 44.44 g
27. 13 mL

## Chapter 13

### ELECTROLYTE SOLUTIONS

*(Page 210)*

1. 372.8 mg
3. 4 mEq
5. 0.298%
7. 200 mEq
9. 180.18 g
11. 20 mL
13. 2.5 mEq per mL
15. 10 mEq per liter
17. 14 mOsmol
19. 20 mEq
21. 4.36 mEq per liter
23. 25 mEq
25. 2.7 mEq
27. 4.5 mEq
    2.25 mOsmol
29. 154 mOsmol
31. 555.5 or 556 mOsmol
33. 4.7 mEq
35. 32 mEq
37. *(a)* 28.08 g
    *(b)* 60 mL
39. 296 mg
41. 24.16 or 24 mEq
43. 16 tablets
45. 713 mL
47. 200.6 or 201 mL

## Chapter 14

### SOME CALCULATIONS INVOLVING PARENTERAL ADMIXTURES

*(Page 221)*

1. 3 mL
3. 1.8 mL
5. 8.3 mg
7. *(a)* 7 mL
    2.5 mL
    *(b)* 2.1 mL per minute
9. 41.7 or 42 drops per minute
11. 1.25 mL per minute
13. 7.5 mL
15. 44.6 mEq
17. 1.1 mL
    52.8 or 53 mg
19. *(a)* 15 mL
    *(b)* 31.1 mmol
21. 40 drops per minute

## Chapter 15

### SOME CALCULATIONS INVOLVING HYDROGEN-ION CONCENTRATION AND pH

*(Page 228)*

1. 10.6
3. 6.22 or 6.2
5. 7.36 or 7.4
7. 2.88 or 2.9
9. 0.0000079 gram-ion per L
11. $3.98 \times 10^{-7}$, or $4.0 \times 10^{-7}$
13. 0.00000063 gram-ion per L

## Chapter 16

### Some Calculations Involving Buffer Solutions

*(Page 235)*

1. 3.86
3. 4.56
5. 5.5
7. 6.91
9. 2.82:1
11. 0.03 unit
13. 8.2 g
    6.0 g

## Chapter 17

### Some Calculations Involving Radioactive Pharmaceuticals

*(Page 243)*

1. 152 days
3. 0.0541 $hour^{-1}$
5. $\lambda = 0.04794\ day^{-1}$
   $T\frac{1}{2} = 14.5$ days
7. $\lambda = 0.01084\ day^{-1}$
   $T\frac{1}{2} = 64$ days
9. 77.3 microcuries
11. 0.17 mL
13. *(a)* 4.7 millicuries
    *(b)* 3.2 mL

## Chapter 18

### Basic Statistical Concepts

*(Page 256)*

1. Mean: 127.8
   Median: 126
   Mode: 125
3. Mean: 100.7
   A.D.: 2.62
   S.D.: 3.22
5. Mean: 5.02
   Median: 5.02
   Mode: 5.05
7. Yes. Since every button has an equal chance of being drawn, every subject has an equal chance of being selected for the experiment.
9. 1:3 in favor of the later check.
11. *(a)* 247.75 or 248 mg
    *(b)* Tablets weighing ±19 mg of the average weight fall within the designated limit. Others do not.

## APPENDIX A

### THERMOMETRY

*(Page 265)*

1. 50°F
3. 39.2°F
5. 25°C
7. 37°C
9. 23°F to 572°F
11. 40°C
13. −40°C
15. 86°F to 95°F
17. 68°F
19. −4° and 14°F
21. 176°F
    179.6°F
23. 198°C
    −111.1°C
25. 4.4°C

## APPENDIX B

### PROOF STRENGTH

*(Page 269)*

1. 102.6 proof gallons
3. 490 proof gallons
5. 8,550 proof gallons
7. 125 wine gallons
9. $118.63
11. $393.30
13. $42.60
15. 36.1 proof gallons

## APPENDIX C

### SOLUBILITY RATIOS

*(Page 274)*

1. 1:5.25, or 1 g in 5.25 mL of water
3. 1:2.67, or 1 g in 2.67 mL of water
5. 5.88% (w/w)
7. 59.5 g
   178.57 or 178.6 mL
9. 1 g in 0.7 mL
11. 1 g in 0.55 mL

## APPENDIX D

### EMULSION NUCLEUS

*(Page 277)*

1. *(a)* 125 g
   *(b)* 250 mL
3. *(a)* 625 g
   *(b)* 1250 mL
5. *(a)* 2 g
   *(b)* 4 mL
7. *(a)* 17.5 g
   *(b)* 35 mL

## APPENDIX E

### HLB System: Problems Involving HLB Values

*(Page 282)*

1. 14.7
3. 10.7
5. 12.2
7. 73% of Tween 40
   27% of Span 40
9. 5.6 g of Span 60
   19.4 g of Tween 20

## APPENDIX F

### Some Calculations Involving the Use of Tablets and Capsules in Compounding Procedures

*(Page 285)*

1. Dissolve 1 tablet in enough distilled water to make 60 mL, and take 10 mL of the dilution.
3. 2500 mL
5. 15 tablets
7. 24 tablets
9. 1.5 tablets
11. 15 tablets
13. 16 granules
15. 14 tablets
17. 1.5 mL
19. 6 capsules

## APPENDIX G

### Some Calculations Involving Units of Potency

*(Page 291)*

1. 0.45 mL
3. 9.6 or 10 minims
5. 400,000 units
7. 4 capsules
9. Dissolve 1 tablet in enough isotonic sodium chloride solution to make 8 mL, and take 3 mL of the dilution.
11. 0.3 mL
13. 17 units
15. 46.9 units

## APPENDIX H

### SOME CALCULATIONS INVOLVING THE USE OF DRY POWDERS FOR RECONSTITUTION

*(Page 295)*

1. 8 mL
3. Dissolve 500,000 units of polymyxin B sulfate in enough sterile distilled water to make 10 mL, and take 3 mL of the dilution.
5. 0.64 mL
7. 0.6 mL

## APPENDIX I

### EXPONENTIAL AND LOGARITHMIC NOTATION

### EXPONENTIAL NOTATION

*(Page 300)*

1. *(a)* $1.265 \times 10^4$
   *(b)* $5.5 \times 10^{-9}$
   *(c)* $4.51 \times 10^2$
   *(d)* $6.5 \times 10^{-2}$
   *(e)* $6.25 \times 10^{-8}$
2. *(a)* 4,100,000
   *(b)* 0.0365
   *(c)* 0.00000513
   *(d)* 250,000
   *(e)* 8695.6
3. *(a)* $17.5 \times 10^7 = 1.75 \times 10^8$
   *(b)* $16.4 \times 10^{-4} = 1.64 \times 10^{-3}$
   *(c)* $6.0 \times 10^0$
   *(d)* $12 \times 10^7 = 1.2 \times 10^8$
   *(e)* $36 \times 10^2 = 3.6 \times 10^3$
4. *(a)* $3.0 \times 10^3$
   *(b)* $3.0 \times 10^{-10}$
   *(c)* $3.0 \times 10^9$
5. *(a)* $8.52 \times 10^4$, or $8.5 \times 10^4$
   *(b)* $3.58 \times 10^{-5}$, or $3.6 \times 10^{-5}$
   *(c)* $2.99 \times 10^3$, or $3.0 \times 10^3$
6. *(a)* $6.441 \times 10^6$, or $6.4 \times 10^6$
   *(b)* $6.6 \times 10^{-3}$
   *(c)* $6.94 \times 10^3$, or $6.9 \times 10^3$

### LOGARITHMIC NOTATION

*(Page 308)*

1. *(a)* 3.3512
   *(b)* 0.7214
   *(c)* 3.8451
   *(d)* 2.2739
   *(e)* $\bar{3}.4675$
   *(f)* $\bar{1}.8600$
   *(g)* 5.3324
   *(h)* $\bar{4}.1373$
   *(i)* 1.8375
   *(j)* 6.7924
2. *(a)* $2.827 \times 10^4 = 28{,}270$
   *(b)* $1.42 \times 10^1 = 14.2$
   *(c)* $2.139 \times 10^0 = 2.139$
   *(d)* $1.29 \times 10^{-1} = 0.129$
   *(e)* $6.154 \times 10^2 = 615.4$
   *(f)* $1.468 \times 10^2 = 146.8$
   *(g)* $1.062 \times 10^0 = 1.062$
   *(h)* $7.766 \times 10^{-3} = 0.007766$
   *(i)* $8.383 \times 10^1 = 83.83$
   *(j)* $1.329 \times 10^{-2} = 0.01329$

3. *(a)* 22,790
   *(b)* 7315
   *(c)* 14.76
   *(d)* 822.6
   *(e)* 17,090
4. *(a)* 7517
   *(b)* 197.6
   *(c)* 0.00517
   *(d)* 35.37
   *(e)* 13.75 or 13.8
5. *(a)* 79.36 or 79.4
   *(b)* 108.5 or 109
   *(c)* 292.8 or 293

## APPENDIX J

### Chemical Problems

*(Page 317)*

1. C: 64.81%
   H: 13.60%
   O: 21.59%
3. Na: 16.66%
   H: 2.92%
   P: 22.45%
   O: 57.97%
5. 1024 g
7. 178.5 or 179 mg
9. 55.2 or 55 mg
11. 530.5 or 531 mg
13. 2.1 g
15. 585 g
17. 66.88 or 66.9 g
19. 571 g
21. 18.2 g
23. 11.8 or 12 g
25. *(a)* 8.59 or 8.6 g
    *(b)* 20.1 g
27. 11.36 or 11.4 g
29. 14.52 or 14.5 g
31. 487.5 or 488 mL
33. 7 liters
    7.69 or 7.7 liters
35. 883 mL

## APPENDIX K

### Some Commercial Problems

*(Page 326)*

1. *(a)* 44.1%
   *(b)* 43.6%
   *(c)* 34.8%
3. $1.93
5. $1,117.20
7. $2.11
9. $99.00
11. $1.28
13. $3.13
15. 78 cents
17. 41.3%
19. $2.75
21. $2.34
23. 2.18%
25. $3.00
27. $3.19

## APPENDIX L

### Graphical Methods

*(Page 337)*

1. 5
   $-1.67$
3. *(b)* $y = -3.7x + 250$
   *(c)* 194.5 mg/5 mL
   *(d)* $-3.7$ mg/5 mL/day
   or $-0.74$ mg/mL/day
5. *(d)* $\log y = -0.028x + 1.78$
   *(e)* 11 days
   39 days
   *(f)* 0.944 $day^{-1}$

## APPENDIX M

### Some Calculations Associated with Drug Availability and Pharmacokinetics

*(Page 351)*

1. 1.75 mL
3. 0.33
5. 25 L
7. 0.408 $hr^{-1}$
9. 12.5%
11. 52.3 mg
    15.8 mg

### Review Problems

*(Page 355)*

1. *(a)* $\frac{1}{104}$ gr
   *(b)* Weigh 150 mg
   Dissolve in water to 10 mL
   Measure 1 mL
3. 13.3%
5. 6.25%
7. Weigh 120 mg
   Add diluent 3480 mg
   Weigh 150 mg
9. 0.06 g
   0.024 g
   3.0 g
   0.12 g
11. 6000 μg
13. 168.75 gr
15. $0.58
17. 2.335 g
19. $0.63
21. 329.5 or 330 mg
23. 0.25 g
25. 6 gr
27. 20 mg
29. *(a)* 160 mg
    *(b)* 96.8 or 97 mg
31. 1,580,000 units
    526,667 units
    5.267 g
33. 56 capsules
35. 42 tablets
37. 21.818 g
39. 62.5 g
    12.5 g
    5 g
    500 g

41. 227 g
 340.5 g
 908 g
 794.5 or 795 mL
43. 7.57 g
 3.785 g
 378.5 mL
 1324 mL
 ad 3785 mL
45. 27.24 g
 13.62 g
 413.14 g
47. 0.791
49. 3704 mL
51. 18.16 or 18 mL
53. 160 mL
55. (*a*) 0.067%
 (*b*) 4.85 gr
 (*c*) 667 μg
 (*d*) 1200 mL
57. 2.4 mL
59. 1.180 g
 0.636 g
61. 4.731 g
63. 4 capsules
 1%
65. 3.3%
 1%
67. 0.03%
69. 120 gr
71. 375 μg
73. 300 mg
75. 1 fluidounce
77. 3.44 mL
79. 80.8 or 81 mL
81. 5 gal, 3 gal, 3 gal, 5 gal or 3 gal, 5 gal, 5 gal, 3 gal
83. 10 g
85. 3.785 g
 2789 mL
87. 2572.7 g
89. 4455 mL
91. 75 mL
93. 15.3%
95. 8000 mL
 4000 mL
97. 77.8 or 79 mL
99. 20,800 mL
101. 43.5 mL
103. 56.2 mL
105. 0.036 g
107. (*a*) 0.273 g
 (*b*) 48 mg
109. 96.747 or 96.7 g
111. 26.3 g
113. 1931.7 g
115. 222.2 g
117. 372.5 g
119. 1 mEq per 100 mL
121. 2.5 mEq
123. 16.8 mEq
125. 67.2 g
127. 1410 g
129. 183.75 g
131. 5.2
133. $6.31 \times 10^{-10}$
135. 4.2
137. 1.7:1
139. 0.4:1
141. 0.83 mL
143. mean 1.4620
 range 0.0060
 average deviation 0.0022
145. mean 4.8 μm
 median 4.75 μm
 mode 4.5 μm
147. (*a*) 77 F
 (*b*) 30 inches
149. No
151. 35.7
153. $712.50
155. 0.075 g
157. 2523.3 or 2523 g
 2523.3 or 2523 mL

159. 1 g in 18.75 mL
161. 236.5 g
     473 mL
163. 27.2 g
     86.3 g
165. 1.2 mL
167. 18 tablets
169. 4 tablets
171. 22.5 tablets
173. 64 drops per minute
175. 55 drops per minute
177. 125 μg
179. 25 drops per minute
181. $0.75
183. $3.42
185. 46.9 mg/5 mL

# *Index*

Reference in *italics* indicates that a term is defined, illustrated, or otherwise explained.

## TABLE OF ATOMIC WEIGHTS[1]

| Name | Symbol | Atomic number | Weight (accurate to 4 figures[2]) | Approximate weight |
|---|---|---|---|---|
| Actinium | Ac | 89 | * | 227 |
| Aluminum | Al | 13 | 26.98 | 27 |
| Americium | Am | 95 | * | 243 |
| Antimony | Sb | 51 | 121.8 | 122 |
| Argon | Ar | 18 | 39.95 | 40 |
| Arsenic | As | 33 | 74.92 | 75 |
| Astatine | At | 85 | * | 210 |
| Barium | Ba | 56 | 137.3 | 137 |
| Berkelium | Bk | 97 | * | 247 |
| Beryllium | Be | 4 | 9.012 | 9 |
| Bismuth | Bi | 83 | 209.0 | 209 |
| Boron | B | 5 | 10.81 | 11 |
| Bromine | Br | 35 | 79.90 | 80 |
| Cadmium | Cd | 48 | 112.4 | 112 |
| Calcium | Ca | 20 | 40.03 | 40 |
| Californium | Cf | 98 | * | 251 |
| Carbon | C | 6 | 12.01 | 12 |
| Cerium | Ce | 58 | 140.1 | 140 |
| Cesium | Cs | 55 | 132.9 | 133 |
| Chlorine | Cl | 17 | 35.45 | 35 |
| Chromium | Cr | 24 | 52.00 | 52 |
| Cobalt | Co | 27 | 58.93 | 59 |
| Copper | Cu | 29 | 63.55 | 64 |
| Curium | Cm | 96 | * | 247 |
| Dysprosium | Dy | 66 | 162.5 | 163 |
| Einsteinium | Es | 99 | * | 252 |
| Erbium | Er | 68 | 167.3 | 167 |
| Europium | Eu | 63 | 152.0 | 152 |
| Fermium | Fm | 100 | * | 257 |
| Fluorine | F | 9 | 19.00 | 19 |
| Francium | Fr | 87 | * | 223 |
| Gadolinium | Gd | 64 | 157.3 | 157 |
| Gallium | Ga | 31 | 69.72 | 70 |
| Germanium | Ge | 32 | 72.59 | 73 |
| Gold | Au | 79 | 197.0 | 197 |
| Hafnium | Hf | 72 | 178.5 | 179 |
| Helium | He | 2 | 4.003 | 4 |
| Holmium | Ho | 67 | 164.9 | 165 |
| Hydrogen | H | 1 | 1.008 | 1 |
| Indium | In | 49 | 114.8 | 115 |
| Iodine | I | 53 | 126.9 | 127 |
| Iridium | Ir | 77 | 192.2 | 192 |
| Iron | Fe | 26 | 55.85 | 56 |
| Krypton | Kr | 36 | 83.80 | 84 |
| Lanthanum | La | 57 | 138.9 | 139 |
| Lawrencium | Lr | 103 | * | 260 |
| Lead | Pb | 82 | 207.2 | 207 |
| Lithium | Li | 3 | 6.941 | 7 |
| Lutetium | Lu | 71 | 175.0 | 175 |
| Magnesium | Mg | 12 | 24.31 | 24 |
| Manganese | Mn | 25 | 54.94 | 55 |

[1]Derived from the table recommended in 1981 by the Commission on Atomic Weights of the International Union of Pure and Applied Chemistry. All atomic weight values are based on the atomic mass of $^{12}C$ = 12.

[2]When rounded off to 4-figure accuracy, these weights are practically identical to the similarly rounded-off weights in the older table based on oxygen = 16.0000.